Disorders of Human Learning, Behavior, and Communication

Ronald L. Taylor and Les Sternberg
Series Editors

Kathryn A. Haring David L. Lovett
Norris G. Haring
Editors

Integrated Lifecycle Services for Persons with Disabilities

A Theoretical and Empirical Perspective

Springer-Verlag
New York Berlin Heidelberg London Paris
Tokyo Hong Kong Barcelona Budapest

Kathryn A. Haring, The University of Oklahoma, Department of Educational Psychology, Norman, OK 73019-0260, USA

David L. Lovett, The University of Oklahoma, Department of Educational Psychology, Norman, OK 73019-0260, USA

Norris G. Haring, University of Washington, Seattle, WA 98105, USA

Series Editors: Ronald L. Taylor and Les Sternberg, Exceptional Student Education, Florida Atlantic University, Boca Raton, FL 33431-0991, USA

With 7 Illustrations.

Library of Congress Cataloging-in-Publication Data
Integrated lifecycle services for persons with disabilities: a theoretical and empirical perspective / [edited by] Kathryn A. Haring, David L. Lovett, and Norris G. Haring.
p. cm. – (Disorders of human learning, behavior, and communication)
Includes bibliographical references and index.
ISBN-13:978-1-4612-7709-5
1. Handicapped–Services for–United States. 2. Handicapped–Education–United States. 3. Handicapped children–Services for–United States. 4. Handicapped children–Education–United States. I. Haring, Kathryn A. II. Lovett, David L. III. Haring, Norris G. 1923- . IV. Series.
HV1553.I55 1992
362.4'048'0973–dc20 91-40745

Printed on acid-free paper.

Softcover reprint of the hardcover 1st edition 1992

Production managed by Dimitry L. Loseff; manufacturing supervised by Jacqui Ashri.
Typeset by Best-set Typesetter Ltd., Chai Wan, Hong Kong.

9 8 7 6 5 4 3 2 1

ISBN-13:978-1-4612-7709-5 e-ISBN-13:978-1-4612-2886-8
DOI: 10.1007/978-1-4612-2886-8

Preface

The field of education is under pressure, both external and internal, to improve the services provided to all students. In American society, and elsewhere, there is a concern that current educational practices fail to adequately prepare many students to be productive citizens. There has been a call for educational services that are more responsive to the needs of students, that use effective educational practices, that involve parents and the local community, and that adequately prepare teachers to assume more professional roles. Over the last several decades special educators have addressed these and other critical issues as they relate to students with disabilities. The knowledge gained from these endeavors can be useful in the reshaping of schools for all students, those with disabilities and those without. Indeed, this information may be useful for services beyond school whether for young children or adults.

This volume has been written to address how people with disabilities can be effectively served in settings with their nondisabled peers. Because many of the students who are not well served by current educational practices have similar needs as students with disabilities, it is anticipated that some of this information may be useful in the discussion regarding the reshaping of educational systems. It is also anticipated that the material presented will help in the design of more effective coordinated systems that serve people with disabilities throughout their lives.

This book is designed to provide the reader with a concept of special education that is expansive and somewhat contrary to traditionally held views. The material describes a theoretical framework that can serve as the basis for the expansion of special education to serve young children and adults as well as school age children and youth. In addition to the theoretical foundation, practical implications arising from this concept are addressed. The book has been designed to (a) review the extant research concerning various special education service delivery systems, (b) develop a philosophical and empirical basis for the lifecycle provision of special services, (c) demonstrate exemplary models for expanding the field of special education, and (d) provide a redefinition of the roles of special educators.

The material presented in this book is not discussed according to specific categories of disability. The delivery of services must be based on the individual's needs. Services should not be delivered according to what is presumed to be appropriate for a person with a particular label. A primary reason for service delivery based on categories is for administrative convenience, not for appropriate individualized education. The allocation of funds, the placement of persons with disabilities, and the preparation and employment of personnel to provide services have been considered more efficiently achieved through the use of categories of disabilities. One of the emphases of this book will be to show that more effective and efficient provision of services can be achieved through the individualization of those services.

Although 68% of students with handicaps in the United States receive some type of regular education services and 93% receive services on regular school campuses (U.S. Department of Education, 1990), regular and special education, in many respects, are two distinct systems (Stainback & Stainback, 1984). Many students in special education are segregated from the mainstream and stigmatized with labels (Lipsky & Gartner, 1989; Wang, this volume). Their opportunities for success in school and later in adult life often are hampered by the segregated nature of the system in which they are served. Few students who are placed into special education ever completely reenter regular education or receive post-secondary education. Many authors have recently called for the total integration of people with disabilities into regular education. The benefits include increased interaction with nondisabled peers while deemphasizing the negative effects of the label *handicapped*. However, there is no assurance that these students will receive an appropriate education in the regular classroom nor that their interaction with nondisabled students will be positive and meaningful. These issues and recommendations for addressing them form a large part of this volume.

Much of the information in this book concerns why and how students with disabilities can be effectively served and integrated in regular education settings. Numerous factors have influenced the philosophy underlying the integration concept. These include legislation and litigation, the development of principles and theory, shifts in philosophical orientation, and research into the efficacy of a service delivery system that has traditionally removed people with disabilities from normal environments. These factors and the issues surrounding them are discussed in the first chapter of this book. Chapter 1 explores the many trends and issues behind the emergence of integration as a critical construct in the provision of special education.

Extensive research has been conducted into the principles of instruction. One of these major theoretical approaches, the applied behavior analysis paradigm, has focused on the development of techniques, data collection, and decision-making rules to guide instructional practice. The fact that new skills can be acquired to fluency by individuals with severely limited cognitive, communicative, and motoric repertoires is well established. A major challenge is in developing new instructional methodologies that enable persons with disabilities to increase their independence in natural settings.

A review of the literature that describes the learning process and the behavioral principles of acquisition, maintenance, and generalization is presented in chapters 2, 3, and 4. Application of these principles and rules into naturally occurring opportunities for instruction in a wide range of settings that may promote integration is also explored. The intent in these chapters is to provide the reader with a brief historical perspective on the development of applied behavior analysis, describe the current limitations of this approach, and suggest innovative practices and concepts that may promote generalization to integrated environments and independence.

Strategies and implications for improving special and regular education efforts, while emphasizing individualized instruction, are delineated in chapter 5. The material presented in this chapter examines these dual systems. Methods for determining the success of students with disabilities and their achievement in learning important skills are also presented.

Chapter 6 explores the basic, essential elements of curriculum for students with disabilities. This chapter discusses the historical precedents within curricular development and the philosophical basis for current curricular requirements. Chapter 6 explores how developments in curriculum reflect changes in theoretical and philosophical viewpoints and practices in the field of special education and implications for services in integrated environments.

Several chapters in this book address the concepts of individualized education and integration at specific ages. Chapter 7 discusses the first years of life of a child with disabilities. The services provided to the child and family in the hospital are described and recommendations for improved services are included. The importance of ensuring smooth transitions from hospital to home and community services is also emphasized.

Chapter 8, on early childhood services, delineates several principles on which exemplary early childhood special education programs should be based. The chapter also describes the results of a recent survey designed to identify best practices in this area. Implications for integrated services and strategies to provide those services are included.

Chapter 9 describes secondary education services for students with disabilities. Much of the emphasis in this chapter focuses on determining functional skills and teaching those skills in community settings. A discussion of the importance of planning and preparing for the transition to adult life is a major focus of this chapter.

Chapter 10 presents information on the methods and results of follow-up research and implications for integrative services. It describes current adult services and provides recommendations for how those services may be improved to increase the independence and integration of people with disabilities.

The last chapter on age specific services (chapter 11) addresses the needs of and existing services for elders with disabilities and how the concept of integration relates to those services. The chapter also provides a detailed discussion of the many issues surrounding the quality of life for individuals with disabilities.

In the first half of this century, parents were usually told to institutionalize their child if disabilities were detected early in life. Professionals told parents that they lacked the necessary skills and knowledge to raise a child with handicaps and that the presence of this child would have drastic, negative effects on the family. Even today, some parents feel that the advice they receive from professionals reflects a similar message—that they are not competent and that the presence of a child with disabilities will be detrimental to their family.

It is evident that professionals can influence initial family perceptions of the child with disabilities. For example, if a parent is approached with the perspective that they have a *disabled* child, treating the disability becomes the entire focus. If approached with the message that they have a *child* who is disabled, the child may be perceived as a child first and second as a person who has a disability that may require specialized services.

Chapter 12 describes the feelings of families toward their children with disabilities and how they view the services they receive. This chapter explores parent involvement in special services received by their children. The chapter discusses the shifts in roles that families have played in affecting change in special education. The material also describes how family needs change over the life span of a child with disabilities.

The final chapter of the book (chapter 13) synthesizes the material previously presented. It examines the implications of present practices to projected future developments in improved delivery of services to people with special needs. Chapter 13 encourages the reader to envision and strive for a comprehensive and integrated system of service delivery for individuals with disabilities. This chapter concludes with a description of what is envisioned as a new role model for professionals in special and regular education. It also includes a discussion of how present systems must change in order to support the development of this new role.

The last several decades have witnessed the improvement of service systems to address the needs of people with disabilities. A main emphasis of these improvements is the recognition of individual rights. In service delivery this has recently focused on individualization and integration. Much more remains to be accomplished to support people with disabilities in becoming participating members of their communities. We hope this book provides some assistance to achieve that goal.

David L. Lovett
Kathryn A. Haring

References

Lipsky, D.K., & Gartner, A. (1989). *Beyond Separate Education Quality Education for All.* Baltimore: Paul H. Brookes.

Stainback, W., & Stainback, S. (1984). A rationale for the merger of special and regular education. *Exceptional Children*, *51*(2), 102–111.

U.S. Department of Education. (1990). *Twelth annual report to Congress on the implementation of the Education of the Handicapped Act.* Washington, DC: Author.

1
Perspectives on Continuous Integrated Services

KATHRYN A. HARING AND DAVID L. LOVETT

Effective service systems are dynamic. They change and develop to meet the needs of society. The purpose and the implementation of effective systems must undergo frequent evaluation to ensure that they adequately address societal concerns. Systems serving people with disabilities are no exception. Recent changes in philosophy, demographics, and the economic structure of society necessitate a reexamination of the theoretical foundations and framework of service systems for people with disabilities. The work presented in this volume is designed to assist in that reexamination. This chapter presents material on the perceived goals of serving people with disabilities; it discusses how one goal, integration, is addressed by existing systems and how that goal may more adequately be addressed in the future.

Complex systems have been developed to serve people with disabilities. Historically, the conceptual basis for these systems and the actual service provision have been topics of debate. One of the most intensely discussed issues in this debate is the degree of integration of people with disabilities into society. Originally, special education was a specifically school-based service available only to certain children with specific disabilities. Currently, school programs in many nations are required to serve students with all types and levels of disabilities. Many educators are required to provide services to preschool-age children; to school-age students; or, in some circumstances, to adults with disabilities. Many of these services are provided beyond the school campus. Thus, special education can no longer be viewed *only* as a school-based educational effort.

To adequately examine the issue of integration it is important to understand what special services are and why they were created. The traditional definition of special education emphasizes the extraordinary assistance deemed necessary to support a learner who is significantly different from peers in the public school system. The basic concept of special education is to provide additional services to students who differ significantly from "normal" in order to maximize each individual's potential. Although these services might be supplied by a number of professionals representing various disciplines (e.g., teachers, psychologists, therapists, and health specialists), the original intent was to help the identified student succeed in only one life dimension—school.

The definition of special education used in this volume is expanded to include services that assist persons with disabilities in every life domain throughout the lifespan. Assistance may be necessary for success across many environments (educational, residential, vocational, and recreational). This assistance may be necessary before and beyond the ages of children who typically receive public school services. For example, recent evidence has emerged that early provision of family and infant services may have long-term beneficial effects (Weiner & Koppleman, 1987). Due to this expanded function of special education the term *special services* more adequately reflects the true nature of lifelong support for people with disabilities. The term *special services* is used to denote special education and encompasses all other forms of assistance not provided to the majority of citizens who act within generally accepted standards. Special services include multidisciplinary, interagency, home, school, and community involvement in service provision.

The vast majority of recipients of special services have mild disabilities. The definitions and labels applied to these individuals include learning disabled, mildly mentally retarded, behaviorally or emotionally disordered, communication disordered, hearing or visually impaired, and other labels that denote mild physical disabilities. The parameters used to identify a child as disabled shift and vary frequently over time and widely between countries, states, provinces, districts, or whatever geographic boundaries separate administrative structures. Thus, myriad definitional problems surround labeling and categorizing people with mild disabilities.

For instructional purposes, it is difficult to separate all of the individuals described as mildly handicapped into specific categories. For example, there is little documented difference related to effective educational practices for students with mild handicaps such as learning disabilities and for a significant proportion of nonidentified low-achieving students (Deshler, Schumaker, Lenz, & Ellis, 1984a, 1984b; Ysseldyke, Algozzine, Shinn, & McGue, 1982). The problems both sets of students encounter are very similar, and many methods that teachers use to instruct each group may be identical. In addition, students with disabilities may actually have a combination of problems or disabilities. For example, a student with learning disabilities may also exhibit some behavior disorders.

Students with learning disabilities are considered to be of average or above-average intelligence and have difficulties in one or more specific academic areas such as reading or mathematics (Hammill, 1990). Students with mild mental retardation are slower to learn in all academic areas than are typical students. They may not master more complex skills or abstract understanding. However, there are many basic academic

Contents

Contributors

Forrest C. Bennett, University of Washington, Seattle, WA 98195, USA.

Catherine G. Breen, University of California at Santa Barbara, Santa Barbara, CA 93106, USA.

**Robert Gaylord-Ross*, Peabody College, Vanderbilt University, Nashville, TN 37212, USA.

Michael J. Guralnick, University of Washington, Seattle, WA 98195, USA.

Ruth N. Gustafson, Edmonds School District, Lynnwood, WA 98036, USA.

Marci J. Hanson, San Francisco State University, San Francisco, CA 94132, USA.

Kathryn A. Haring, University of Oklahoma, Norman, OK 73019, USA.

Norris G. Haring, University of Washington, Seattle, WA 98105, USA.

Thomas G. Haring, University of California at Santa Barbara, Santa Barbara, CA 93106, USA.

Craig H. Kennedy, University of California at Santa Barbara, Santa Barbara, CA 93106, USA.

Susan Lehr, Syracuse University, Syracuse, NY 13210, USA.

* deceased

Kathleen A. Liberty, Department of Education, University of Canterbury, Christchurch, New Zealand.

David L. Lovett, University of Oklahoma, Norman, OK 73019, USA.

Thomas B. Pierce Jr., University of Nevada at Las Vegas, Las Vegas, NV 89154, USA.

Stephen Richards, Florida Atlantic University, Boca Raton, FL 33431, USA.

Margaret C. Wang, Temple University, Center for Research in Human Development and Education, Philadelphia, PA 19122, USA.

abilities they can develop, and they benefit from social interaction with peers who are less disabled or nondisabled. Students with behavior disorders, in many cases, can perform the tasks required of them in regular education classes. However, their lack of appropriate social skills and the frequent inappropriate social interactions they exhibit hinder their academic progress. These students need a program designed to promote their education and to provide them with skills that will help them control their behavior. All of these individuals, and those with other types of disabilities, may require some special services. These services primarily include various adaptations of materials or instructional techniques. Other special services might include the use of various technological devices or related services such as speech or physical therapy.

There are two basic premises underlying this discussion of special services. First, individualization is paramount. No two people are identical in ability or limitation. Uniqueness should be valued and considered in determining the type of special services and how those services are provided. To support the ever changing needs of the individual, these services should be available throughout the life cycle. The second premise is that all people should have the opportunity to participate in society. Thus, services for people with disabilities should be provided, whenever possible, in generic environments where people without disabilities are served. This also means that services should be designed to enhance the abilities of individuals and to assist in promoting their independence. A discussion and rationale for each premise are presented below.

Individualized Integrated Services

In the early development of special education, programs were created according to categories of handicapping conditions. The assumption was that each disabling condition required a specific educational perspective and instructional methodology. Systems with advanced services provided separate schools for those who were mentally retarded, deaf, blind, physically handicapped, mentally ill, or emotionally disturbed. Institutions were built to exclude individuals with the most severe impairments from society. A general belief existed that it was better for society, and perhaps better for individuals with disabilities, to provide services in segregated settings.

These unique services were considered to be most efficiently provided in separate centralized locations. Recent literature has suggested that this separate and centralized provision of services is not the most beneficial or efficient system (Lipsky & Gartner, 1989). Developments in service delivery have promoted the concept of provision of services in environments that the individual would attend if nondisabled. Several models of services in generic environments have been proposed and implemented

(Stainback & Stainback, 1984; Lipsky & Gartner, 1989). For example, a student with mental retardation may be educated in the same school and even in the same class as his nondisabled peers.

Individuals are placed into categories primarily based on the results of an assessment using standardized tests. Such tests have been questioned as to their validity—Do they test what they purport to test?—and their reliability—Are they accurate? (Salvia & Ysseldyke, 1988). The assessment of a person's type or level of disability is, for the most part, irrelevant to the delivery of effective services. For example, the labeling of a student as learning disabled provides little help to the teacher in designing an instructional program. Tests should be designed so that assessment information can assist in the development of a specific individualized service delivery program. If the assessment is designed to plan individualized services, there is little need for the use of disability categories to determine the components of an appropriate education program. Special education is designed to provide individualized services by planning a specific program to meet the needs of each student. Evaluations should be designed to assist in the development of these specific programs.

One major purpose of special services is to provide the individual with the necessary skills to participate in the mainstream. In this case, *mainstream* means the normal course of life. For example, in a school setting the mainstream is the regular classroom. Any attempt to fit people with disabilities into categories that isolate them from others is counterproductive to appropriate service delivery. Such categorization impedes an individual's right to educational, residential, and vocational experiences in the mainstream of life. Integrated lifecycle services should be available to all who are disabled.

When provided adequate support and an individualized education that emphasizes the training of functional skills (i.e., skills that prepare students to cope with and solve persistent life problems, live successfully in the community, and communicate their needs and desires), individuals will be better prepared to succeed in integrated environments (Kelly & Vergason, 1985). Through the implementation of such programs, students with disabilities can be served in the "neighborhood" school. The neighborhood school, or home school, has been defined as the school attended by same-age nondisabled children in the immediate neighborhood. Acceptance in the community is enhanced if students are able to access their neighborhood while learning the necessary social, recreational, and mobility skills to function within it. Attending school with nondisabled peers increases the probability of interaction, both structured and casual.

There is a value in serving students with disabilities in their home and neighborhood. Unfortunately, this value has not been reflected by past, and many current, placement patterns. Significant numbers of students with disabilities, particularly those with severe or low-incidence handicaps, still are educated in segregated schools (Danielson & Bellamy, 1989; Haring, K.A., Farron-Davis, Zeph, Goetz, & Sailor, in press; McDonnell & Hardman, 1989). In this case, *segregated* refers to services provided in facilities, or programs, designed primarily to serve people with disabilities. Segregated schools, for example, have their own campuses. Other models of segregation include special classes in separate wings on regular school grounds. Some segregated structures involve a cluster of special education classes grouped on a regular campus. These configurations describe a "side-by-side" or cluster model, in which concentrations of students with disabilities are placed in separate sections of regular schools (Thomason & Arkel, 1980). The major problem with this model is that it defies natural proportion (the distribution of people with disabilities within the general population). That is, more people with disabilities are grouped together than would normally be distributed in a school population. Such grouping hinders both meaningful interaction between students who are disabled and their peers and the complete social development of the individual with disabilities (Brown et al., 1989).

Many variables affect the placement of students with disabilities. As previously described, special services were traditionally provided in environments where a sufficient number of students with disabilities could be grouped. Students with severe and/or low-incidence disabilities were transported from a large number of neighborhoods to the location of a special class or school. The common practice of categorical grouping removed most special education students from the school they would attend were they not disabled. Prevalence figures (Haring, N.G., & McCormick, 1990) indicate that no more than 10% of the population is classified as disabled and receives special education services (U.S. Department of Education, 1990). Research on the characteristics, numbers, and placement of students with severe disabilities (Haring, K.A., et al., in press) suggests that approximately 8% of those identified as disabled are actually severely disabled (defined as persons with severe or profound mental retardation that is frequently concurrent with other behavior, health, sensory, or orthopedic handicaps). Therefore, to achieve a natural proportion, an elementary school with 500 children could, at most, serve 50 children with disabilities, 4 of whom might be labeled severely disabled. Fortunately, there are too few children with severe disabilities to make up a class in each school. Therefore, special provisions must be made to ensure that students with severe disabilities receive an appropriate education while having the opportunity to interact meaningfully with their nondisabled peers.

Because a majority of students with disabilities are mildly involved, most schools have a class for them. Typically, these are resource rooms that daily serve up to 35 children for an hour or more. Usually these services are provided by "pulling out" the student from the regular classroom (Hagerty & Abramson, 1987). It is presumed that these students can be served in the regular classroom but need special help best provided in isolated settings. For students with severe disabilities, the class is most likely to be self-contained where a small number of children (6–12) spend the entire day. The limitations of this service delivery model will be discussed later.

To serve all students in their neighborhood school, teachers must individualize instruction and teach a wide variety of students. Most regular and many special educators are not trained to provide this service (Ysseldyke, Thurlow, Wotruba, & Nania, 1990). To achieve this goal, teachers should be trained to use a variety of instructional techniques and be prepared to adapt curricula to meet the needs of individual students. In addition, related services should be provided by itinerant therapists acting as consultants, preferably in the classroom.

People who support the continuance of segregated services argue that equipping every school to serve students with disabilities is not only costly but also highly impractical. In reality, adaptations needed for specific types of disabilities—such as braille for people with visual impairments, sign language, computerized communication boards, and wheelchairs—are relatively rare (Lewis & Doorlag, 1987). Those individuals who do require adaptations and prosthetics should be instructed to use them in natural environments. Society must accept the use of adaptive equipment to ensure that schools are accessible to students with physical disabilities, to provide buses with wheelchair lifts, and to be willing to attempt to understand augmentative forms of communication.

Some believe that to provide services to individuals with disabilities in mainstream settings will isolate these individuals from their peers with similar disabilities. However, opportunities for interaction between individuals who have similar disabilities can be provided so that experiences may be shared. These interactions can take place both within and outside the service location. Many organizations currently exist that provide avenues for support to families and individuals with disabilities. Adequate support, a cornerstone of appropriate special services, includes promoting interaction between all people, including those who have disabilities and those who do not. These interactions are critical for the support needed in the mainstream be it in the home, school, or community.

Research and Evaluation

A large body of research exists that examines the learning characteristics of, and effective practices for serving, persons with disabilities (Haring, N.G., & McCormick, 1990). Much of the existing research focuses on the systematic use of behavioral technology to promote learning. Studies of the effectiveness of applying the principles of behavior analysis to the problems of students with learning and behavior disorders have been conducted over the last 25 years (Anderson-Inman, Walker, & Purcell, 1984). There is no doubt that the use of behavioral techniques can bring about significant improvements in the social and academic performance of individuals who are disabled (Tawney & Gast, 1984). However, most research has been conducted in special education settings such as experimental or laboratory schools, self-contained (full-day) special classes, or in pull-out programs for remediation that use resource rooms. Strategies are needed to promote the use of this knowledge in integrated settings. Special educators are now being challenged to develop strategies to help transfer skills from special settings into integrated settings, and to apply behavioral principles in regular classrooms and natural environments. Such strategies will help students succeed while in school and when they become adults. (See chapters 3 and 4, on behavior analysis, in this volume.)

As special education services have expanded throughout the past century, so have researchers' interest in measuring the outcomes or efficacy of such programs. There have been many discussions about, and several attempts to determine the effectiveness of, special education services (Tawney & Gast, 1984). The decision of how and what to measure to determine effectiveness depends, to a large extent, on the perceived goals. One perceived goal of special education is to prepare the student to reenter regular education programs. To determine the efficacy of special education to achieve this goal, the number of students reentering and their success in regular education might be analyzed. On the other hand, if the purpose of special education is seen as to teach certain functional skills, then the student's progress toward learning the desired skills would be measured. One factor that recently has been of much concern is the large number of students, particularly special education students, who drop out of school (Edgar, 1987). Thus, another measure of special education effectiveness might focus on the number of students with disabilities who graduate or "age out" of special education. Throughout this book these goals, as related to the effectiveness of special services, are examined.

Many educators feel that the purpose of education is to prepare students, whether disabled or nondisabled, to succeed as adults. Follow-up studies are the most common measure used to determine the adult adjustment of individuals who have left school. Most recent follow-up studies have painted a dismal picture for adults with disabilities (Haring, K.A., & Lovett, 1990). High unemployment or underemployment and poor adjustment to the adult world are common features of their lives. G. Thomas Bellamy (1987), former director of the Office of Special Education Programs in the United States stated,

> Special education is successful, we believe, when a person leaving school has: (a) a job or access to further schooling, together with the skills to succeed in these

situations independently or with affordable support; (b) a home, and the skills to live there with affordable support; (c) a network of friends; and (d) choices about the first three. This focus on the products of special education gives a long-range perspective to our concern for effectiveness. Its challenge for quality improvement, given the results of recent follow-up studies, is to review the conventional wisdom in special education, and make any changes in curriculum, procedures, materials, location, staffing, coordination with other agencies, and so on, that increases the chance students have of obtaining valued adult lifestyles.

This statement expresses what many believe to be the expected final outcome of special education. That is, special education is designed to increase the possibility that individuals with disabilities will become participating members of society. A possible interpretation of follow-up research results would imply that the quality of school-based special education programs is inadequate. However, any conclusive interpretation of follow-up literature is difficult because it is not possible to determine whether the problems individuals with disabilities encounter are the result of poor special education or the lack of adequate adult services. (See chapter 10 in this volume, on adult services, for a detailed discussion of these services.)

One might also conclude that, given the recent expansion of special education programs, Bellamy's (1987) expectations are stringent and unrealistic. Is it a realistic goal to help *all* individuals, even those with the most severe disabilities, become valued members of their community? At this time, American society and other societies have decided in the affirmative—all people should have the opportunity to participate as equals.

Clearly, the results of follow-up research and other types of research to determine the effectiveness of special education are inconclusive. However, results of follow-up data imply that providing special education services only to persons of school age is insufficient. The need for special education does not necessarily diminish after secondary school. Individuals who required special services in school may need special services as adults. This potential need has resulted in the expansion of the concept of special education to include continuous (lifecycle) services available to people with disabilities no matter what their age. These services should help integrate individuals with disabilities into the same homes, schools, and work places they would access were they not disabled so that they may become true participating citizens of their communities.

Upon reflection, it seems shortsighted to have assumed that effective school-based special education programs would develop students who could live independently in the community. Students with disabilities may require intense and long-term assistance in order to benefit from school. It is reasonable to believe that similar interventions are needed in order to assure that these individuals benefit from living and working in society as adults.

Life-Long Services

The field of special education should be extended from its original goal of primarily providing services to school-age persons. Special educators must now embrace an umbrella concept for the provision of services continuously from birth to death. This necessitates viewing people with disabilities of all ages as citizens who are entitled to receive the support they need to reach their fullest potential as members of the community. In practice, this means that specialized, developmental, and educational interventions are necessary for (a) infants and toddlers who have been identified as having handicaps or who are at risk for delay due to prematurity, congenital anomalies, and neurological or other damage at birth; (b) preschoolers and school-age children with disabilities; (c) adults with disabilities who need special services to help them adjust successfully in work and in the community; and (d) senior citizens with disabilities who require support to enable them to enjoy their later years as participating members of the community.

Age-Specific Services

Innovative models of service delivery provide support services to enhance the accessibility of natural environments. These models are based on the concept that regardless of the type, severity, or multiple nature of people's disabilities, individuals benefit from living in their home and working within their community, and they have a right to do so. Research indicates that even people with the most severe disabilities can learn to initiate and maintain social interactions with nondisabled peers (Haring, T.G., Breen, Pitts-Conway, Lee, & Gaylord-Ross, 1987). In addition, the lives of nondisabled people may be enriched by consistent, meaningful interaction with those who are disabled. For example, co-workers have stated their greater appreciation of people with disabilities after having an opportunity to work with them (Gaylord-Ross, Lee, Johnston, & Goetz, in press). However, the development of meaningful interaction may require increased awareness by people without disabilities. For example, it may be necessary to provide information to help them understand the abilities and needs of people with disabilities.

The role of special educators should expand to dimensions consistent with the recent expansion of the field. These professionals should be prepared to provide training to increase the awareness level of, and the ability for meaningful interaction by, school and community members who are nondisabled. In addition, special educators must be prepared to provide services in a variety of school, home, and community settings. That is, not only should they know how to teach in classrooms, but they should also be able to work with families and provide instruction in community environments. It is apparent that providing training within the school setting does not ensure that the skills will generalize into other situations (Haring, N.G., 1988; Liberty & Michael, 1985). School-based special education personnel must facilitate the generalization of skills into nonschool situations and into environments in which the student is anticipated to live in the future. They must be able to analyze subsequent environments and communicate and collaborate with the family, agency personnel, service providers, or caretakers who are responsible for the continued competence of the individual who is disabled. The special educator has become increasingly responsible for the overall adjustment of people with disabilities. (Chapters 6 and 9 of this volume, on curricular concerns and secondary education, respectively, provide a more detailed discussion of these topics.)

Early Childhood Services

Over the past few decades, as the perceived value of specialized education increased, a consensus developed that providing more intense services at earlier ages would enhance benefits. In recent years, research has demonstrated that early intervention (the provision of special education to children from birth to age 5 with developmental delays or at significant risk for disability) dramatically improves children's physical, cognitive, and social abilities, while minimizing the effects of existing and potential disabilities (Weiner & Koppleman, 1987). In the United States, public law mandated that access to education could not be denied on the basis of disability (the Education for All Handicapped Children Act of 1975, Public Law 94–142). This legislation was broadened in 1986 (Public Law 99–457) to provide states with financial incentives and guidelines that encourage further expansion of programs serving the population from birth to age 5.

Persons at significant risk for, or clearly challenged with, disabilities should be identified as early as possible (ideally at birth). Every effort should be made to assess and meet the needs of individuals with disabilities and their families. Early intervention services can be provided in the home, in regular preschools, and in day-care centers. Because the services can be provided in generic settings, the segregation of preschool-age children who are at risk or disabled is simply not justifiable. Chapters 7 and 8 of this volume, on early intervention and early childhood services, respectively, provide information on child identification, best practices for serving these children, concepts for ensuring integrated services, and methods for providing support to families.

School-Age Services

When children reach school age, it becomes the responsibility of the special educator to provide services within the public school. Special services should be provided in the regular classroom whenever possible.

Special educators can be trained to consult and collaborate with regular educators, parents, related service staff, and other caregivers to ensure that the child receives appropriate services. The goals and objectives that are identified by this team should address the need for generalization to home and community environments. When all significant individuals are involved, including the student, a plan can be developed that identifies strengths and needs and is designed to provide the support and training the student requires for success. As students with disabilities progress through the school system, it is necessary for them to have opportunities to develop vocational; social; daily living (housekeeping, shopping, grooming, etc.); recreational; and community mobility skills. The special educator is becoming increasingly responsible for providing these opportunities and for training corresponding skills. (Several chapters in this volume address these issues in greater detail.)

The motivating factors that prompted research into instructional technology (applied behavior analysis) to remediate significant developmental delays simultaneously spawned various special education curricula. Many misguided curricula were based on the assumption that prescribed activities could compensate for (or restore) neurological deficits (Spitz, 1986). These curricula were founded on the belief that damage to the central nervous system (often undetectable in children with mild handicaps) resulted in disrupted neurological processing and a myriad of disabilities. Practical applications of this theory prescribed activities such as drawing lines between objects or engaging in certain motor activities as essential precursors to advanced development. Medical technology cannot detect most impairments in neurological processes or improvements in such processes. Therefore, the basis for these approaches was inadequate and results could not be substantiated (Spitz, 1986).

These are extreme examples, and most pioneers in the field did not seek to capitalize on people's hopes and dreams through promises with misguided applications of theory. However, such questionable practices as those mentioned above hindered the development and application of effective methods of instruction. By emphasizing these inadequate approaches and convincing parents that their techniques were worthwhile, some curriculum educators deflected time, energy, and resources from promising techniques.

In many ways, early materials and methods reflected a "teach-and-pray" or "dump-and-hope" philosophy. When a nonfunctional skill is taught in hopes that it will improve future abilities, such as prevocational training on nut-and-bolt sorting to promote employability, teach-and-pray thinking is at work. Another example of this philosophy is to teach children to discriminate shapes in order to improve visual perception and thereby enhance reading skills. Clearly, teaching students with learning impairments skills that are nonfunctional or only useful in the classroom sacrifices precious instructional time.

The dump-and-hope model involves a pull-out approach and has been widely applied in public schools in the United States (Hagerty & Abramson, 1987). This occurs when the individual is removed from the regular environment, taught to be proficient in isolated skills, and returned to the original (or in some cases a more complex community or vocational) setting without necessary support for maintenance or generalization of the newly acquired skills. If in fact the individual returns to the mainstream environment, this "method" often results in his or her failure to succeed in that setting (Hagerty & Abramson, 1987). A program that emphasizes training of functional skills needed in future environments (including regular classrooms) and provides support to individuals as they move into new settings will enhance the likelihood of success. (See chapter 6 in this volume, on curricular concerns, for a detailed discussion of these issues.)

Adult Services

School system personnel have become increasingly responsible for collaborating with adult service providers to ensure a smooth transition from secondary school to adult life. Traditional postschool programs exclusively serve adults with more severe disabilities in segregated residences and workshops. Segregating adults with disabilities prevents them from being assimilated into their community. It is impossible to be a fully participating member of society if one works and lives in isolation. In addition, individuals with more mild disabilities (e.g., learning disabilities) rarely have received services to help them as adults.

Adult special services are expanding to meet the complex, multi-environmental needs of individuals who have graduated from or exited special education. For example, supported employment services for people with severe disabilities and postsecondary support services for people with learning disabilities have become more common. Ongoing support is typically required to maintain adults with more severe disabilities in vocational and residential situations. As adults with disabilities become senior citizens, special services are required to ensure a high quality of life in integrated settings. These types of services and the issues surrounding their implementation are discussed at length in chapters 10 and 11, on adult services and elders with disabilities, respectively.

Integration

The needs of persons with disabilities are best met initially within the family, educationally within the neighborhood school, and socially and vocationally within the immediate community. The role of professionals in special education should be to ensure that adequate resources are available for maintaining individuals with disabilities within the systems they would access were they not disabled. Special educators should possess the skills to develop collaboration with families and other professionals to design and implement programs that promote meaningful interactions and success for people with disabilities.

Simply put, integration is the placement of individuals with disabilities in environments where nondisabled individuals are served. However, true integration is more than this. Support should be available to promote success in the integrated environment. In addition, methods should be employed to encourage meaningful interactions between people with disabilities and those without. People with disabilities should receive training to develop appropriate social skills. People without disabilities should become aware of the strengths and needs of people with disabilities. When this training and information are provided, the opportunities for meaningful interactions are enhanced.

It must be remembered that in true integration individuality is not lost. Each individual is unique and his or her special nature should be appreciated. Diversity is beneficial to society. Each individual has value and brings worth to all interactions. Special services can be designed to enhance each person's strengths and value in interactions. These services should create opportunities for worthwhile interaction that will help promote the growth of all individuals.

This concept of integration is based on two modifications in the traditional role of the family and school in providing special education. First, the family is viewed as a critical component of early intervention. Service is provided directly to the family and the individual with disabilities. The needs of the family are assessed and addressed. The family is perceived as an active partner in program decision making and implementation. This shift in the family role necessitates changes in the skills required of special educators. Teachers should be trained to encourage family involvement and to increase communication between the home and school or other service settings. They must be aware of the needs of individuals in the home as well as at school. Teachers of young children are expected to assist in assessing family needs and incorporating them into the educational plan. To strengthen this support, all teachers need to be knowledgeable about available social services. They must serve as resource guides for families that require medical, financial, or emotional support that the special education program cannot provide.

Second, special educators must be skilled in providing support and consultation to regular educators so that children with disabilities can be maintained in the neighborhood school in optimal contact with nondisabled peers. In this regard the special educator acts as a consultant, providing expertise and information about resources to the regular educators. This knowledge may include methods for adapting curricula or alternative instructional techniques.

The secondary school special educator is expected to link families with adult service providers. For example, the teacher should work closely with organizations that provide employment opportunities and support for job success. Special educators at the secondary level also should be knowledgeable about the social and vocational environment into which the student will move after leaving school. This, too, is a new dimension of their role. Special educators must increase their abilities to communicate and cooperate with families and with a wide variety of professionals to meet the expanded responsibilities. An understanding of the methods of collaboration and a thorough knowledge of the community will help in achieving these goals. (See chapter 10 of this volume, on adult services, for an elaboration on these topics.)

System Paradigm

To make integrated lifecycle services a reality, collaboration between numerous social service agencies and disciplines is necessary. For example, in order to provide an orderly transition from public high school to the community, a number of agencies (schools, adult service programs, and government agencies) must cooperate and coordinate their efforts. Goals concerning vocational, residential, and social adjustment should be set by school personnel in conjunction with family and community members for adolescents with disabilities. To ensure a successful transition, adult service providers should participate in this goal-setting process. The school must be provided with sufficient information about adult services to design a program that prepares students to meet the expectations of community agencies. Personnel in adult service programs need to be informed about school training programs and the skills of special education graduates. Thus, personnel who work with special education graduates can then be better prepared to meet their needs. As discussed earlier, similar collaborative relationships are needed at the early childhood level to assure that movement between the hospital, infant, preschool, and school programs is systematic and smooth.

Effective collaboration can be achieved by (a) holding interagency meetings for planning, (b) developing a cooperative agreement that specifies each agency's roles and responsibilities, (c) increasing staff members' ability to share information and resources, and (d) providing personnel with the time and support to attain this cooperation and coordination (Schindler-Rainman & Lippitt, 1980).

Analysis of Service Delivery

Many chapters of this volume include discussions of the historical development of special services. An examination of the components of service delivery in the United States from a historical perspective may assist educators in other nations to avoid the development of programs and facilities that are counterproductive to the provision of comprehensive services. Information presented through this examination can help prevent developments such as large-scale institutionalization and segregation into schools and vocational facilities that serve only people with disabilities. Special educators in nations that have established service systems in place may use this analysis to enhance their perspective and plan for future change. The concept of collaboration among agencies toward meeting mutual goals can be extended to include an international perspective. Professionals and agencies from different countries can work together to develop the principles of model service delivery systems. For example, countries, such as Sweden, that provide innovative community living options and unique adult employment services can share their ideas and models with those nations, such as the United States, that are experiencing difficulty providing high-quality integrated adult services.

Systems Change

Special service providers should be knowledgeable about the theories of, and strategies to improve, the service systems in which they work. To develop an integrated lifelong special service system, special service professionals must become collaborative change agents. That is, they should be able to determine goals for improving the system and to work with other professionals to achieve those goals. The concept of systems change in special services is a recent development. It is based on the concept that for large-scale innovation and improvement in special service delivery to take place, the systems by which people with disabilities are served must change. As public policy shifts from a segregated to an integrated model through which to provide special services, the well-established systems that provide segregated services are affected and forced to change. Special educators, families, communities, and social service organizations are presently engaged in a transformation of the paradigm, or pattern, of service delivery (Kuhn, 1970; Skritic, 1987). In the original paradigm, people with disabilities were treated as a uniquely separate group whose deficits were best remediated in specialized settings isolated from the rest of society. A new paradigm based on the concept of the integration of people with disabilities is currently emerging.

For a new paradigm to emerge, it must possess two characteristics: (a) a theoretical grounding sufficiently unprecedented to attract a committed group of adherents away from competing models, and (b) adequate open-endedness so that a myriad of problems remain to be solved by that newly redefined group of researchers and practitioners (Kuhn, 1970). In the field of special services, the newly redefined group is promoting a change in the traditional systems. It is forcing the personnel within these systems to change their perceptions of individuals with disabilities. The new paradigm disallows categorizing people by handicapping condition and placing them in a predetermined set of treatment conditions on that basis. In this way of thinking, segregated facilities and service delivery systems are unacceptable because they are exclusionary. Obviously, many issues must be resolved to implement such a change. New systems must be developed that can adequately serve all individuals in integrated settings. The material presented here is designed to elaborate on this new theoretical concept, propose changes in service delivery systems, and provide examples of system change strategies.

A number of effective strategies to promote systems change have emerged recently. One is the development of model demonstration sites where *best practices* in integrated schools are implemented. Providing site visits for people who are resistant to integration is very persuasive. Often people are fearful of innovation if they have never seen the new concepts implemented. After they see an idea in practice, their perspective on what is possible is broadened. A second strategy toward systems change is to use technical assistance to teach educators, administrators, parents, and other service providers the skills necessary to operate in new settings. The primary characteristic of technical assistance is the provision of expert consultation. One technical assistance method is a peer-to-peer training approach. This occurs when one person with knowledge and similar background provides training to another, for example, pairing a resistant parent with an advocating parent, or a principal of a segregated school with a principal of a regular school that serves students with disabilities. This method has been shown to be highly successful in bringing about changes in educational service delivery systems.

When developing a strategy for systems change, it is important to establish planning teams. Planning teams are necessary at the individual school level. Participation and communication by all interested parties is imperative if positive change is to take place. At a minimum, planning-team membership should include regular and special teachers and administrators, parents, paraprofessionals, and related service providers. The school site team is responsible for completing an assessment in which areas of strength and areas of needed improvement are addressed. This needs assessment generates a written integration plan in which goals and objectives, timelines, responsible personnel, and criteria for completion are specified. An initial objective may be to make the school physically accessible through ramps and restroom modifications. The plan should also address the following questions:

1. What type of disability awareness or other training will be provided to the staff and nondisabled students?
2. What methods will be utilized to assure that students with disabilities are included in all aspects of the school?

generalization (3rd. ed.). (U.S. Department of Education, Contract No. 300–82–0364). Seattle, WA: University of Washington, College of Education.

Lipsky, D.K., & Gartner, A. (1989). *Beyond separate education quality education for all*. Baltimore: Paul H. Brookes.

McDonnell, A.P., & Hardman, M.L. (1989) The desegregation of America's special schools: Strategies for change. *Journal of the Association for Persons with Severe Handicaps*, *14*(1), 68–74.

Salvia, J., & Ysseldyke, J.E. (1988). *Assessment in special and remedial education* (4th ed.). Boston: Houghton Mifflin.

Schindler-Rainman, E., & Lippitt, R. (1980). *Building the collaborative community: Mobilizing citizens for action*. Riverside, CA: University of California Extension.

Skritic, T. (1987). An organizational analysis of special education reform. *Counterpoint*, *8*(2), 15–19.

Spitz, H.H. (1986). *The raising of intelligence: A selected history of attempts to raise retarded intelligence*. Hillsdale, NJ: Erlbaum.

Stainback, W., & Stainback, S. (1984). A rationale for the merger of special and regular education. *Exceptional Children*, *51*(2), 102–111.

Tawney, J.W., & Gast, D.L. (1984). *Single subject research in special education*. Columbus, OH: Charles E. Merrill.

Thomason, J., & Arkell, C. (1980). Educating the severely/profoundly handicapped in the public schools: A side-by-side approach. *Exceptional Children*, *47*, 114–122.

U.S. Department of Education, Special Education Programs (1990). *Twelfth annual report to Congress on the implementation of the Education of the Handicapped Act*. Washington, DC: Author.

Weiner, R., & Koppleman, J. (1987). *From birth to 5: Serving the youngest handicapped children*. Alexandria, VA: Capital.

Ysseldyke, J.E., Algozzine, B., Shinn, M.R., & McGue M. (1982). Similarities and differences between low achievers and students classified as learning disabled. *Journal of Special Education*, *16*, 73–85.

Ysseldyke, J.E., Thurlow, M.L., Wotruba, J.W., & Nania, P.A. (1990). Instructional arrangements. *Teaching Exceptional Children*, *22*(4), 4–8.

2
Social Competence Issues in the Integration of Students With Handicaps

Ruth N. Gustafson and Norris G. Haring

Introduction

As we explore the many issues involved in integration, it is important that we also take an integrative approach to expanding our knowledge base. Toward that end, in addition to studying the special education literature, we have looked to the literature on social competence and peer relationships. Although the latter does not focus on students with handicaps per se, it is nonetheless a rich source of theories, data, and hypotheses pertinent to the examination of issues and concerns in the integration of such students. In view of this, the current chapter will review relevant research on mainstreaming practices and consider potential problems and solutions from a social competence perspective. Our goals are (a) to provide the reader with an overview of the basic issues and concerns involved in the selection, preparation, and placement of students with handicaps in mainstream settings; (b) to present a social competence perspective, based on a multifaceted theoretical frame of reference, from which to consider these issues and concerns; and (c) to provide some suggestions for addressing them.

Trend Toward Increasing Integration

In 1954, when the U.S. Supreme Court handed down its landmark decision in *Brown v. Board of Education*, it marked the beginning of a series of movements to eliminate separateness in education, not only for students of different racial and ethnic backgrounds, but for those of different intellectual, social, and physical abilities as well. In particular, the subsequent passage of Public Law 94–142, the Education for All Handicapped Children Act of 1975, has had a profound impact on public education in the United States. With its mandate that students with handicaps be provided with a free, appropriate education within the "least restrictive environment," Public Law 94–142 was the driving force behind the development of "mainstreaming" as an educational service delivery model for students with handicaps, and as such it has had significant ramifications for both regular education and special education programs.

In a more recent move to further reduce the segregation of students with handicaps, the Office of Special Education and Rehabilitative Services within the Department of Education issued what has come to be called the Regular Education Initiative (REI) or General Education Initiative (GEI). This statement calls for a partnership between regular and special education to "serve as many children as possible in the regular classroom" (Will, 1986, p. 20), and proponents of this move have piloted some promising models for service delivery (Wang, Gennari, & Waxman, 1985).

Furthermore, some educators have called for at least part-time integration of all students, including those with severe and profound disabilities (Haring & Billingsley, 1984), and others have called for the merger or total elimination of the dual systems of regular education and special education to be replaced by a single new system carefully designed to accommodate the educational needs of *all* students (e.g., Gartner & Lipsky, 1987; Stainback & Stainback, 1984).

However, the move toward a merger of special education and regular education has not been uniformly well-received. (See Davis, 1989, for a discussion.) Regular educators are already under pressure to increase the academic performance of the students they now serve, and there are concerns that the addition of students with handicaps would have a negative impact on overall academic achievement. Other concerns include the lack of preparation and resources in regular education. In view of this, a number of educators have argued that such a move is too far-reaching and premature and would undo many of the gains that have been made in the education of students now served in separate programs (e.g., Braaten, Kauffman, Braaten, Polsgrove, & Nelson, 1988; Bryan, Bay, & Donahue, 1988; Fuchs & Fuchs, 1988a; Hallahan, Keller, McKinney, Lloyd, & Bryan, 1988; Kauffman, Gerber, & Semmel, 1988; Keogh, 1988; Schumaker & Deshler, 1988).

Social Competence Concerns

Concurrent with the changes in education since the passage of Public Law 94–142, there has been a significant increase in the study of childhood social competence. Sparked by growing recognition of the importance of peer relationships to children's cognitive and social development as well as their general socialization (Hartup, 1970, 1983), researchers are continuing to address and refine an extensive body of literature indicating that experiences with peers provide a forum for the development of important social interaction skills, are important to the developing child's sense of security and support, and contribute to the development of his or her self-concept (Bukowski & Hoza, 1989; Ladd, 1989; Parker & Gottman, 1989). Furthermore, evidence that poor peer relationships in childhood affect later problems such as juvenile delinquency in adolescence (Roff, Sells, & Golden, 1972) and emotional mental health problems in adulthood (Cowen, Pederson, Babigian, Izzo, & Trost, 1973) has led to the conclusion "that poor peer relations are centrally involved in the etiology of a variety of emotional and social maladjustments" (Hartup, 1983, p. 167). The strength and consistency of these findings are such that a lack of competence in establishing and maintaining satisfactory relationships with peers has come to be cause for concern.

This has particular significance for the move toward increasing integration because many students with handicaps in mainstream settings are not well accepted by their nonhandicapped peers (Sabornie, 1985; Taylor, Asher & Williams, 1987), and some educators are concerned that mainstreaming efforts "are likely to result in increased social isolation and more restrictive social environments unless provisions are made to train handicapped children in the social skills necessary for effective social interaction and peer acceptance" (Gresham, 1982, p. 423).

Mainstreaming: An Overview

Definitions, Assumptions, and Implications

Defined as the "temporal, instructional and social integration of exceptional children with normal peers" (Kaufman, Gottleib, Agard, & Kukic, 1975, p. 40), mainstreaming is intended to facilitate the academic and social growth of students with handicaps by providing them with equal access to both human and material school resources of the regular classroom setting, most importantly including "constructive interaction with non-handicapped peers" (Johnson & Johnson, 1980, p. 90). Research on the importance of peer relationships lends support to the intent of the mainstreaming movement, but the constructive influence of peer relationships depends to a large degree on the quality of those relationships.

In practical terms, mainstreaming refers to the practice of placing children with handicaps in regular classrooms with nonhandicapped peers for some portion of the school day. This means that students with handicaps who were previously taught in segregated classrooms are moved into regular classrooms for the first time or returned to regular classrooms where they had previously been unsuccessful. This often occurs with little or no preparation or support for the student, the new teacher, and/or the new classmates. At the same time, many students with handicaps or other special needs who would previously have been pulled out of regular education classrooms because of cognitive, academic, or social-behavioral problems are remaining in those classrooms with varying levels of support. This assumes that physical proximity will foster acceptance, participation, and the modeling of positive behaviors (Gresham, 1982; 1984). Unfortunately, however, although physical proximity is clearly a necessary condition for mainstreaming, it satisfies only the temporal integration aspect. It is not, by itself, a sufficient condition for constructive interaction (Johnson & Johnson, 1980), and it in no way assures positive instructional and/or social integration outcomes (Gresham, 1984).

Placement Issues

The selection and preparation of students for mainstreaming placement has been identified as a key issue in education (Hundert, 1982), and the increasing press toward merging special and regular education programs highlights its importance. Many school districts continue to offer a full range of services along the continuum from full-time education in a segregated facility to full-time placement in a regular classroom, but others have a limited range of options. In addition, criteria for recommending one type of placement rather than another and for preparing a child to be successful in that placement remain unclearly specified (Salend, 1984) and have sometimes been criticized for favoring administrative, economic, or compliance needs over the needs of the students themselves (Hersch & Walker, 1982; Hundert, 1982).

Review of the literature indicates that there is a clear lack of explicit, reliable criteria for making decisions in the assessment, placement, and mainstreaming of students with handicaps (Olson & Midgett, 1984; Ysseldyke et al., 1983), but there are consistent indications that behavior is a significant factor in these decisions (Hersch & Walker, 1982; Kavale & Andreassen, 1984; Salend & Lutz, 1984; Wilkes, Bireley, & Schultz, 1979). Sarason and Doris (1978, cited in Hersch & Walker, 1983) have suggested that class placement is based not on a student's diagnosis but on the degree to which the student is disturbing to the teacher and students in the regular classroom, and Gresham (1983) has called specifically for the use of social skills assessment in mainstreaming placement decisions. Consistent with this, Gustafson (1989) found significant differences in teachers' behavioral ratings of students in self-contained placements versus those in mainstream placements for more or less than half the school day, and suggested that there may be a threshold of behavioral readiness related to whether or not a student needs the support and structure of a self-contained placement or can handle the less-restrictive placement of being "home-based" in a regular classroom.

Palmer (1980) has gone a step further in emphasizing the importance of "functional characteristics" including impulsivity, attentional problems, temperamental behavioral patterns, and motivational problems that might foster and/or exacerbate behavior and learning problems, and he has suggested that attention be given to these behavioral dimensions in addition to students' academic and social skills. Gustafson's (1989) finding that impulsivity showed a strong effect on placement status of students with mild handicaps as well as on teacher ratings of mainstreaming readiness and success, above and beyond the contribution of age, IQ, and achievement variables, lends strong support to this recommendation.

Still others have argued for the importance of considering the social and instructional characteristics of potential receiving classrooms, including teachers' expectations, tolerances, and attitudes, and have suggested that efforts be made to match students with handicaps with regular program teachers and classroom situations on the basis of these variables (Hersch & Walker, 1982; Hundert, 1982; Palmer, 1980; Walker, 1986). Interestingly, studies have found that both regular and special education teachers place a higher priority on student behaviors oriented toward teacher control, compliance, and classroom discipline than on the peer interaction behaviors and social skills that would seem most important to successful social integration (Cartledge, Frew, & Zacharias, 1985; Walker, 1986; Walker & Lamon, 1985).

At the same time, however, Cartledge et al. (1985) found that regular education students placed a higher priority on such interpersonal behaviors as informal conversation and play or sport skills. These findings are consistent with the notion that there are two major tasks that contront a handicapped student in a mainstream setting: (a) adjustment to the teacher's standards and expectations for academic performance and compliance with classroom rules, and (b) adjustment to a peer group of largely nonhandicapped students with a potentially different set of norms and expectations (Walker et al., 1982). Both of these tasks need to be considered in preparing for and evaluating successful mainstreaming placement. If we fail to consider both of them and consider only the teacher's standards, we may succeed in achieving instructional integration but will continue to fall short of the goal of social integration, which is central to the purpose of mainstreaming.

Outcomes

Not only are placement criteria unclear for students with handicaps, but the results of outcome research are also mixed. In a widely cited article, Gresham (1982) reviewed over 30 studies from 1970 to 1980 pertaining to the social integration outcomes for mainstreamed students with handicaps. No preparation or training had been provided for the mainstreamed students in these studies, and the collective findings indicated that (a) nonhandicapped children interacted less or more negatively with handicapped children in mainstream environments; (b) handicapped children were poorly accepted by their nonhandicapped peers; and (c) handicapped children did not automatically model the behavior of their nonhandicapped peers.

Yoshida (1986) has concluded that the "current literature provides little support for the continued implementation of this [mainstreaming] policy" (p. 17). Citing three different definitions of mainstreaming, he states that one of the problems for evaluation is the lack of clearly defined goals and objectives for mainstreaming. Zigler and Hall's (1986) conclusion is that, at least with regard to students with mental retardation, the current outcome data are at best contradictory and inconclusive, and the authors strongly urge that "social competence must be our ultimate criterion for the evaluation of programs for the handicapped" (p. 5).

Madden and Slavin's (1982, 1983) reviews of mainstreaming research led them to observe that although mainstreamed students with mild academic handicaps (MAHs) are often found to be less accepted and more rejected than their nonhandicapped peers, they nonetheless have better self-esteem, make fewer self-deprecating comments, and have more appropriate behavior than similar students in special classes. Madden and Slavin (1983) concluded that for these students "belonging may be the most important goal" (p. 557), and indeed, a recent panel of learning disabled adults who graduated from public school special education programs in the 1970s unanimously reported a painful sense that they did not belong.[1] For Madden and Slavin (1982), the conclusion was that "special programming within the context of regular class placement holds the greatest potential for improving academic and social-emotional outcomes for MAH students" (pp. 29–30).

Since then, Wang and Birch (1984) have compared the effects of full-time mainstreaming with resource room placement of primary grade students with mild handicaps on student achievement, perceived competence, and overall classroom process. They found results favoring the mainstream placement on all measures. It is important to note, however, that this "mainstream" classroom was specially designed to accommodate the learning needs of exceptional children according to the Adaptive Learning Environments Model (ALEM). This model employs a curriculum that combines direct instruction in basic skills, supported by criterion-referenced assessment and systematic recordkeeping, with open-ended activities designed to foster self-responsibility, inquiry learning, and social cooperation. Instruction is individualized, and each student is expected to progress through the curriculum at his or her own pace. The physical arrangement allows students to work individually and in small and large groups while teachers circulate among them providing individual feedback and tutoring as well as small- and large-group instruction. Self-management skills are specifically taught, and students are responsible for planning and carrying out both self-selected and teacher-assigned

1. Panel discussion, State Conference of the Learning Disabilities Association of Washington, 1989, Seattle, WA.

tasks within an agreed-upon time frame. The model includes a family involvement component to facilitate integration of experiences at home and in school, and it is supported by special educators and support personnel available for consultation, in-service assistance, and diagnostic and instructional assistance (Wang, 1980; Wang, Rubenstein, & Reynolds, 1985). Although the Wang and Birch (1984) results provide an indication of what may be possible given adequate support, they cannot be generalized to the majority of mainstream classroom, where such accommodations have not been made. Furthermore, this and other evaluations of the ALEM have not been uniformly accepted (e.g., Fuchs & Fuchs, 1988a, 1988b).

Methodological issues have also contributed to mixed results in the outcome literature. Many of the outcome studies have used sociometric measures, both peer nomination and peer rating measures, which are vulnerable to a negative bias due to lack of familiarity between the rater and the ratee (Hartup, 1983; Sabornie, 1985). One study that controlled for this factor (Sabornie, 1983, cited in Saborine, 1985) found that sociometric status differences in high school students with learning disabilities (LDs) were nonsignificant. Subsequent findings in a study by Coben and Zigmond (1986) support the importance of considering acquaintance as a factor. Using positive and negative peer nominations and a forced-choice peer rating scale to indicate acceptance, tolerance, rejection, or "don't know him/her" with 43 self-contained LD students and 137 regular program students in their mainstream classes, Coben and Zigmond found that the LD students were both less popular and less rejected on the nominations. On the rating scale, however, the LD students were similar to the regular students in tolerance and rejection ratings but received significantly fewer acceptance ratings and significantly more "don't know" ratings.

It should also be remembered that students with handicaps, like their nonhandicapped peers, are a heterogeneous groups, and not surprisingly, their acceptance and popularity are related to the same characteristics that correlate with sociometric status in children in general, that is, physical attractiveness, friendliness and sociability, academic achievement, IQ, athletic ability, and (negatively) aggressiveness and antisocial behavior. For example, a few studies of students classified as LD have looked beyond overall group means and found subgroups of LD students to be as well liked on some sociometric measures as their nonhandicapped peers (Gottleib, Levy, & Gottleib, 1986; Perlmutter, Crocker, Cordray, & Gorstecki, 1983; Prillaman, 1981).

The Gottleib et al. (1986) study is of particular interest because it included observational data in unstructured play behavior (lunch recess) as well as sociometric ratings of the LD and non-LD students in third, fourth, and fifth grades. Although the LD students did play alone more than the non-LD students, data collected on frequency and type of play (sensorimotor, symbolic, games with rules); size of group; and frequency of neutral and/or aggressive play showed no significant differences between the two groups. There was a significant correlation between roster-and-rating sociometric rating and isolate play, and the LD students were lower on same-sex ratings, but this was primarily the result of LD girls being rated very negatively by non-LD girls. Opposite-sex ratings were not significantly different. Of particular importance, however, was the finding that two thirds of the LD sample had average ratings and played with others to the same extent as non-LD children, whereas a subset of one third of the LD students was responsible for all of the statistically significant differences.

Siperstein, Bopp, and Bak (1978) used peer nominations for "like best," "best athlete," "smartest," and "best looking" in a study of fifth- and sixth-grade LD and non-LD students. They found that academics, athletic ability, and appearance all correlated with popularity, but appearance showed the strongest correlation. LD students were significantly less popular, and none were nominated as "smartest," but they were also no more rejected than non-LD students and were equally as likely as non-LD students to be nominated for athletics or appearance.

Studies of parent ratings (McConaughy & Ritter, 1986) and teacher ratings (McKinney, 1984) have also shown significant social and behavioral variability in learning disabled students, and La Greca (1981) has argued for increased recognition of the fact that social relationships are not problematic for all students identified as learning disabled.

In a study of attitudes of nonhandicapped fourth- and sixth-grade children toward peers with mental retardation, Siperstein and Bak (1986) used audiotapes and photographs to present students varying in academic competence and physical appearance (e.g., Down's syndrome features). They found that physical appearance had a negative effect when students were presented as academically competent, but that academic incompetence was a stronger factor than physical appearance alone. They also found that nonhandicapped students generalized their perception beyond the information given; for example, if a student was presented as academically incompetent, he or she was also perceived as socially incompetent and unhappy. However, when a behavior component was added by showing the students engaged in aggressive, withdrawn, or prosocial behavior, prosocial behavior was found to ameliorate academic incompetence and physical stigma.

When Taylor et al. (1987) studied the social adaptation of mainstreamed fourth, fifth, and sixth graders with mild retardation, they found them to be more rejected, dissatisfied, and socially anxious than regular education students matched on race and socioeconomic status. At the same time, however, not all students with retardation were classified as rejected, and those who were fell into two distinct groups: externalizers (high in aggressive and/or disruptive behavior) and internalizers (high in shy/avoidant behavior).

Mildly handicapped students are clearly a heterogeneous population, both within and across handicapping categories, and a basic premise of this chapter is that their individual differences play a significant role in their acceptance and adjustment in mainstream settings. Furthermore, it is suggested that a social competence perspective provides a useful frame of reference from which to examine those differences when mainstreaming is considered.

A Social Competence Perspective

Definitions

Although there is considerable consensus about the importance of social competence and considerable interest in promoting its healthy development in all children, there has been much less agreement about its definition. Proposed definitions have ranged from some so broad that they have obscured the boundary between social competence and other competencies and attributes to those that have been so narrow and exclusive in focus that they prompted one reviewer to comment, "One would readily compare attempts to define social competence to the proverbial tale about the blind men who study the elephant" (Meichenbaum, Butler, & Gruson, 1981, p. 37).

In addition, although many researchers have referred to *social competencies* and *social skills* interchangeably and have used *social competence* to refer to a specific cluster of skills and characteristics, at least one has argued that social competence and social skills are distinctly different constructs (McFall, 1982). In this view, social competence is defined as a value-based, situationally determined judgment by another, whereas social skills are the specific underlying processes that enable an individual to function in a socially competent manner.

In line with the more inclusive view of social competence as a multifaceted construct comprised of a range of specific skills and characteristics, several authors have noted the need for an integrative approach to defining it (e.g., Furman, 1984; Greenspan, 1981; Meichenbaum et al., 1981). The hallmark of these more integrative definitions is their recognition of the contributions of cognitive, affective, and behavioral factors to competent social functioning. Although authors may vary in the degree to which they emphasize one or another of these areas, they have in common an appreciation of the interactive influence of all three and an understanding of the inadequacy of any definition that focuses exclusively on a single one.

One author who has proposed a more integrative definition (Greenspan, 1981) has suggested that much of the confusion in the social competence literature stems from the fact that writers and researchers have used at least three different approaches to the task of defining social competence. The first, the "outcome-oriented" approach, is exemplified by McFall's (1982) definition in that it focuses on judgments of success or failure in attaining a relevant goal. For children, this is usually conceptualized in terms of peer acceptance or popularity and is generally operationalized as sociometric status. This sociometric approach yields a global index of social competence and has the advantage of minimizing culturally biased or adultocentric attributions about what constitutes socially competent behavior. However, its usefulness in an applied setting is limited to serving as a screening device, an outcome evaluation tool, or an index of the social validity of other elements assumed to contribute to social competence. It is not helpful in diagnosing contributing factors that might then become the focus of intervention. The latter purpose is better served by the second ("content-oriented") and third ("skill-oriented") approaches.

The content-oriented approach focuses on specific behavioral traits or characteristics believed to contribute to socially successful outcomes. As such, it emphasizes personality characteristics (e.g., internalizing, externalizing) or affective-behavioral predispositions (e.g., anxiety, impulsivity) that may mediate the performance of socially competent behavior, but it fails to give adequate attention to the social-cognitive skills that likewise contribute to competent social functioning. The latter, which Greenspan (1981) refers to as social awareness skills, are the focus of the skill-oriented approach. This approach has received considerable attention in recent years but is often still not adequately integrated with the content-oriented approach.

In our view, such an integrated approach is mandatory, and we define social competence as a multifaceted construct comprised of cognitive, affective, and behavioral factors. The frame of reference for the current chapter draws on models of social competence and social information processing developed by Greenspan (1981) and Dodge (1986), respectively. These models were selected because of their complementary nature in (a) providing a "whole child" perspective, including factors from the affective, behavioral, and cognitive domains, and in (b) outlining and ways in which specific social-cognitive skills may contribute to social competence outcomes.

Greenspan's Model

Consistent with the current concerns, Greenspan's (1981) model of social competence grew out of his interest and experience in special education and his conclusion that social competence is a crucial factor in determining whether or not handicapped individuals can function successfully in normal roles and settings. Intended primarily as a "heuristic device" to provide a framework for efforts toward understanding, evaluating, and facilitating social competence in children, this model clearly delineates the multidimensional nature of social competence.

Couched within his hierarchical model of personal competence, which also includes physical competence and adaptive intelligence (a combination of what he calls practical and conceptual intelligence), Greenspan's (1981) tripartite model of social competence includes the components of social awareness, temperament, and character. Social awareness refers to the individual's understanding of how to be effective in interpersonal situations and as such has a more cognitive emphasis than the behaviorist construct of social skills. Temperament and character, on the other hand, refer, respectively, to the physiological and emotional individual difference variables that also have an impact on social outcomes and can contribute to our understanding of the competence/performance question.

Although Greenspan (1981) considered all three components to be equally important in determining an individual's general level of social success or failure, he focused most on the more cognitive social awareness component with its constituent elements of social sensitivity (including role-taking and social inference); social insight (including social comprehension, psychological insight, and moral judgment); and social communication (including referential communication and social problem solving). In his view, this component is the one most amenable to educational interventions. Figure 2.1 provides a visual representation and description of each component and its constituent elements according to this model.

Although Greenspan (1981) speculated briefly about a hierarchical relationship among the social inference, social sensitivity, and social communication elements of his social awareness component, he stopped short of clearly specifying the exact nature of the relationship among them. The social information processing model outlined by Dodge (1986) provides a useful and complementary elaboration, and it highlights the dynamic interactive character of social relationships.

Dodge's Model

First formulated as a way to conceptualize individual differences in aggressive behavior, Dodge's (1986) model attempts to "describe how children process social information in order to respond in social settings" (p. 82). The model begins with the encoding and interpretation of a set of social cues but specifies that this is influenced by the child's "biologically determined set of response capabilities" (p. 83) analogous to the tem-

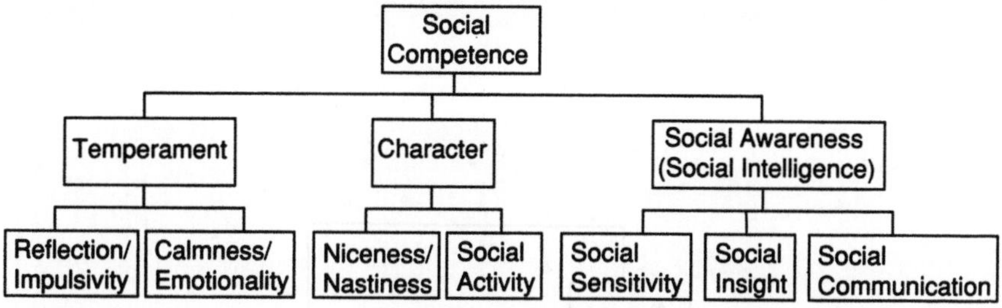

Temperament	The quality of the child's physiological and autonomic response to social stimuli and situations.
Reflection/impulsivity	The ability to focus sustained attention and to not act without thinking.
Calmness/emotionality	Generalized mood or affective orientation (positive or negative), frustration tolerance, emotional stability.
Character	The quality of the child's moral response to social stimuli and situations (i.e., his or her overt behavior).
Social activity/inactivity	The child's degree of assertiveness and ability to enjoy social interactions (gregariousness).
Niceness/nastiness	The child's degree of cooperativeness, responsibility, and demonstrated concern for others.
Social awareness	The child's understanding of how to be effective in interpersonal situations.
Social sensitivity	"What is happening?" The ability to label accurately the meaning of a social object or event at a given moment in time; includes role-taking.
Social insight	"Why is it happening?" The ability to understand the processes underlying social events and to make evaluative judgments about such events; includes social comprehension, psychological insight, and moral judgment.
Social communication	"What do I do?" The ability to understand how to intervene effectively in interpersonal situations and influence successfully the behavior of others; includes referential communication and social problem solving.

FIGURE 2.1. Greenspan's (1981) model of childhood social competence.

Based on S. Greenspan, (1981).

perament component of Greenspan's (1981) model, and a "data base" or "memory store of past experiences which predispose the child toward a particular goal or way of responding" (Dodge, 1986, p. 83). The latter is congruent with Greenspan's character component and encompasses what others have referred to as motivation (Furman, 1984) or expectancies

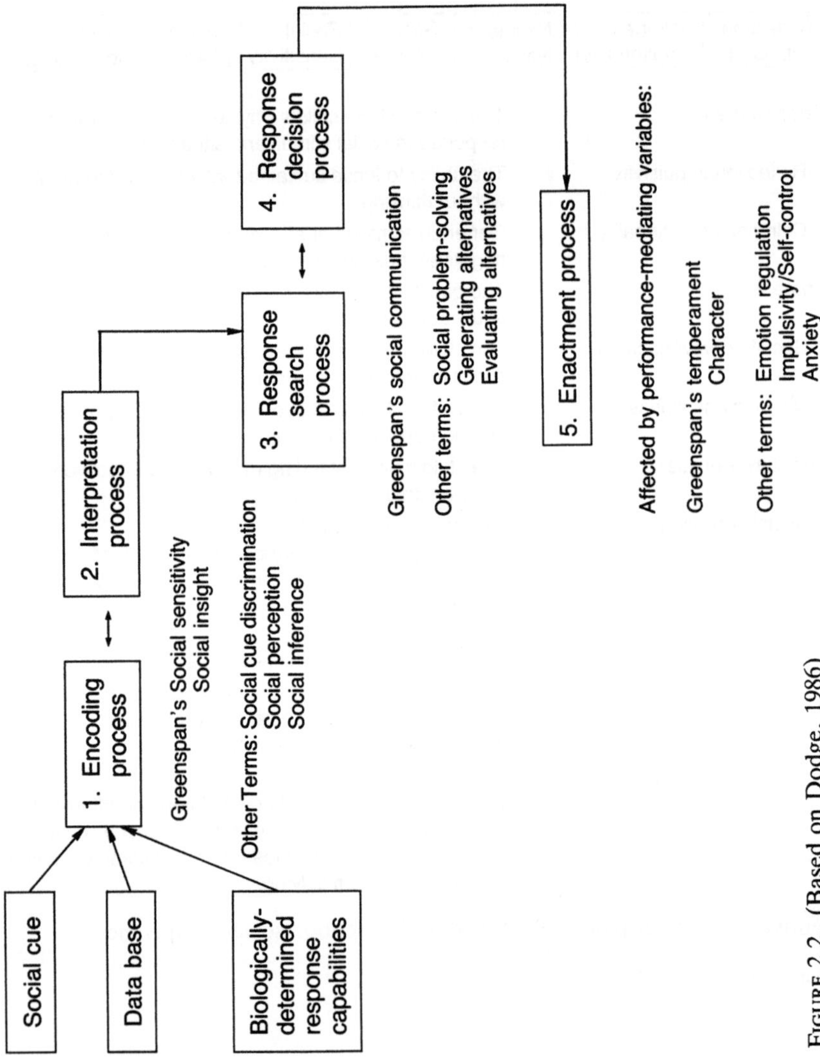

FIGURE 2.2. (Based on Dodge, 1986)

(Meichenbaum et al., 1981). It also clearly raises the issue of children's social goals as an important area of consideration. This is an area that we believe to be significant and will address further below. The social information processing skills in Dodge's model themselves reflect Greenspan's social awareness skills of social sensitivity, social insight, and social communication but are more clearly delineated and sequentially organized. Figure 2.2 presents a basic outline of Dodge's model along with the specific terminology used by Greenspan and other terms frequently used to describe the pertinent social information processing skills.

Encoding and Interpretation

Faced with a set of social cues, the child's first two steps are to encode the information and interpret it in light of past experiences. These two steps are interrelated in a reciprocal fashion and together describe components of the skill areas of social sensitivity and social insight (Greenspan, 1981), alternatively referred to in much of the literature as social cue discrimination, social perception, and social inference. The efficiency and accuracy with which these two steps are accomplished help determine the perceived competence and appropriateness of the child's eventual response. Deviant responses might occur, for example, if a child responds impulsively without attending to all of the available information, if he or she misinterprets cues or misidentifies his or her own or another's feelings, or if he or she has a cognitive bias that skews his or her interpretation of those cues.

As Morrison and Bellack (1981) concluded in their review, "regardless of the magnitude of response skill, the individual cannot perform effectively if he/she does not adequately receive and process the relevant interpersonal stimuli" (p. 70). The studies they reviewed involving children indicated a positive relationship between social perception and social adjustment or appropriate interpersonal behavior, and a positive relationship between social perception and age and IQ. They also found that emotionally disturbed and learning disabled children did less well on measures of social perception than their normal age peers and that situations involving stressful emotions were particularly difficult for poorly adjusted students to interpret accurately. The literature is replete with studies and reviews of social perception deficits in children with mild handicaps (Axelrod, 1982; Bachara, 1976; Bruno, 1981; Bryan, 1977; Dickstein & Warren, 1980; Gerber & Zinkgraf, 1982; Pearl & Cosden, 1982; Schumaker & Hazel, 1984; Wallbrown, Fremont, Nelson, Wilson, & Fischer, 1979; Weiss, 1984; Wong & Wong, 1980), but most of these have not reported or have not analyzed IQ data.

Among those studies that have included IQ data, the results have been inconsistent. La Greca (1981) reviewed studies of role-taking and found nonsignificant differences when 7- to 10-year-old students in LD and normal groups were equivalent on IQ. Horowitz (1981) also found no differences in role-taking in third and fourth graders when IQ was covaried out, and Cartledge, Stupay, and Kaczala (1986) found no differences in empathy when subjects were matched on IQ. On the other hand, Pearl and Cosden (1982) found that sixth-, seventh-, and eighth-grade LD students were significantly less able to "read" feelings and intentions from video segments than their non-LD counterparts, and the significance held even after IQ was covaried out. Gerber and Zinkgraf (1982) studied matched groups of second- and fifth-grade LD and non-LD students and reported significant differences on the Test of Social Inference, but one might question the use of a receptive vocabulary test (Peabody Picture Vocabulary Test) as an adequate measure of IQ.

Weiss (1984) studied aggressive and nonaggressive LD and non-LD black inner-city boys, ages 11 to 15, and found that both aggressive and nonaggressive LD boys who viewed videotapes and heard audiotaped descriptions of unrehearsed interactions (friendly, fighting, and "horse-play") were more likely than aggressive and nonaggressive non-LD boys to judge the interactions as unfriendly; however, group differences accounted for only 5% of the variance. Comparison of aggressive and nonaggressive groups (across LD and non-LD classifications) yielded no significant differences. Although IQs for non-LD boys were not reported, LD group means ranged from 85 to 89, suggesting that IQ may have been a factor in the LD/non-LD differences.

Social perception has also been implicated in peer acceptance and popularity (Dodge, Murphy, & Buchsbaum, 1984; Gottman, Gonso, & Rasmussen, 1975; Kurdek & Krile, 1982); social withdrawal (Waterman, Sobesky, Silvern, Aoki, & McCaulay, 1981); social adjustment (Morrison & Bellack, 1981; Rothenberg, 1970); and aggressive behavior (e.g., Dodge, 1980a, 1980b; Dodge & Frame, 1982; Dodge et al., 1984; Dodge & Newman, 1981; Dodge, Pettit, McClaskey, & Brown, 1986).

In one study of intention-cue detection, Dodge et al. (1984) showed videotaped vignettes of social provocations to kindergarten, second-, and fourth-grade children identified by peer nominations as popular, average, neglected, and rejected. Neglected and rejected, as well as younger, children were found to make more errors than popular and average, as well as older, children. Prosocial and accidental intentions were most often misidentified, and errors were biased toward hostile attributions. Hostile intentions were the most easily identified across all groups. In addition, when the students were shown the same vignettes again later and asked what they would do if the depicted provocation happened to them, responses varied directly as a function of the perceived intention identified in the earlier viewing and not as a function of the actual intention portrayed. When perceived intent was the same, probable behavioral responses varied as a function of sociometric status. Regardless of perceived intent, the popular group was more likely to ask for clarification and less likely to respond with aggression than the other three groups. A grade effect for probable response was also reported.

Dodge (1983, 1986; Dodge et al., 1986) also found a significant relationship between perceived intention and second-, third-, and fourth-grade children's identification by their teachers as severely aggressive and socially rejected versus nonaggressive and socially average. Compared to matched controls, aggressive children were less accurate in interpreting prosocial intentions and made errors in the direction of presumed hostility. In addition, the proportion of errors biased toward hostility was significantly related to actual aggressive responses when subjects were presented with an actual provocation in the laboratory setting. A significant relationship was also found for these subjects between interpretation of hostile intention in a videotaped group-entry analogue situation and actual classroom behavior (proportional duration of solitary inappropriate behavior and antisocial peer interaction; proportional failure of group entry tactics).

Taken together, the reviewed studies underscore the importance of encoding and interpretation in social adjustment and behavior and suggest the need to consider these skills in the selection, preparation, and ongoing support of students with handicaps in mainstream settings.

Goals

Along with the presenting social cues, the child's personal history stored as memories in his or her "data base" comprises an important initial element in Dodge's (1986) model, and it is in this context that the child's social goals are formulated. It should be noted that for his own part, Dodge (1986; Dodge et al., 1986) has not suggested assessing goals separately, noting that the transient nature of a child's goals and their reciprocal interaction with his or her processing of social information makes them difficult to measure. Others, however, have argued convincingly that goals can and should be considered separately in studies of social competence skills (Gustafson, 1989; Renshaw, 1981; Renshaw & Asher, 1982, 1983, 1985; Rubin & Krasnor, 1986; Taylor & Asher, 1984a, 1984b). Unlike many of the hypothetical situations presented in studies of social problem solving, real-life interpersonal situations are often ambiguous, and it is up to the child to determine his or her own goal in each situation.

Children have been shown to have a variety of social goals (Renshaw, 1981; Renshaw & Asher, 1982, 1983; Rubin & Krasnor, 1986) that are presumed to have a strong influence on the strategies they select, their implementation of those strategies, and their appraisals of the outcomes (Rubin & Krasnor, 1986). Furthermore, goals very across situations (Gustafson, 1989; Rubin & Krasnor, 1986; Renshaw, 1981; Renshaw & Asher, 1982, 1983) and are related to sociability (Rubin & Krasnor,

1986) and sociometric status (Asher & Renshaw, 1981; Renshaw, 1981; Renshaw & Asher, 1982, 1983; Taylor & Asher, 1984b). Rubin and Krasnor, for example, observed free-play interactions of matched same-sex preschool and kindergarten children identified as "isolates" or "sociables" and found that the isolates tended to choose "safer" goals, which were less assertive, less costly, and also less effective than the goals chosen by their sociable playmates.

Taylor and Asher (1984a) have proposed that a tendency to pursue maladaptive goals may account for some of the interpersonal difficulties that children with mild retardation have with their nonretarded peers. In addition, Asher and Renshaw (1981) have suggested that some of the positive outcomes of earlier studies in which children were coached in friendship-making skills may have been a function of modifying the children's goals. One specific example is the Oden and Asher (1977) study in which discussions, coaching, and debriefing sessions all focused on "what makes it fun to play a game with another person" (p. 499), thus emphasizing "having fun" as an important goal in playing with peers.

In a study of 8- and 9-year-old and 11- to 13-year-old LD and non-LD students, Oliva and La Greca (1988) found that older children and non-LD children used more sophisticated and more appropriate goals than did younger children or LD children. Strategy differences were not related to the LD versus non-LD distinction, but they were related to age, with older children offering friendlier strategies. The authors concluded that LD students may be aware of what to do but may lack understanding of the reason or goal behind the behavior and may thus find it difficult to adjust to the changing demands of social interaction.

In a study of fourth-, fifth-, and sixth-grade students with mild handicaps, Gustafson (1989) found that self-contained students had a similar lack of sophistication and/or prosocial orientation relative to their mainstreamed peers. Specifically, students in self-contained classrooms gave fewer prosocial goals and more hostile and avoidant or "help-seeking" goals than did same-age students matched on IQ and achievement who were "home-based" in regular classrooms. Self-contained students were also more often unable to articulate any meaningful goal or rationale for a strategy they had proposed, and there was a significant positive relationship between teacher ratings of mainstreaming readiness and goals that focused on being accommodating and taking the perspective of the other child. This is consistent with descriptions of successful group entry behavior as first determining the group's frame of reference and then presenting oneself as sharing that frame of reference or using "low-risk" tactics that avoid calling attention to oneself (Dodge, Schlundt, & Schocken, 1983; Putallaz, 1983; Putallaz & Gottman, 1981).

Parkhurst and Asher (1986) have identified a variety of ways in which children's goals may be problematic. A lack of prosocial goals, for example, may result in a child's failing to attend to significant social cues (e.g., his or her companion's bored expression) or pursuing a singular goal (e.g., to win) at the expense of another that would be more relationship-enhancing (e.g., to make sure everyone has fun). Similarly, pursuit of situationally inappropriate goals, such as carrying on a conversation with a friend who is trying to study or talking to friends when they're trying to pay attention to the teacher or trying to watch a movie, may result in some negative reactions. In studying this area, Parkhurst and Asher (1986) have concluded that

A comprehensive account of social competence will require attention not only to children's social strategies and social behavior but to motivational aspects of social life as well. The goals children pursue, the kinds of orientations they adopt to social situations, will have tremendous impact on their ultimate social adjustment. (p. 200)

Taking this into consideration, the teaching of strategies or social behavioral skills may need to occur within a context that also includes the teaching of situationally appropriate goals. Deciding on a goal is already a part of many programs designed to teach social problem-solving skills (e.g., Elias, 1983; Greenberg, Kusche, Gustafson, & Calderon, in press; Weissberg, Gesten, Leibenstein, Doherty-Schmid, & Hutton, 1980). It appears, however, that the considerable emphasis placed on teaching the evaluation of strategies in these programs should also be directed toward the evaluation of goals.

In addition, Gustafson's (1989) finding that self-contained students had more avoidant and hostile goals than did their mainstreamed peers and that avoidant goals were related to ratings of maladaptive behavior suggests that even when appropriate social behaviors are taught, their actual use may be limited by children's goals. Although the process by which goals are developed is not fully understood, memories of past experiences play an important role (Dodge, 1986). Suggestions that negative expectations and stereotypes may contribute to the social rejection of low sociometric status children (Bierman & Furman, 1984) and behaviorally disordered students in mainstream settings (Hollinger, 1987) are pertinent here. Such attitudes are apt to yield negative experiences for those children, and one could expect that they might then be inclined toward hostile or avoidant goals. Indeed, this seems to have been the experience for at least some learning disabled students.[2]

This line of reasoning suggests that preparation for successful mainstreaming should include activities that will not only teach appropriate social skills and social goals to the students with handicaps but will also address the attitudes of the new peer group. Hollinger (1987) has sug-

2. Panel discussion, State Conference of the Learning Disabilities Association of Washington, 1989, Seattle, WA.

gested that social skills training be extended to include nonhandicapped peers, and Bierman and Furman (1984) have found that a combination of coaching and peer involvement with superordinate goals is effective not only in teaching appropriate behaviors but also in changing peer attitudes and the children's self-perceptions of social efficacy. They concluded that the provision of superordinate goals increased peer interaction and thereby increased the opportunity for improved behaviors to be recognized and reinforced. This suggests that a combination of coaching and inclusion in cooperative group activities with members of the new peer group might be an effective mainstreaming preparation strategy.

Response Search and Response Decision

The third and fourth steps in Dodge's (1986) model involve response search or generation and response decision, referred to by others as accessing and selecting strategies (Rubin & Krasnor, 1986). These steps are also interrelated and have been extensively studied. In addition, they are subject to skill deficits or biases in the preceding two steps, and are shaped by the child's unique goals.

Early studies of social problem solving with children examined the number of alternatives generated to solve hypothetical social problems and the number of means suggested to achieve prespecified ends; results indicated that these quantitative indicators were related to social adjustment (Spivack & Shure, 1974; Spivack, Platt, & Shure, 1976), but subsequent research has produced considerable evidence that the quality of the alternatives generated (e.g., Fischler & Kendall, 1985, cited in Kendall, 1986; Krasnor & Rubin, 1981; Richard & Dodge, 1982; Rubin & Krasnor, 1986) and the child's flexibility in the face of obstacles (Elias et al., 1978; Rubin & Krasnor, 1986) show a stronger relationship to social adjustment and sociometric status.

Ladd and Oden (1979) studied the relationship between peer acceptance and children's ideas about how to be helpful to another child. Third- and fifth-grade children were interviewed about how to help a child depicted as being teased or yelled at by peers or having difficulty with schoolwork in class. Although a wide range of solutions was suggested, there was considerable consensus as well, and unpopular children were more apt to give unique or situationally inappropriate responses than were their popular agemates.

Asher and Renshaw (in Renshaw, 1981) presented popular and unpopular kindergarten children with situations involving initiating and maintaining relationships with other children and dealing with conflicts with peers. They also found a great deal of consensus and went on to examine the ideas suggested exclusively by popular and unpopular children. In general, the unpopular children's exclusive strategies were aggressive, hostile, and less effective, whereas the strategies suggested exclusively by the popular group were prosocial, more apt to include persuasion or social norms, and more effective.

Rubin and his colleagues have conducted a series of studies examining the relationship between sociometric status, observed social play, and social problem solving in young children (e.g., Rubin, 1982; Rubin & Daniels-Beirness, 1983; Rubin, Daniels-Beirness, & Bream, 1984; Rubin, Daniels-Beirness, & Hayvren, 1982; Rubin & Krasnor, 1986). Taken together, they have demonstrated significant, albeit low to moderate, correlations between observations of sociable versus isolate behavior and the quality and flexibility of solutions offered to hypothetical object acquisition and friendship initiation situations. Although withdrawn children have been more apt to suggest passive, unassertive strategies or strategies involving adult intervention (Rubin, 1982; Rubin et al., 1984; Rubin & Krasnor, 1986), the researchers have found no consistent indication that socially withdrawn children are deficient in social-cognitive skills. They have concluded that the difficulty these children have in actual social problem-solving situations is indicative of a lack of confidence (Rubin & Krasnor, 1986). Socially rejected children, however, proposed a higher percentage of antagonistic and assertive strategies to confrontation situations and showed less flexibility after failure (Rubin & Daniels-Beirness, 1983; Rubin et al., 1982).

Richard and Dodge (1982) presented aggressive, isolated, and popular second- and fifth-grade boys with hypothetical situations involving peer conflict and friendship initiation. Popular boys generated more solutions than did aggressive or isolate, boys who did not differ. Most boys in all groups gave effective solutions first, but the popular boys continued to give effective solutions, whereas the subsequent solutions offered by the others were aggressive and ineffective. In contrast to the differences found in their production of strategies, however, the groups did not differ when asked to evaluate solutions on the basis of effectiveness.

Kendall and Fischler (1984) assessed the social problem-solving skills, IQ, behavior adjustment, and actual interpersonal problem-solving behavior in a laboratory situation of 150 families with a son or daughter aged 6 to 11. Using the standard quantitative scoring method, they found no relationship between problem-solving skills and social adjustment or actual problem-solving behavior. In a subsequent analysis using a qualitative scoring system (Fischler & Kendall, 1985, cited in Kendall, 1986), they did find a relationship between appropriateness of solutions and consistency across situations and the children's social adjustment. This relationship held even after controlling for IQ.

Renshaw's (1981; Renshaw & Asher, 1983) study of children's goals and strategies, described earlier, also supports the importance of qualitative analysis of children's strategies and demonstrates differences related to both sociometric status and age. In general, whereas both older and younger children suggested a high proportion of friendly strategies across the four situations presented, older children were more accommodating and polite. Along the assertiveness dimension, older children were more apt to suggest using verbal persuasion, whereas the strategies offered by younger children were more apt to be hostile or rejecting. With regard to sociometric status, strategy difference varied across situations and goals but suggested a picture of low-status children as lacking confidence in their problem resolution strategies and more apt to suggest submissive or avoidant strategies than their higher status peers.

In a video-presented peer group entry situation, Dodge et al. (1986) found a significant relationship between proportion of nonaggressive solutions generated and nonendorsement of passive responses by kindergarten and second-grade children and ratings of their competence and success in an actual peer group entry situation. In his study of response to peer provocation in second-, third-, and fourth-grade severely aggressive and social rejected versus nonaggressive and socially average children, Dodge (1986; Dodge et al., 1986) found no differences in quantity of responses generated, but did find that aggressive children generated a higher proportion of aggressive responses and were less likely than were average children to endorse competent responses. In addition, proportion of competent responses generated, proportion of aggressive responses generated, and endorsement of aggressive responses each contributed significantly to prediction of the child's aggressive behavior in response to an actual peer provocation.

Although the response search and response decision processes have not been widely studied in children with disabilities, some studies have suggested that children with learning disabilities may endorse socially appropriate responses when asked what they should do (Bursuck, 1983) but may make less socially acceptable choices when asked what they actually would do in hypothetical situations (Schumaker & Hazel, 1984). Consistent with this, Gustafson (1989) found that self-contained and mainstreamed students with mild handicaps did not differ on strategy preference or endorsement tasks or when asked for strategies to attain a predetermined prosocial goal, but they did differ when asked to generate both the strategy and the goal. Specifically, although strategies were not more hostile for the self-contained students, these students did give more avoidant or help-seeking strategies and fewer prosocial strategies than did their mainstreamed peers. This apparent tendency toward avoidance is similar to the tendency of isolates to choose "safer" strategies that are less assertive, less costly, and less effective than those chosen by more popular children (Rubin & Krasnor, 1986).

Also in Gustafson's (1989) study, special education teachers' ratings of their students' mainstreaming readiness and regular education teachers' ratings of their students' mainstreaming success were negatively related to use of avoidant or help-seeking strategies. In addition, readiness ratings were positively related to use of outgoing strategies and negatively related to use of hostile strategies. Interestingly, there was one notable difference between ratings by special education teachers (readiness) and ratings by regular education teachers (success) in that the latter showed a positive relationship to assertive as opposed to accommodating strategies. This led to the tentative suggestion that there might be a differential level of acceptance or valuation of assertiveness versus accommodation in regular education versus self-contained contexts.

Enactment and the Competence/Performance Issue

The final step in Dodge's (1986) model is the enactment, or the actual behavioral response. This step is affected not only by the child's accuracy, efficiency, and skill in the preceding steps but also by the child's ability to execute the response in a competent fashion. If, for example, the child's chosen response is to join a group of children, but he or she lacks peer-group entry skills (Dodge et al., 1983; Putallaz, 1983; Putallaz & Gottman, 1981), the result may be unsuccessful.

It is at the point of enactment, too, that the competence/performance issue becomes most obvious, and self-control and emotion regulation play an important role (Gresham, 1981, 1982). Consistent with Palmer's (1980) identification of "functional characteristics," Asher and Hymel (1981); Gresham (1981, 1984, 1986); Kendall (1986); Schumaker and Hazel (1984); and Urbain and Kendall (1980) have emphasized the need to distinquish between competence and performance deficits in social skills, and this takes on particular importance if one's purpose for assessing the social skills is to plan some kind of intervention.

In this regard, Gresham (1984, 1986; Elliott, Gresham, & Heffer, 1987) identified four types of social skill deficits using a two-dimensional grid that considers the presence or absence of an "emotional arousal response" (i.e., anxiety, anger, or impulsivity) and the presence or absence of the skill itself within the child's behavioral repertoire (i.e., whether or not the child knows how to perform the skill). The four types of deficits thus identified are (a) social skill deficits, that is, a basic lack of social skills; (b) social performance deficits, in which skills have been acquired but are performed infrequently because of a lack of motivation or limited opportunity; (c) self-control skill deficits, in which the child's acquisition of a specific skill has been impeded by an emotional arousal response (e.g., extreme social anxiety may preclude a child's development of conversation or play skills); and (d) self-control performance deficits, in which the skill is within the child's repertoire but is infrequently or inconsistently performed because of an emotional arousal response such as anxiety, anger, or impulsivity. In other words, some children may be able to respond quite adequately to hypothetical-reflective assessments of competence in the earlier processing steps and may even be able to adequately role-play the desired skills, but their lack of self-control or high level of anxiety may interfere with their demonstration of these skills in day-to-day social encounters. Consistent with this, Kendall (1986) has suggested that impulsive children may skip prematurely to the enactment step without adequate response search and evaluation. Anxious and impulsive children may therefore be less successful in, or perceived as less ready for, a mainstreaming setting than those who are less anxious or whose self-control skills are better developed.

With regard to anxiety, Gustafson (1989) found no significant effects for self-contained versus mainstreamed students and no relationship to teacher ratings of mainstreaming readiness or success. This may be due to the measure used, the Revised Children's Manifest Anxiety Scale (RCMAS), which assesses chronic general anxiety (trait anxiety). It may be that the anxiety more apt to interfere with competent social functioning is more socially specific (i.e., state anxiety). Support for this comes from a subsequent study on the Social Anxiety Scale for Children (SASC) (La Greca, Dandes, Wick, Shaw, & Stone, 1988). This 10-item self-report scale contains two factors: fear of negative evaluation (FNE) and social avoidance and distress (SAD). In a study of 287 second-through sixth-grade students, a moderate positive correlation was found between this measure of social anxiety and the chronic manifest anxiety measured by the RCMAS. Of greater interest, however, was the finding that the SASC was able to detect peer status group differences, with neglected children reporting the greatest level of social anxiety and controversial children reporting the lowest level. As in Gustatson's (1989) study, administration of the RCMAS at the same time showed no significant group differences. In a related study that addressed the anxiety factor through a self-perception questionnaire it was found that mainstreamed students with mild retardation reported greater anxiety about game situations with peers and more dissatisfaction with their social relationships in school than their nonretarded classmates (Taylor et al., 1987).

With regard to impulsivity, Gustafson (1989) found that teacher ratings on the Self-Control Rating Scale were significantly higher (indicating poorer self-control) for self-contained than for matched mainstreamed students; and among mainstreamed students, ratings were higher for those mainstreamed less than half the school day than for those who spent more than half the day in a regular classroom setting. Impulsivity ratings were also strongly related to teacher ratings of mainstreaming readiness and success. Perhaps more significant, however, was the fact that impulsivity made a significant contribution to the prediction of readiness, placement, and success in the presence of all other social competence variables. Goals and strategies also contributed to placement and to ratings of mainstreaming readiness, but impulsivity made the only significant contribution to ratings of mainstreaming success. The overriding significance of impulsivity suggests that, regardless of social-cognitive abilities, adequate self-control may be a prerequisite for successful placement in a mainstream setting, and that the self-control skills of children with mild handicaps warrant particular attention. Social skills training that teaches students a repertoire of appropriate behaviors, even training that includes the identification of appropriate goals and strategies, may not provide sufficient preparation for mainstreaming if the student lacks self-control. Kendall (1986) has asserted the impulse control is the first step in social problem solving, and Bernfeld and Peters (1986) have suggested that training should focus on the "implementation of available social-cognitive skills rather than on the knowledge of these skills, per se" (p. 226).

Facilitating Successful Mainstreaming

It should be clear from the foregoing discussion that successful mainstreaming placement, including social and instructional as well as temporal integration, is considerably influenced by the entering child's level of social competence. In view of this, it is not surprising to see special educators' current level of interest in social skills training. It should also be clear, however, that careful consideration of a child's readiness in this regard requires an understanding of the multidimensional nature of social competence and should not be limited to any single dimension. A promising new approach to identifying problem areas is Gresham and Elliott's (1990) Social Skills Rating System. This system uses self-ratings as well as ratings by teachers and parents at the preschool, elementary, and secondary levels, and has been normed on both handicapped and nonhandicapped students. It includes five subscales of social skills (cooperation, assertion, responsibility, empathy, and self-control); three subscales of problem behaviors (internalizing problems, externalizing problems, and hyperactivity); and a general rating of academic competence. Taken together, these measures are designed to facilitate identification of social skills strengths, performance deficits, and acquisition deficits, as well as specific problem behaviors that may interfere with the acquisition or performance of social skills. Suggestions are also included for linking the results with appropriate behavioral interventions. In addition to providing some normative information on the identified factors, it includes a number of items that address the areas of social anxiety (e.g., shows anxiety with children, is easily embarrassed) and social-cognitive skills (e.g., compromises in conflicts, ends disagreements calmly) and might thus serve to identify students with possible deficits in those areas. These might then be further explored through additional ratings, direct observation, role play, or structured interviews.

Just as assessment techniques should be multidimensional, any programming planned to improve social competence should also take cognitive, affective, and behavioral factors into account. Although it is well beyond the scope of this chapter to provide a comprehensive review of prevention and/or intervention programs and related research, we will present a brief overview of the kinds of programs available.

To date, the majority of programs for training in this area have been behavioral in focus, emphasizing either operant or social-learning techniques. The former are generally focused on manipulation of consequences through carefully designed behavior management programs to increase the frequency of desirable target behaviors and decrease the frequency of undesirable behaviors, but manipulation of antecedents such as arranging seating or encouraging peer initiations to promote positive interactions is also often used (Elliott & Gresham, 1987; Gresham, 1985).

Social-learning techniques, on the other hand, involve the use of such strategies as specific instruction in the target behaviors, modeling, coaching, role play, and feedback and reinforcement. Some effective examples include coaching programs designed to teach conversation skills (Bierman, 1986); the skills of asking questions, giving directions, and offering support or encouragement (Ladd, 1981); and game-playing skills (Oden & Asher, 1977). Examples of published programs are Goldstein et al.'s (1980) *Skillstreaming the Adolescent* McGinnis et al.'s (1984) *Skillstreaming the Elementary School Child*, and Walker et al.'s (1983) *A Curriculum for Children's Effective Peer and Teacher Skills (ACCEPTS)*. The first two present 60 and 50 prosocial skills, respectively, in a single-lesson format and are intended for use with any students whose classroom or social behavior is problematic. The latter was specifically designed to teach students with mild or moderate handicaps a set of 28 behavioral skills to prepare them for successful adjustment in mainstream settings. All three programs include guidelines for selecting and teaching specific skills as well as some suggestions to encourage generalization, an essential component of any training program (Weissberg, 1985). Two important limitations in these and other primarily behavioral programs, however, are (a) their failure to specifically address the issue of self-control or emotional arousal as it applies to either the acquisition or the performance of the specified behaviors and (b) their lack of attention to the social-cognitive skills that are a significant component of social competence.

With regard to self-control, most approaches to training include a combination of cognitive-behavioral and social-learning techniques. These involve the use of modeling and rehearsal to teach the student to use verbal self-instruction as he or she goes through the basic steps of problem solving, beginning with a reminder to "stop and think." One example of this is Kendall and Braswell's (1985; Kendall, Padewar, Zupan, & Braswell, 1985) treatment program for impulsive children. This 16-session program not only teaches a stop-and-think strategy for cognitive (academic) tasks but also, consistent with our multidimensional model, includes training in recognizing emotions and social problem solving. The program begins with the introduction of five steps, which the student is instructed to put in his or her own words and say out loud when approaching a task or a problem. The steps involve identifying what the problem is ("What am I supposed to do?"), looking at every option presented ("Look at all the possibilities"), concentrating ("Focus in"), making a decision ("Pick an answer"), and double-checking to see if the decision is correct ("Check out your answer"). Through a process of modeling, practice, and response-cost contingencies that carries throughout the entire program, the student is encouraged to use the steps as he or she goes through a series of tasks of varying type and complexity. The first eight lessons begin with paper-and-pencil tasks such as following directions, solving arithmetic problems, and performing word searches, followed by more social activities such as playing board games. In the second half of the program, the focus becomes more interpersonal, and tasks include recognizing feelings, evaluating possible courses of action in terms of emotional and behavioral consequences, thinking about hypothetical problem situations, and considering and acting out possible solutions to some personally relevant problems. Throughout the program, all sessions also include generalization training through homework activities called Show That I Can (STIC) tasks.

Another approach to self-control training is Schneider and Robin's (1978) Turtle Technique, which teaches students to cue themselves to stop and think through a specific behavioral response. This approach begins with a story about an impulsive and unhappy little turtle who receives some sage advice from the oldest and wisest turtle in town. The advice is to not react immediately when he feels upset, but rather to pull himself into his shell and calm down first, and then to think carefully about what to do next. After listening to the story and acting it out, students are taught (or develop) a behavioral signal to represent "pulling into one's shell." Then, through modeling, practice, and reinforcement, they are encouraged to use the signal whenever they are upset as a reminder to calm down and think. This approach also includes some training in social problem-solving skills, but that is not the primary focus of either program.

Programs that do focus primarily on social problem-solving (SPS) skills or interpersonal cognitive problem-solving (ICPS) skills are indebted to the early prevention work of Spivack and Shure (1974; Sprivack et al., 1976). Although specific programs vary in the number and specificity of the problem-solving steps they teach, they all have in common some training in encoding and interpretation (feelings identification, problem identification); response search and response selection (generation of alternatives, evaluation of consequences, selection of a solution); and enactment (means–ends thinking to implement the choice). The more comprehensive programs have a developmental orientation to allow for differences in cognitive development, language skills, and affective understanding, and also include a strategy for self-control, consideration, and evaluation of goals; steps for overcoming obstacles; and specific activities to enhance generalization. One example is Greenberg et al.'s (in press) *PATHS (Providing Alternative THinking Strategies) Curriculum* which presents an extensive set of developmentally sequenced and hierarchically organized lessons designed to teach self-control, emotional understanding, and interpersonal problem solving to special-needs children in the elementary school. Additional programs developed by Elias (1983) and Weissberg et al. (1980) have shown promise both as primary prevention programs and as interventions with aggressive, maladjusted, and seriously emotionally disturbed children.

One final type of approach for facilitating successful adjustment in the mainstream involves working to make the mainstream environment itself more conducive to success. Specific strategies might include structuring cooperative learning activities (Johnson & Johnson, 1980) and teaching collaborative skills (Putnam, Rynders, Johnson, & Johnson, 1989); using coaching techniques and involving nonhandicapped peers as partners in structured practice sessions (Bierman & Furman, 1984); or teaching social skills to the entire mainstream class. Another promising strategy is developing a "circle of friends" (Forest & Lusthaus, 1989) for the mainstreamed student. This involves a set of activities to sensitize the nonhandicapped students in the mainstream setting and to enlist some of them to form a support network for the mainstreamed student. Circles thus formed are facilitated by a trained adult; are informal, open, and entirely voluntary; and have as their sole purpose to nurture the development of genuine, reciprocal, caring, and supportive relationships.

Ideally, as students with handicaps are increasingly integrated into the mainstream, programs addressing their social competence needs will likewise become an integral part of the services provided. It is critical, however, that these not just be another form of "pull-out" program. Although some specific skills may be most efficiently taught in individual or small-group sessions, the overall program must include carefully planned strategies for generalization and maintenance, including active involvement of classroom teachers, other staff, and nonhandicapped peers. For more information about the types of interventions discussed here, the reader is referred to (a) Gresham (1986), Elliott et al., (1987), and Michelson, Sugai, Wood, and Kazdin (1983) for behavioral approaches; (b) Kendall and Braswell (1985), for cognitive-behavioral treatment; (c) Ladd and Mize (1983) for cognitive-social learning approaches; and (d) Gesten, Weissberg, Amish, and Smith (1987) and Pellegrini and Urbain (1985) for social problem-solving training.

Summary

In 1986, Madeline Will, then assistant secretary of the Office of Special Education and Rehabilitation Services, proposed a partnership between regular and special education to increase, to the fullest extent, the number of students with handicaps to be included in regular classrooms in the schools throughout the nation. This statement was received wholeheartedly by many of the professionals in special education. Some educators have gone so far as to recommend a total elimination of the dual systems of regular education and special education to form a single comprehensive system appropriately organized and administered to educate all students.

This position is not shared totally by regular educators or by all special educators. Many general education teachers argue that the pressures of large classes, students with behavior problems, and the emphasis on greater academic achievement are already extremely demanding. Adding one more instructional problem would be overwhelming. In addition, there are concerns that adding children with handicaps would increase the already high teacher stress level. Finally, many general education teachers express a concern about their lack of professional preparation to teach students with disabilities.

Since the mid-1970s, greater emphasis has been placed on teaching social skills competence. Social competence has been seen as important to building positive social interaction between students with handicaps and their nonhandicapped peers. By contrast, poor peer relationships in childhood can be associated with dropping out of school, juvenile delinquency, and emotional and social/behavior problems. This research has provided the basis for associating social competence with the maintenance of positive social relationships with peers and adults. Students experiencing mild to moderate learning and behavior disabilities are by far the greatest number of students now being integrated in general education. It is reasonable to assume that if these students are responsive to social skill development, their positive social experiences in regular classrooms will be substantially increased.

The ideology that students with learning and behavior disabilities should be placed in regular classrooms offers many practical advantages. Social interactions gained by experiences with nonhandicapped peers outweigh by far the administrative convenience of social segregation. However, placement is an important consideration. The indiscriminate, unplanned placement of students with disabilities in regular classes can create major problems, both for the students involved as well as for nonhandicapped peers. Some school districts have followed completely the General Education Initiative (GEI) without consideration for the severity of learning and behavior disabilities. The literature does not provide systematic strategies for guiding the placement process; nevertheless, social behavior skills seem to be a major determinant in how much of the school day a student is placed in the regular classroom or, in some districts, whether or not he or she is placed there at all.

Students with learning and behavior disabilities are a heterogeneous population, and their individual differences contribute significantly to their acceptance by peers and teachers in regular education. Among these characteristic differences demonstrated by students with disabilities, the most pervasive determinant is social behavior, which strongly suggests that intervention programs designed to increase social competency should facilitate the process of mainstreaming these students successfully.

We have defined social competence as a multifaceted construct comprised of cognitive, affective, and behavioral factors. In keeping with this comprehensive approach to the definition, we have drawn on models of social competence and social information processing developed by Greenspan (1981) and Dodge (1986), respectively.

These models have advantages over several others available because they are complementary in (a) providing a "whole child" perspective, including factors from the affective, behavioral, and cognitive domains; and in (b) outlining the ways in which specific social-cognitive skills may contribute to social competence outcomes.

The Greenspan (1981) social competence model is particularly "teacher friendly," and is also very appropriate in terms of its applicability to at-risk students and students with learning and behavior disabilities. The model defines social competence as consisting of three major components: temperament, character, and social awareness. By temperament, Greenspan refers to reflection/impulsivity and calmness/emotionality. Character relates to social activity/inactivity and niceness/nastiness. Social awareness refers to social sensitivity, social insight, and social communication.

Using these dimensions as basic references in comparing children with emotional disturbance and learning disabilities with normal same-age peers, children with disabilities perform less well on measures of social perception and situations involving stressful emotions. Particular difficulties are encountered by these students in interpreting social cues accurately. Students with learning disabilities are significantly less able to discern feelings and intentions of others.

Severely aggressive, externalizing students are less accurate in interpreting positive social intentions and make a greater number of errors toward presumed hostility. Further, the proportion of errors slanted toward hostility is significantly related to actual aggressive responses. One might well conclude that skills in encoding (perceiving) and interpreting social cues and responding appropriately are very important and need to be considered in the selection and arrangement of experiences for students with handicaps in mainstream settings.

Apparently, students with handicaps placed in self-contained classrooms have more avoidant and hostile social goals than do their peers who are in regular classrooms. Avoidant goals are related to ratings of maladaptive behavior, which suggests that even when appropriate social behaviors are taught, they may not be generalized (Haring, 1988). Negative expectations and stereotypes may contribute to the social rejection of low sociometric status children and students with behavior disorders in mainstream settings. These negative attitudes are very likely to result in aversive experiences for these children, and it is reasonable to expect such experiences to influence them toward hostile or avoidant goals. The preparation, then, for successful mainstreaming should include activities that will not only teach appropriate social skills and social goals, but also address the attitudes of their nonhandicapped peer group.

Recommendations

1. The placement of students with behavior disorders and learning disabilities in general education settings is necessary, but this process must be carefully planned and systematically implemented.
2. Placement must be assisted and supported by information gained through multidimensional assessment of the social competence of students who are to be placed in regular education.
3. The relationship between the level of social competence demonstrated and the prospect of successful social adaptation to integrated classroom placement and subsequent performance is significantly high as to warrant attention to social skill training to facilitate integration.
4. Social skill training programs designed to improve social competence should include cognitive, affective, and behavioral components.
5. Broader, more comprehensive strategies designed toward building social competence appear to be more effective where cognitive behavior intervention is used. Strategies such as specific instruction in target social behavior, modeling, peer coaching, role play, and feedback and reinforcement are especially effective.
6. Self-control, a cognitive behavior critical to social adaptability, can be improved significantly. Approaches effective in increasing self-control include a combination of cognitive-behavioral and social-learning techniques. These involve the use of modeling and rehearsal, student self-instruction, and learning the basic steps in problem solving.
7. Nonhandicapped peers display a significantly higher level of acceptance of students with handicaps who make appropriate social responses. It is crucial to teach a range of socially acceptable responses and to structure opportunities for generalization of those behaviors so they will be observed and acknowledged by the nonhandicapped peers.

References

Asher, S.R., & Hymel, S. (1981). Children's social competence in peer relations: Sociometric and behavioral assessment. In J.D. Wine & M.D. Smye (Eds.), Social Competence (pp. 125–157). New York: Guilford.

Asher, S.R., & Renshaw, P.D. (1981). Children without friends: Social knowledge and social skill training. In S.R. Asher & J.M. Gottman (Eds.), *The development of children's friendships* (pp. 273–296). New York: Cambridge University Press.

Axelrod, L. (1982). Social perception in learning disabled adolescents. *Journal of Learning Disabilities*, *15*, 10–13.

Bachara, G.H. (1976). Empathy in learning disabled children. *Perceptual and Motor Skills*, *43*, 541–542.

Bernfeld, G.A., & Peters, R. DeV. (1986). Social reasoning and social behavior in reflective and impulsive children. *Journal of Clinical Child Psychology*, *15*, 221–227.

Bierman, K.L. (1986). Process of change during social skills training with preadolescents and its relation to treatment outcome. *Child Development*, *57*, 230–240.

Bierman, K.L., & Furman, W. (1984). The effects of social skills training and peer involvement on the social adjustment of preadolescents. *Child Development*, *55*, 151–162.

Braaten, S., Kauffman, J.M., Braaten, B., Polsgrove, L., & Nelson, C.M. (1988). The regular education initiative: Patent medicine for behavioral disorders. *Exceptional Children*, *55*, 21–27.

Bruno, R.R. (1981). Interpretation of pictorially presented social situations by learning disabled and normal children. *Journal of Learning Disabilities*, *14*, 350–352.

Bryan, T.H. (1977). Learning disabled children's comprehension of nonverbal communication. *Journal of Learning Disabilities*, *10*, 501–506.

Bryan, T., Bay, M., & Donahue, M. (1988). Implications of the learning disabilities definition for the regular education initiative. *Journal of Learning Disabilities*, *21*, 23–28.

Bukowski, W.M. & Hoza, B. (1989). Popularity and friendship: Issues in theory, measurement, and outcome. In T.J. Berndt & G.W. Ladd (Eds.), *Peer relationships in child development* (pp. 15–45). New York: Wiley & Sons.

Bursuck, W.D. (1983). Sociometric status, behavior ratings, and social knowledge of learning disabled and low achieving students. *Learning Disability Quarterly*, *6*, 329–339.

Cartledge, G., Frew, T., & Zacharias, J. (1985). Social skill needs of mainstreamed students: Peer and teacher perceptions. *Learning Disability Quarterly*, *8*, 132–140.

Cartledge, G., Stupay, D., & Kaczala, C. (1986). Social skills and social perception of learning disabled and nonhandicapped elementary school children. *Learning Disability Quarterly*, *9*, 227–234.

Coben, S., & Zigmond, N. (1986). The social integration of learning disabled students from self-contained to mainstream elementary school settings. *Journal of Learning Disabilities*, *19*, 614–618.

Cowen, E.L., Pederson, A., Babigian, H., Izzo, L.D., & Trost, M.A. (1973). Long-term follow-up of early detected vulnerable children. *Journal of Consulting & Clinical Psychology, 41*, 438–446.
Davis, W.E. (1989). The regular education initiative debate: Its promises and problems. *Exceptional Children, 55*, 440–446.
Dickstein, E.B., & Warren, D.R. (1980). Role-taking deficits in learning disabled children. *Journal of Learning Disabilities, 13*, 378–382.
Dodge, K.A. (1980a). Attributional bias in aggressive children. In P.C. Kendall (Ed.), *Advances in cognitive-behavioral research and therapy*. New York: Academic.
Dodge, K.A. (1980b). Social cognition and children's aggressive behavior. *Child Development, 51*, 162–170.
Dodge, K.A. (1986). A social information processing model of social competence in childhood. In M. Perlmutter (Ed.), *Cognitive perspectives on children's social and behavioral development* (pp. 77–125). Hillsdale, NJ: Erlbaum.
Dodge, K.A., & Frame, C.L. (1982). Social cognitive biases and deficits in aggressive boys. *Child Development, 53*, 620–635.
Dodge, K.A., Murphy, R.R., & Buchsbaum, K. (1984). The assessment of intention-cue detection skills in children: Implications for developmental psychopathology. *Child Development, 55*, 163–173.
Dodge, K.A., & Newman, J.P. (1981). Biased decision making processes in aggressive boys. *Journal of Abnormal Psychology, 90*, 375–379.
Dodge, K.A., Pettit, G.S., McClaskey, C.L., & Brown, M.M. (1986). Social competence in children. *Monographs of the Society for Research in Child Development, 51*(2, Serial No. 213).
Dodge, K.A., Schlundt, D.G., Schocken, I., & J.D. (1983). Social competence and children's sociometric status: The role of peer group entry strategies. *Merrill-Palmer Quarterly, 29*, 309–336.
Elias, M.J. (1983). Improving coping skills of emotionally disturbed boys through television-based social problem solving. *American Journal of Orthopsychiatry, 53*, 61–72.
Elias, M.J., Lareen, S.W., Zlotow, S.P., & Chinsky, J.H. (1978). *An innovative measure of children's cognitions in problematic interpersonal situations*. Paper presented at the American Psychological Association, Toronto, Canada.
Elliott, S.N., Gresham, F.M., & Heffer, R.W. (1987). Social-skills interventions: Research findings and training techniques. In C.A. Maher & J.E. Zins (Eds.), *Psychoeducational interventions in the schools* (pp. 141–159). New York: Pergamon.
Forest, M. & Lusthaus, E. (1989). Promoting educational equality for all students: Circles and maps. In S. Stainback, W. Stainback, & M. Forest (Eds.), *Educating all students in the mainstream of regular education* (pp. 43–57). Baltimore: Paul H. Brookes.
Fuchs, D., & Fuchs, L.S. (1988a). Evaluation of the adaptive learning environments model. *Exceptional Children, 55*, 115–127.
Fuchs, S., & Fuchs, L.S. (1988b). Response to Wang and Walberg. *Exceptional Children, 55*, 138–146.
Furman, W. (1984). Issues in the assessment of social skills in normal and handicapped children. In T. Field, J.L. Roopnarine, & M. Segal (Eds.), *Friendships in normal and handicapped children*. Norwood, NJ: Ablex.

Gartner, A., & Lipsky, D.K. (1987). Beyond special education: Toward a quality system for all students. *Harvard Educational Review*, *57*, 367–395.

Gerber, P.J., & Zinkgraf, S.A. (1982). A comparative study of social-perceptual ability in learning disabled and nonhandicapped students. *Learning Disability Quarterly*, *5*, 374–378.

Gesten, E.L., Weissberg, R.P., Amish, P.L., & Smith, J.K. (1987). Social problem-solving training: A skills-based approach to prevention and treatment. In C.A. Maher & J.E. Zins (Eds.), *Psychoeducational interventions in the schools* (pp. 26–45). New York: Pergamon.

Goldstein, A.P., Sprafkin, R.P., Gershaw, N.J., & Klein, P. (1980). *Skillstreaming the adolescent*. Champaign, IL: Research Press Company.

Gottlieb, J., Levy, L., & Gottlieb, B.W. (1986). The play behavior of mainstreamed learning disabled children. In C.J. Meisel (Ed.), *Mainstreaming outcomes, controversies, and new directions*. Hillsdale, NJ: Erlbaum.

Gottman, J., Gonso, J., & Rasmussen, B. (1975). Social interaction, social competence and friendship in children. *Child Development*, *46*, 709–718.

Greenberg, M.T., Kusche, C.A., Gustafson, R.N., & Calderon, R. (in press). *The PATHS (Providing Alternative THinking Strategies) Curriculum*. Seattle, WA: University of Washington Press.

Greenspan, S. (1981). Defining childhood social competence: A proposed working model. In B.K. Keogh (Ed.), *Advances in special education* (Vol. 3, pp. 1–39). Greenwich, CT: JAI Press.

Gresham, F.M. (1981). Social skills training with handicapped children: A review. *Review of Educational Research*, *51*, 139–176.

Gresham, F.M. (1982). Misguided mainstreaming: The case for social skills with handicapped children. *Exceptional Children*, *48*, 422–433.

Gresham, F.M. (1983). Social skills assessment as a component of mainstreaming placement decisions. *Exceptional Children*, *49*, 331–336.

Gresham, F.M. (1984). Social skills and self-efficacy for exceptional children. *Exceptional Children*, *51*, 253–261.

Gresham, F.M. (1985). Best practices in social skills training. In A. Thomas & J. Grimes (Eds.), *Best practices in school psychology* (pp. 181–192). Kent, OH: National Association of School Psychologists.

Gresham, F.M. (1986). Strategies for enhancing the social outcomes of mainstreaming: A necessary ingredient for success. In C.J. Meisel (Ed.), *Mainstreaming handicapped children: Outcomes, controversies and new directions* (pp. 193–218). Hillsdale, NJ: Erlbaum.

Gresham, F.M., & Elliot, S.N. (1990). *Social skills rating system*. Circle Pines, MN: American Guidance Service.

Gustafson, R.N. (1989). An examination of the relationship between social competence and mainstreaming readiness, placement and success in mildly handicapped students (Doctoral dissertation, University of Washington, 1988). *Dissertation Abstracts International*, *50*, 627A.

Hallahan, D.P., Keller, C.E., McKinney, J.D., Lloyd, J.W., & Bryan, T. (1988). Examining the research base of the regular education initiative: Efficacy studies and the adaptive learning environments model. *Journal of Learning Disabilities*, *21*, 29–35.

Haring, N.G. (Ed.). (1988). *Generalization for students with severe handicaps: Strategies and solutions*. Seattle, WA: University of Washington Press.

Haring, N.G., & Billingsley, F.F. (1984). Systems-change strategies to ensure the future of integration. In N. Certo, N. Haring, & R. York (Eds.), *Public school integration of severely handicapped students: Rational issues and progressive alternatives* (pp. 83–105). Baltimore: Paul H. Brookes.

Hartup, W.W. (1970). Peer interaction and social organization. In P. Mussen (Ed.), *Carmichael's manual of child psychology* (Vol. 2). New York: Wiley.

Hartup, W.W. (1983). The peer system. In E.M. Hetherington (Ed.), *Handbook of child psychology: Socialization, personality, and social development*. New York: Wiley.

Hersch, R.H., & Walker, H.M. (1982). *Great expectations: Making schools effective for all students*. Paper presented at the Conference on Public Policy and the Special Education Task of the 1980s, Racine, WI.

Hollinger, J.D. (1987). Social skills for behaviorally disordered children as preparation for mainstreaming: Theory, practice, and new directions. *Remedial and Special Education*, *8*, 17–27.

Horowitz, E.C. (1981). Popularity, decentering ability, and role-taking skills in learning disabled and normal children. *Learning Disability Quarterly*, *4*, 23–30.

Hundert, J. (1982). Some considerations of planning the integration of handicapped children into the mainstream. *Journal of Learning Disabilities*, *15*, 73–80.

Johnson, D.W., & Johnson, R.T. (1980). Integrating handicapped students into the mainstream. *Exceptional Children*, *47*, 90–98.

Kauffman, J.M., Gerber, M.M., & Semmel, M.I. (1988). Arguable assumptions underlying the regular education initiative. *Journal of Learning Disabilities*, *21*, 6–11.

Kaufman, M., Gottlieb, J., Agard, J., & Kukic, M. (1975). Mainstreaming: Toward an explication of the construct. In E.L. Meyer, G.A. Vergason, & R.J. Whelan (Eds.), *Alternatives for teaching exceptional children*. Denver, CO: Love.

Kavale, K., & Andreassen, E. (1984). Factors in diagnosing the learning disabled: Analysis of judgmental policies. *Journal of Learning Disabilities*, *17*, 273–278.

Kendall, P.C. (1986). Comments on Rubin and Krasnor: Solutions and problems in research on problem solving. In M. Perlmutter (Ed.), *Cognitive perspectives on children's social and behavioral development* (pp. 69–76). Hillsdale, NJ: Erlbaum.

Kendall, P.C., & Braswell, L. (1985). *Cognitive-behavioral therapy for impulsive children*. New York: Guilford.

Kendall, P.C., Padawer, W., Zupan, B. & Braswell, L. (1985). In P.C. Kendall & L. Braswell (Eds.), *Cognitive-behavioral therapy for impulsive children* (pp. 179–209). New York: Guilford.

Kendall, P.C., & Fischler, G.L. (1984). Behavioral and adjustment correlates of problem-solving: Validational analyses of interpersonal cognitive problem-solving measures. *Child Development*, *55*, 879–892.

Keogh, B.K. (1988). Improving services for problem learners: Rethinking and restructuring. *Journal of Learning Disabilities*, *21*, 19–22.

Krasnor, L.R., & Rubin, K.H. (1981). Assessment of social problem-solving in young children. In T. Merluzzi, C. Glass, & M. Genest (Eds.), *Cognitive assessment*. New York: Guilford.

Kurdek, L.A., & Krile, D. (1982). A developmental analysis of the relation between peer acceptance and both interpersonal understanding and perceived social self-competence. *Child Development*, *53*, 1485–1491.

Ladd, G.W. (1981). Effectiveness of a social learning method for enhancing children's social interaction and peer acceptance. *Child Development*, *52*, 171–178.

Ladd, G.W. (1989). Toward a further understanding of peer relationships and their contributions to child development. In T.J. Berndt & G.W. Ladd (Eds.), *Peer relationships in child development*. New York: Wiley & Sons.

Ladd, G.W., & Mize, J. (1983). A cognitive-social learning model of social-skill training. *Psychological Review*, *90*, 127–157.

Ladd, G.W., & Oden, S. (1979). The relationship between peer acceptance and children's ideas about helpfulness. *Child Development*, *50*, 402–408.

La Greca, A.M. (1981). Social behavior and social perception in learning disabled children: A review with implications for social skills training. *Journal of Pediatric Psychology*, *6*, 395–416.

La Greca, A.M., Dandes, S.K., Wick, P., Shaw, K., & Stone, W.L. (1988). Development of the social anxiety scale for children: Reliability and concurrent validity. *Journal of Clinical Child Psychology*, *17*, 84–91.

Madden, N.A., & Slavin, R.E. (1982). *Count me in: Academic achievement and social outcomes of mainstreaming students with mild academic handicaps*. Baltimore: Center for Social Organization of Schools.

Madden, N.A., & Slavin, R.E. (1983). Mainstreaming students with mild handicaps: Academic and social outcomes. *Review of Educational Research*, *53*, 519–569.

McFall, R.M. (1982). A review and reformulation of the concept of social skills. *Behavioral Assessment*, *4*, 1–33.

McConaughy, S.H., & Ritter, D.R. (1986). Social competence and behavioral problems of learning disabled boys aged 6–11. *Journal of Learning Disabilities*, *19*, 39–45.

McGinnis, E., & Goldstein, A.P. (1984). *Skillstreaming the elementary school child*. Champaign, IL: Research Press Company.

McKinney, J.D. (1984). The search for subtypes of specific learning disabilities. *Journal of Learning Disabilities*, *17*, 43–50.

Meichenbaum, D., Butler, L.,& Gruson, L. (1981). Toward a conceptual model of social competence. In J.D. Wine & M.D. Smye (Eds.), *Social competence* 36–60. New York: Guilford.

Michelson, L., Sugai, D.P., Wood R.P., & Kazdin, A. (1983). *Social skills assessment and training with children: An empirically based handbook*. New York: Plenum.

Morrison, R.L., & Bellack, A.S. (1981). The role of social perception in social skill. *Behavior Therapy*, *12*, 69–79.

Oden, S.L., & Asher, S.R. (1977). Coaching children in social skills for friendship making. *Child Development*, *48*, 495–506.

Oliva, A.H., & La Greca, A.M. (1988). Children with learning disabilities: Social goals and strategies. *Journal of Learning Disabilities*, *21*, 301–306.

Olson, J., & Midgett, J. (1984). Alternative placements: Does a difference exist in the LD populations? *Journal of Learning Disabilities*, *17*, 101–103.

Palmer, D.J. (1980). Factors to be considered in placing handicapped children in regular education classes. *Journal of School Psychology*, *18*, 163–171.

Parker, J.G., & Gottman, J.M. (1989). Social and emotional development in a relational context: Friendship interaction from early childhood to adolescence. In T.J. Berndt & G.W. Ladd (Eds.), *Peer relationships in child development*. New York: Wiley & Sons.

Parkhurst, J.T., & Asher, S.R. (1986). Goals and concerns: Implications for the study of children's social competence. In B.B. Lahey & A.E. Kazden (Eds.), *Advances in clinical child psychiatry* (Vol. 8, pp. 199–228). New York: Plenum.

Pearl, R., & Cosden, M. (1982). Sizing up a situation: LD children's understanding of social interactions. *Learning Disability Quarterly*, *5*, 371–373.

Pellegrini, D.S., & Urbain, E.S. (1985). An evaluation of interpersonal cognitive problem-solving training with children. *Journal of Child Psychology and Psychiatry*, *26*, 17–41.

Perlmutter, B.F., Crocker, J., Cordray, D., & Gorstecki, D. (1983). Sociometric status and related personality characteristics of mainstreamed LD adolescents. *Learning Disability Quarterly*, *6*, 20–30.

Prillaman, D. (1981). Acceptance of learning disabled students in the mainstream environment: A failure to replicate. *Journal of Learning Disabilities*, *14*, 344–346.

Putallaz, M. (1983). Predicting children's sociometric status from their behavior. *Child Development*, *54*, 1417–1426.

Putallaz, M., & Gottman, J.M. (1981). An interactional model of children's entry into peer groups. *Child Development*, *52*, 986–994.

Putnam, J.W., Rynders, J.E., Johnson, R.T., & Johnson, D.W. (1989). Collaborative skill instruction for promoting positive interactions between mentally handicapped and nonhandicapped children. *Exceptional Children*, *55*, 550–557.

Renshaw, P.D. (1981). *Social knowledge and sociometric status: Children's goals and stratetgies for peer interaction* (Doctoral dissertation, University of illinois, 1981). *Dissertation Abstracts International*, *42*, 3081A.

Renshaw, P.D., & Asher, S.R. (1982). Social competence and peer status: The distinction between goals and stratetgies. In K.H. Rubin & H.S. Ross (Eds.), *Peer relationships and social skills in childhood* 376–395. New York: Springer-Verlag.

Renshaw, P.D., & Asher, S.R. (1983). Children's goals and strategies for social interaction. *Merrill-Palmer Quarterly*, *29*, 353–374.

Renshaw, P.D., & Asher, S.R. (1985). The study of children's social goals: A reply to Gresham's commentary. *Merrill-Palmer Quarterly*, *31*, 105–109.

Richard, B.S., & Dodge, K.A. (1982). Social maladjustment and problem-solving in school-aged children. *Journal of Consulting and Clinical Psychology*, *50*, 226–233.

Roff, M., Sells, S.B., & Golden, M.M. (1972). *Social adjustment and personality development in children*. Minneapolis: The University of Minnesota Press.

Rothenberg, B.B. (1970). Children's social sensitivity and the relationship to interpersonal competence, intrapersonal comfort, and intellectual level. *Developmental Psychology*, *2*, 335–350.

Rubin, K.H. (1982). Social and social-cognitive developmental characteristics of young isolate, normal, and sociable children. In K.H. Rubin & H.S. Ross (Eds.), *Peer relationships and social skills in childhood* 353–374. New York: Springer-Verlag.
Rubin, K.H., & Daniels-Beirness, T. (1983). Concurrent and predictive correlates of sociometric status in kindergarten and grade one children. *Merrill-Palmer Quarterly*, *29*, 337–352.
Rubin, K.H., Daniels-Beirness, T., & Bream, L. (1984). Social isolation and social problem-solving: A longitudinal study. *Journal of Consulting and Clinical Psychology*, *52*, 17–25.
Rubin, K.H., Daniels-Beirness, T., & Hayvren, M. (1982). Social and social-cognitive correlates of sociometric status in preschool and kindergarten children. *Canadian Journal of Behavioral Science*, *14*, 338–348.
Rubin, K.H., & Krasnor, L.R. (1986). Social-cognitive and social behavioral perspectives on problem solving. In M. Perlmutter (Ed.), *Cognitive perspectives on children's social and behavioral development* (pp. 1–68). Hillsdale, NJ: Erlbaum.
Sabornie, E.J. (1985). Social mainstreaming of handicapped students: Facing an unpleasant reality. *Remedial and Special Education*, *6*, 12–16.
Salend, S.J. (1984). Factors contributing to the development of successful mainstreaming programs. *Exceptional Children*, *50*, 409–416.
Salend, S.J., & Lutz, J.G. (1984). Mainstreaming or mainlining: A competency based approach to mainstreaming. *Journal of Learning Disabilities*, *17*, 27–29.
Schneider, M., & Robin, A. (1978). *Manual for the Turtle Technique*. Unpublished manuscript, State University of New York at Stony Brook, Department of Psycholgoy.
Schumaker, J.B., & Deshler, D.D. (1988). Implementing the regular education initiative in secondary schools: A different ball game. *Journal of Learning Disabilities*, *21*, 36–42.
Schumaker, J.B., & Hazel, J.S. (1984). Social skills assessment and training for the learning disabled: Who's on 1st and what's on 2nd? Part 1. *Journal of Learning Disabilities*, *17*, 422–431.
Siperstein, G.N., & Bak, J.J. (1986). Understanding factors that affect children's attitudes toward mentally retarded peers. In C.J. Meisel (Ed.), *Mainstreaming handicapped children: Outcomes, controversies and new directions*. Hillsdale, NJ: Erlbaum.
Siperstein, G.N., Bopp, M.J., & Bak, J.J. (1978). Social status of learning disabled children. *Journal of Learning Disabilities*, *11*, 98–102.
Spivack, G., Platt, J., & Shure, M. (1976). *The problem-solving approach to adjustment*. San Francisco: Jossey-Bass.
Spivack, G., & Shure, M. (1974). *Social adjustment of young children*. San Francisco: Jossey-Bass.
Stainback, W., & Stainback, S. (1984). A rationale for the merger of special and regular education. *Exceptional Children*, *51*, 102–111.
Taylor, A.R., & Asher, S.R. (1984a). Children's goals and social competence: Individual differences in a game-playing context. In T. Field, J.L. Roopnarine, & M. Segal (Eds.), *Friendships in normal and handicapped children*. Norwood, NJ: Ablex.

Taylor, A.R., & Asher, S.R. (1984b). *Children's interpersonal goals in game situations*. Paper presented at the meeting of the American Educational Research Association, New Orleans, LA.

Taylor, A.R., Asher, S.R., & Williams, G.A. (1987). The social adaptation of mainstreamed mildly retarded children. *Child Development*, *58*, 1321–1334.

Urbain, E.S., & Kendall, P.C. (1980). Review of social-cognitive problem-solving interventions with children. *Psychological Bulletin*, *88*, 109–143.

Walker, H.M. (1986). The AIMS (Assessments for Integration into Mainstream Settings) assessment system: Rationale, instruments, procedures, and outcomes. *Journal of Child Clinical Psychology: Special Issue on Social Skills in Children and Adolescents*.

Walker, H.M., & Lamon, W.E. (1985). A comparative analysis of the social behavior standards and expectations of samples of Australian and U.S. teachers. *Journal of Special Education*.

Walker, H.M., McConnell, S., Holmes, D., Todis, B., Walker, J.L., & Goldenn, N. (1983). *A curriculum for children's effective peer and teacher skills (ACCEPTS)*. Austin, TX: Pro-Ed Publishers.

Walker, H.M., McConnell, S., Walker, J.L., Clarke, J.Y., Todis, B., Cohen, G., & Rankin, R. (1982). *Initial analysis of the ACCEPTS curriculum: Efficacy of instructional and behavioral management procedures for improving the social adjustment of handicapped children*. (Available form the Center on Human Development. Clinical Services Building, University of Oregon, Eugene, OR 97403).

Wallbrown, F.H., Fremont, T.S., Nelson, E., Wilson, J., & Fischer, J. (1979). Emotional disturbance or social misperception? An important classroom management question. *Journal of Learning Disabilities*, *12*, 645–648.

Wang, M.C. (1980). Adaptive instruction: Building on diversity. *Theory Into Practice*, *19*, 122–128.

Wang, M.C., & Birch, J.W. (1984). Comparison of a full-time mainstreaming program and a resource room approach. *Exceptional Children*, *51*, 33–40.

Wang, M.C., Gennari, P., & Waxman, H.C. (1985). The adaptive learning environments model: Design, implementation, and effects. In M.C. Wang & H.J. Walberg (Eds.), *Adapting instruction to individual differences* (pp. 191–235). Berkeley, CA: McCutchan.

Wang, M.C., Rubenstein, J.L., & Reynolds, M.C. (1985). Clearing the road to success for students with special needs. *Educational Leadership*, *43*, 62–67.

Waterman, J.M., Sobesky, W.E., Silvern, L., Aoki, B., & McCaulay, M. (1981). Social perspective-taking and adjustment in emotionally disturbed, learning disabled, and normal children. *Journal of Abnormal Child Psychology*, *9*, 133–148.

Weiss, E. (1984). Learning disabled children's understanding of social interactions of peers. *Journal of Learning Disabilities*, *17*, 612–615.

Weissberg, R.P. (1985). Designing effective social problem-solving programs for the classroom. In B.H. Schneider, K.H. Rubin, and J.E. Ledingham (Eds.), Children's peer relations: Issues in assessment and intervention (pp. 225–242). New York: Springer-Verlag.

Weissberg, R.P., Gesten, E.L., Leibenstein, N.L., Doherty-Schmid, K., & Hutton, H. (1980). *The Rochester social problem-solving (SPS) program: A training manual for teachers of 2nd–4th grade children*. Rochester, NY: University of Rochester.

Wilkes, H.H., Bireley, M.K., & Schultz, J.J. (1979). Criteria for mainstreaming the learning disabled child into the regular classroom. *Journal of Learning Disabilities*, *12*, 46–51.

Will, M.C. (1986). Educating children with learning problems: A shared responsibility. *Exceptional Children*, *52*, 411–415.

Wong, B.Y.L., & Wong, R. (1980). Role-taking skills in normal achieving and learning disabled children. *Learning Disability Quarterly*, *3*, 11–18.

Yoshida, R. (1986). Setting goals for mainstreaming programs. In C. J. Meisel (Ed.), *Mainstreaming handicapped children: Outcomes, controversies and new directions*. Hillsdale, NJ: Erlbaum.

Ysseldyke, J.E., Thurlow, M., Graden, J., Wesson, C., Algozzine, B., & Deno, S. (1983). Generalizations from five years of research on assessment and decision making: The University of Minnesota Institute. *Exceptional Education Quarterly*, *4*, 75–93.

Zigler, E. & Hall, N. (1986). Mainstreaming and the philosophy of normalization. In C.J. Meisel (Ed.), *Mainstreaming handicapped children: Outcomes, controversies and new directions*. Hillsdale, NJ: Erlbaum.

3
Philosophic Foundations of Behavior Analysis in Developmental Disabilities

THOMAS G. HARING, CRAIG H. KENNEDY, AND CATHERINE G. BREEN

Introduction

A review of potential evolutionary paths for behavior analysis will be conducted by assessing the implications of four distinctly different means of "understanding" the world. These "world views" are derived from the work of philosopher and aestheticist Stephen C. Pepper. Pepper's writings, in particular his 1942 publication, *World Hypotheses: A Study in Evidence*, have undergone a renaissance among behavioral scientists in recent years (e.g., Hayes, Hayes, & Reese, 1988; Lerner, Hultsch, & Dixon, 1983; Morris, 1988; Rosnow & Georgoudi, 1986). Pepper's work is of particular interest to the current analysis because he presents the thesis that there are several *distinct*, *autonomous*, and *relatively adequate* world views that are used in understanding and structuring our experiences. These world hypotheses provide us with frameworks with which to assess various paths along which behavior analysis, and the technologies derived from it, may change in the 1990s and beyond.

World hypotheses offer a way to organize our experience of the world, our theories, and our research questions. All observation and analysis is grounded in some preconceived theory. Even data collection is not atheoretic. The scientific process of observation requires us to define categories within which to code or fit observations (whether quantitative or qualitative). These codes, or categories that describe the sequence of events within the natural environment, are driven by theories, constructs, paradigms, world views, or even social biases and prejudices (e.g., Gould, 1981). The natural environment presents "streams" of multiple stimuli within which an individual's responses are embedded (Schoenfeld & Farmer, 1970). Determining which aspects of this ongoing stream to code as relevant to analysis (or irrelevant) is inherent to science. A world view selects certain types of behavior–environment interrelations as fundamental to analysis and others as less relevant. The procedures developed within a technology, the data that are accepted to help solve problems, and the conceptual tools used to analyze data will differ substantially across world hypotheses because each world view selects different aspects of the environment as relevant.

In describing these theories, we begin with the premise that each of Pepper's world views has something unique and significant to offer developing technologies in the area of instruction for learners with disabilities. We will review examples of research that exemplify the use of behavioral analyses from each of these frameworks (i.e., the four world hypotheses). We will then attempt to elucidate potential future paths for developing support technologies in terms of the types of research questions and objectives that could be developed by adopting each world view. In the following sections of this chapter we will review the sorts of questions that behavior analysis might be able to answer within each of the four frameworks of Pepper's world views.

The Four World Views

Pepper (1942) summarizes four world views: mechanism, organicism, formism, and contextualism. According to Pepper, most philosophies and scientific theories can, at a broad level, be classified according to one of these four world views. Pepper's work offers a metatheory to examine philosophic and scientific theories. For example, according to Hayes et al. (1988) some theories of behavior analysis, evolutionary biology, ethology, economics, and cultural anthropology are closely related because they represent, at a broad level, the same world view (in this case contextualism). These theories, because they share the same basic postulates of contextualism, are highly related even though they deal with vastly different subject matter. Each world view has a "root metaphor" that provides a simple model to aid in understanding that viewpoint. In addition to having a root metaphor, world views posit distinct standards of proof, or what constitutes evidence that a given proposition is true or false. What Pepper attempted to do was to strip all theories and philosophies of their details to leave the fundamental essences and tenets of each theory.

A Mechanistic Behavior Analysis

The root metaphor for mechanism is the machine. Within this world view, the functioning of a system is understood in terms of inputs and outputs and in terms of the functioning of the individual parts comprising the machine. A set of inputs of a certain type, when acting on parts connected in a certain way, deterministically produces a set of outputs.

Within a mechanistic world view, the whole is defined by its parts. Understanding how the parts fit together and work is the key to understanding any system within this perspective. After an understanding is gained of how the parts of a machine operate, given the same inputs, the machine should operate in a highly predictable fashion. This deterministic feature of mechanism is also consistent with the goals of behavioral analysis, that is, the prediction and control of behavior, as described by the following operant relation:

$$\text{Stimulus} \rightarrow \text{Response} \rightarrow \text{Consequence}$$

where the repeated presentation of a stimulus in the presence of an established consequence will predict the occurrence of a behavior. Indeed, the theoretical analysis of the importance of determinism as a central tenet of behavior analysis is an active area of philosophical inquiry (Baldwin, 1988). Although behavior analysis has long been labeled as a purely mechanistic theory by proponents of its conceptual rivals (e.g., Chomsky, 1959; Gardner, 1985), this characterization of modern behavioral analyses has been contested by many behavior analysts (e.g., Morris, 1988; Shimp, 1989). Although many behavioral theorists have argued that mechanism is not consistent with several fundamental tenets of behavior analysis, it is clear that the bulk of the applied research in special education is entirely consistent with a mechanistic world view.

Mechanism as a Basis for Behavior Analysis

Many features of mechanism are consistent with basic tenets of behavior analysis: (a) Functional as well as topographic definitions of behavior can be defined from this perspective; (b) in analyzing learning problems, the task is typically broken into smaller parts (a process of reduction that is central to mechanism); and (c) the concepts of prediction and control of behavior (central tenants of behavior analysis) are consistent with a mechanistic world view. That is, mechanism is deterministic and, given an adequate definition of the parts of a machine and the laws under which they operate, we ought to be able to predict and control the outcomes of the system.

Implications for Instruction

The use of task-analytic instruction is an example of how mechanism is used within a behavioral framework. In task analysis, the steps needed to engage in a skill are systematically broken down into component steps (Bellamy, Horner, & Inman, 1979; Cuvo & Davis, 1983; Haring, T. G., & Kennedy, 1988). Each step can be taught, with the final product of learning each step being the ability to perform the skill sequence. The skill sequence is understandable in total from an analysis of the component parts. In solving new problems via task analysis, goals are defined, and a series of steps is determined to achieve each goal.

Many critiques of behavior analytic instructional procedures are actually critiques of mechanistic demonstrations. For example, Peck, Schuler,

Tomlinson, Theimer, and Haring (1984) refer to such procedures as being *stripped of context*. For example, in teaching language skills from earlier behavioral models (e.g., Guess, Sailor, Rutherford, & Baer, 1968), students are placed at a table within a classroom (because context is considered irrelevant, or even inimical, to learning the skills). Response rate or "motivation" is maintained, not through naturally occurring consequences, but through indirect response-reinforcer relations (cf. Saunders & Sailor, 1979; Williams, Koegel, & Egel, 1981) such as delivery of tokens, objects, or edible rewards. Thus, reinforcement comes to control or predict subsequent responding. The use of these earlier language training programs is no longer recommended because the students' ability to extend their responses to naturally occurring contexts, consequences, and interactions proved too limited. Most current attempts to teach language are highly contextualized, with instruction being embedded in the natural flow of events across a day (e.g., Goetz, Gee, & Sailor, 1985; Haring, T.G., Neetz, Lovinger, Peck, & Semmel, 1987; Warren & Kaiser, 1988).

Task-analytic methods of instruction have also been criticized because they do not take into consideration the full range of demands in the natural environment (Brown, Evans, Weed, & Owen, 1987). Brown et al. point out the following problems when task analysis is applied mechanistically:

1. The beginning and ending of behavioral chains are arbitrary. That is, different task analyzers might begin or end a chain at different points. For example a cooking task analysis might begin with the step "Go to the kitchen" or "Get out the ingredients." Brown et al. point out that an ideal starting point for a chain is some critical event that would naturally cue the beginning of the chain.

2. Task analysis is of limited scope. A task analysis generally only includes those steps necessary to independently perform a task. However, many other responses and skills (such as communicative competence in a setting, or solving problems that might arise) can be critical to competent performance but are not included in the analyses.

3. Task analysis rarely deals with generalization. Natural environments present an entire range of people, objects, and variation in events that occur. A task such as washing the dishes should not be considered mastered unless a learner can generalize across the natural range or variation in contexts that occurs with the task, such as changes in the type of soap available or the type of faucet to regulate temperature.

Brown et al. (1987) suggest that the model of instruction be expanded to include the following additional components: (a) student initiation of the task across the range of natural conditions that occasion it; (b) preparation for the task; (c) the monitoring of the quality and tempo of engaging in the task; (d) problem solving around variable task parameters; and (e) correct termination of the task. We concur with Brown et al. that these are desirable modifications to the basic process of task analysis. However, from a philosophic perspective, the addition of these procedures does not fundamentally change the basis of instruction. These processes (initiation, preparation, monitoring, and termination) are themselves analyzable as steps in the task-analytic process. For example, when teaching problem-solving skills that might be needed when performing a task-analyzed chain of responses, it is possible to develop subtask analyses that teach solutions to specific problems that have been noted to arise at specific points in the chain. In the mechanistic metaphor, this is equivalent to having a repair manual for problems that might trouble the machine. An important point is that there is nothing in Brown et al.'s suggestions that is inherently different from the primarily mechanistic nature inherent in task analysis. They provide a mechanistic extension of the analysis to better cope with the demands of the real world.

Strengths and Limitations

Many of the achievements of behavior analysis over the last decade are directly due to a model of behavior analysis that is consistent with mechanism in Pepper's (1942) system. There have been many challenges to the seemingly dominant role that this world view has had on special education (e.g., Skrtic, 1988). One of the most important critiques of this model has been that it has a tendency to analyze solely the primary qualities of performance (such as rate or accuracy of performance) and to de-emphasize secondary qualities (such as people's perceptions of interventions and the behavioral changes that they induce).

Extending the mechanistic analysis to be more inclusive is the major way that traditional behavior analysis has adapted to changes in instructional requirements. As new areas of instruction are identified, the power and established effectiveness of task analysis can be expected to continue making significant contributions. For example, as new goals have been established to extend instruction from classroom, community, home, and vocational settings, this technology has been able to solve problems posed by these new demands. Although we expect mechanistic applications of behavior analysis to continue to generate important contributions, the critical question is: Are there areas of current or future need for which a solely mechanistic analysis will be insufficient in generating needed technologies? There are several areas of concern for which mechanistic behavior analysis will have difficulty providing solutions.

Friendships and Social Networks

As the field of special education evolves with new values, the outcomes that are newly identified will provide a challenge to existing quantitative (and scientific) research strategies (e.g., Peck & Furman, 1990). One example of this involves friendship. Friendships, and the social networks that emerge from them, are now considered to be primary educational outcomes rather than hoped-for side effects of intervention and programming. However, the creation of friendships may not be amenable to simple sequences of responses (such as approach, greet, initiate play, and terminate). Instead, the development of friendships is based on an ongoing, complex set of processes such as creating opportunities for interaction; teaching social skills that facilitate interactions; and providing organizational and social support to maintain relationships. Although mechanistically based behavioral analysis can assist in some of these processes (e.g., social skill instruction), it offers little guidance for other components.

More Complex Developmental Tasks

Task analysis and systematic instruction are ideally suited to identify responses and sequences of responses as they occur in temporal order. Task analysis is not designed to study or analyze the development of more complex repertoires that might demand interrelated skills. A purely mechanistic assessment would not identify this relationship as necessary.

Many students with severe and profound disabilities need instruction in skills that underlie basic development and responsiveness to the environment rather than discrete training on daily living skills. Holvoet (1989), for example, reports that traditional behavioral training efforts to teach persons with profound handicaps to communicate verbally have been largely ineffective. These techniques have typically involved attempts to increase rates of vocalization and then to shape these vocalizations into more complex verbalizations. It is not clear that this failure is due to problems in breaking down speech into smaller and smaller components, according to the instructional logic from mechanistic behavior analysis. Analyzing the child's current repertoire of prelinguistic responses and shaping these into more prelinguistic communicative responses (though still nonverbal) is a more promising approach (e.g., Peck et al., 1984). This approach represents a departure from mechanistic behavior analysis because the normal developmental sequence of communication is considered as the template for selecting responses for intervention.

Environmental Effects on Social Perceptions

Increasing importance is being placed on the effects of the physical appearance of the environment on the interactions between persons with and without disabilities (Wolfensberger, 1983). The selection of age-appropriate and culturally appropriate activities, schedules, modes of dress, and instructional procedures can have a significant impact on the attitudes that typical community members have concerning the abilities and social characteristics of people with disabilities and consequently can affect the success or failure of integration efforts. The analysis of these factors entails a more qualitative assessment of culturally based characteristics than is found when applying a strict mechanistic analysis.

Effects of Context on Resulting Behavior Change

The mechanistic model has been critiqued for being decontextualized. That is, interventions developed from this world view have not been well referenced to the demands of the natural environment. An intervention can fail because the sociological characteristics of the environment do not support the resultant behavior change or provide opportunities to actually use a newly taught skill. It is frequently observed that skills that have been taught remain unused and are eventually forgotten because the adults in the child's environment rarely provide the child opportunities to use the skills (Horner, Williams, & Knobbe, 1985). Thus, it is important to assess the attitudes and behavioral patterns of other key individuals in a student's life to ensure that the environment will support the skills being taught. This introduces a set of value-based criteria into instructional planning that go beyond the analysis of the discrete aspects of a mechanistic instructional technology. In addition, an intervention that does not consider the broader characteristics of the *natural* context can fail because the natural context presents demands that were not considered.

In summary, we have provided support for the application of a mechanistic world view to current best instructional practices, including the breaking down of a task into its component parts, the precise definition of a behavior, and the establishment of prediction and control of behavior through the modification of the relations between the components of the model. Although the basis for a great number of current practices can be supported by a mechanistic world view, we have also identified four areas that would be difficult to accommodate within a purely mechanistic analysis. In creating friendships and supporting social interactions, there are variables that require measurement and interventions that are not purely mechanistic, such as the qualitative measure of the strength of friendships. When instruction is extended to persons with the most severe disabilities, many of the procedures that are developed from task analysis to teach independent living skills are not relevant to the instructional needs of this population. In this example, the development of complex repertoires such as language (a) is dependent on development in other areas, (b) necessitates the analysis of complex interactions across other skills, and (c) requires an analysis of the relationships between skills that are acquired and the motivational characteristics of the environment. A mechanistic behavioral analysis will not provide a sufficient foundation for many of the upcoming challenges facing special education.

A Formistic Behavior Analysis

The root metaphor for formism is similarity. Formistic theories are systems used to separate or discriminate differences between objects, with the ultimate purpose being to categorize and classify. As an analysis of the components of formism will show, several tenets of behavior analysis are consistent with this world view. In addition, two major branches of instructional research closely related to behavior analysis—direct instruction (Engelmann & Carnine, 1982) and general case programming (Bellamy, Horner, & Inman, 1979)—are primarily formistic systems.

Formism generates a powerful analytic tool: the concept of classes. The class of blue things includes the sky today, water, a bluejay, the pad for the "mouse" by my computer, and a book on my desk. Classes themselves can be organized into classification systems; for example, living things, animals, mammals, dogs, golden retrievers, and a particular golden retriever named Judy comprise a system of classes moving from the most inclusive (living things) to one particularization (Judy). Classification carried to the limit always produces a single particularization. Classification is the major analytic system that formism contributes.

In formism, the criterion for truth relates to the formation of scientific laws. It is the aim of science to discover laws and investigate the regularities in nature. Formism is inductive—observations are gathered to determine regularities, laws, or norms of nature. After laws are formulated through inductive reasoning, they are further tested to study the regularity of nature. The regularity of nature (and the truth of a particular law) is further established when specific observations act as described by the law. Pepper (1942) uses the example of gravity, specifically, a lead ball dropped from some height. In this example, there are the physical masses of the earth and ball; their spatial relationship to each other (e.g., the height of the ball); and their temporal relationship (e.g., the instant at which the ball is dropped). These entities participate within the law of gravity. This law describes the motion of the ball as having a specific acceleration in a straight line to the earth. The law describes and regulates the times, distances, and velocities of the ball at each moment of its descent. The falling ball is simply one example, or particularization, of the class of objects that obey the law of gravity. The truth criterion for formism is the degree of similarity between a description (such as a quantitative law of nature) and its object of reference.

Formism as a Basis for Behavior Analysis

Inductive Truth Criterion

A major area of compatibility between formism and behavior analysis is that both theories share a common truth criterion based on inductive logic and the correspondence between laws derived from inductive logic and observation of natural phenomena. Behavior analysis, too, has derived basic laws of learning that are continually tested under novel circumstances.

Stimulus and Response Classes

The definition of classes is central to behavior analysis. In his classic paper, "The Generic Nature of the Concepts of Stimulus and Response," Skinner (1935) proposed that response classes be defined on a functional basis. In defining a response class, a topographical definition (or a formistic definition) would include the pattern of muscular responses inherent in the class. From Skinner's perspective, defining response classes topographically is misleading because a diverse array of topographically dissimilar responses can function in the same way. By social convention, a gestural wave of the hand or the words "Good morning" both function equally as greeting responses, yet they share no common response topographies.

Skinner's (1935) analysis of stimulus classes is also based on a functional definition. After a response has been trained, the experimenter can test a wide variety of stimuli that vary from the original training stimulus to determine to which novel stimuli the organism will respond. The class of novel stimuli is usually much larger than the class of stimuli that were trained initially. Thus, the stimuli to which the response has generalized are members of the same stimulus class as the original training stimuli and, like responses in a response class, are functionally substitutable or interchangeable.

As reviewed above, the major analytic tool of formism is categorizing particulars into classes. Formistically determined classes, however, are of a fundamentally different sort than functionally determined classes. In formistically determined classes, groupings are created on the basis of observed similarities. For example, an easy chair looks in many ways like a desk chair (i.e., they share qualities such as arms, padded cushions, etc.). However, a challenge to this classification system arises when we consider a beanbag chair. The beanbag chair shares few, if any, discernible qualities with the other two chairs, yet it can function interchangeably with the prior two examples. From Skinner's (1935) definition of a stimulus class, the beanbag chair does not pose a problem because it is functionally equivalent (if, in fact, a person responds to the beanbag chair in an equivalent manner to other chairs).

Implications for Instruction

In spite of this fundamental difference in how classes are defined, formistic instructional theories that combine elements from behaviorally based teaching and formistic class definitions have been developed very successfully. General case programming (Albin & Horner, 1988; Bellamy et al., 1979) and direct instruction (Becker, Engelmann & Thomas, 1975; Engelmann & Carnine, 1982) have generated a powerful and well-replicated instructional system using this perspective. The composition of response and stimulus classes inherent to general case programming is based on a structural analysis of qualities that are formistic. That is, specific examples from an instructional universe are selected for instruction based on their shared observable response or stimulus qualities. However, general case programming is also consistent with behavior analysis and Skinner's (1935) functional definitions of response classes. This is evident in the final step in the process when the response class that has actually been taught is compared to the initial formistically determined structural class and modified through additional instruction to include examples that are functionally, however, not structurally similar. In fact, this final step is consistent with the truth criterion for formism (correspondence theory), where the validity of the abstract class produced through structural analysis is compared to the natural observation of the functional class learned by the student. A close match between the response class actually acquired and the structural analysis provides a test of the validity for the structural analysis. If there are errors in responding within the functionally acquired response class at this point in instruction, the structural class is retained as the template to determine the course of instruction. Instruction continues until the functional class displayed by the student matches the structural class determined through logical analysis of the similarity across particulars.

Strengths and Limitations

Formism is limited in many of the same ways that mechanistic behavior analysis is limited. Formistic analyses will have difficulty with problem solving that cannot be fit into the training of one particular class or the teaching of one particular concept. As reviewed before, friendship and social networks are more comprehensive than can be analyzed as a chain of responses or component responses, as mechanism would provide, or as a class of responses, as formism is well suited for. In addition, formistic analysis is not well suited to analyze the interrelationships across related sets of responding (e.g., Haring, T.G., 1985) or more complex developmental tasks, such as language development. For instance, from a formistic analysis the functional relationship between pointing at an object to request it and verbalizing a request is not obvious, yet from a functional perspective these responses can be equivalent. In early acquisition of language, this more functional perspective is demonstrably more effective.

Formism is, however, well suited for adapting instruction to the needs of the environment and for studying generalization within natural contexts. General case programing provides a means for studying contextual variation and provides a training strategy for exposing students to this variation. Thus, as special education becomes more concerned with responding in natural environments, a formistic behavior analysis can be expected to contribute new instructional programs of great effectiveness.

Formism is well suited to studying and teaching generalization. The procedures in general case programing represent a powerful technology for promoting generalization. In addition, a formistic behavior analysis can be fit to meet the demands of contextual variation that are generated by natural environments. Indeed, formism is superior to a mechanistic behavior analysis in programming generalization and contextually sensitive behavior change, because of the strong analytic system provided by the structural analysis of classes.

Formism is also superior to a mechanistic analysis when concept learning is the focus of instruction. In formism, a concept is equivalent to a class. Thus, a formistic behavior analysis provides a model for defining classes and designing interventions to teach classes.

In summary, as with mechanism, a formistic behavioral analysis can be expected to contribute important technological packages to meet future instructional needs. However, its limitations argue strongly that this world view, like mechanism alone, may not be sufficient.

An Organicismic Behavior Analysis

The root metaphor for organicism is the developing organism. Of the four world views, organicism is the least compatible with behavior analysis. Many of the fundamental tenets of the organicismic world view conflict directly with a behavioral world view. There are few examples of integration or synthesis between these two approaches.

The components of organicism consist of *steps* (or stages) involved in the organic process. The steps of development ultimately lead to an *organic structure*. In Piaget's (1952) theory of cognitive development, formal operational thought (the ability to reason symbolically) is the ultimate achievement of the earlier stages in cognitive development. Furthermore, the observable responses that comprise the early stages, or the final stage, are reflections (or appearances) generated by the much more fundamental reality of the structures attained through development. For behavior analysis, which concentrates on observable behaviors, this assumption of the primacy of nonobservable internalized structures that function to direct development is a fundamental incompatibility.

Organicism as a Basis for Behavior Analysis

It is unclear that a logically consistent integration of the organicismic world view with behavior analysis is possible. To have such an integration, behavior analysis must be stripped of its theoretical assumptions and tenets and used solely as a technology. In so doing, the procedures and interventions developed through behavior analysis are used to facilitate an organic process. The targets for intervention, dependent variables, and judgments of the validity of intervention are determined from the frame of reference of organicism. Of necessity, the basic philosophic tenets of behavior analysis are largely ignored in this synthesis. In addition, a synthesis between behavior analysis and organicism does not leave that world view unscathed. In the syntheses to be reviewed, the stagelike progression of skills implied by organicism is typically retained, but the internal direction of organic structures is frequently omitted from these syntheses. This is because the user of this synthetic theory is implicitly acknowledging that an external technology is effective (and needed) in promoting the change that is desired.

In the early 1970s, Bricker and Bricker (e.g., Bricker & Bricker, 1970; Vincent, Bricker, & Bricker, 1973) developed a model of intervention that coupled Piaget's (1952) theory of child development with the procedural tools of behavior analysis. Within this system, Piaget's theory was used as the world view to select instructional objectives. For example, in teaching early language responses, responses indicating object permanence were first trained to facilitate receptive language development. Although behavioral procedures such as two-choice discrimination training formats were employed, these formats were interpreted to be procedures to affect basic developmental functions such as secondary circular reactions. In this synthesis, behavior analysis is retained as a powerful technology to structure and evaluate interventions, but the goals of interventions are derived from developmental theory.

Another attempt to integrate behavior analysis (interpreted procedurally) with the world view of organicism is evidenced in the work of Cohen and Haring (1979). These authors surveyed scales of normal development to identify sequences of responses through which developing children pass. The resulting products of this analysis were referred to as developmental pinpoints. The developmental pinpoints were observable responses from normal developmental sequences organized in linear order. The pinpoints corresponded to the emergence of the ability to engage in these responses. The developmental pinpoints were used in designing interventions and instructional goals. This model was synthetic because the methods of intervention were based on behavior analysis procedures.

Strengths and Limitations

The most serious threat to the validity of an organicismic behavior analysis in developmental disabilities is the powerful role that normal developmental sequences play in determining instruction. From organically based theories, a basic tenet is the integrative function of development through stages. The sequence of moving through stages is assumed to be linear and invariant. This assumption is open, of course, to empirical investigation and validation. That is, it can be directly determined through measurement whether children with developmental disabilities pass through stages and substages in the same invariant sequences as typically developing children. Although presently there are far too few data for a definitive answer to this question, some studies suggest that the development of persons with severe and profound disabilities does not proceed in sequences that are the same as those observed in typical development (e.g., Macpherson & Butterfield, 1988; Ravish, 1987). In many cases, this difference concerns uneven development across different areas of "cognitive" development (e.g., object permanence often is developmentally more advanced than verbal imitation). In addition, this difference can entail skipping steps that were presumed to be necessary in order to reach subsequent steps. Finally, even if research shows that persons with disabilities develop according to preset sequences, it does not follow logically that these preset sequences are the most efficacious means of attaining skill development.

An organicismic world view assumes that the normal developmental sequence controls what can be learned. This is clearly a limiting assumption for persons with mental retardation and other developmental disabilities. If a 15-year-old person has attained a level of development that is equivalent to that of a normally developing 4-year-old, this model assumes that the responses to be taught to that 15-year-old should be selected from the responses that a 4-year-old is capable of making. This assumption is not valid because powerful intervention procedures (e.g., task analysis) offer alternative processes of acquisition that allow persons with very low developmental ages to learn skills far beyond those predicted by normal developmental sequences. Organicismic interventions in developmental disabilities run the risk of underpredicting what can be accomplished through interventions.

There are, however, some areas of research that show potential for this world view. In particular, the passage of recent federal legislation (Public Law 99–457) requires states to develop instructional programs for children with disabilities between the ages of 3 and 5 by the 1990–91 school year. The new law also encourages states (through financial incentives) to develop programs for eligible children from birth through 3 years of age. This establishment of programming for young children and infants will require a reassessment of organicismic models. When intervention is planned for young children and infants, the primary goal of intervention is to promote development, particularly of language skills, motor skills, and cognitive skills. A fine-grained understanding of development will be critical in conducting these programs. In contrast, a reliance on task-analyzed independent living skills is not relevant to intervention with infants.

This new area of service delivery will require a closer look at an organicismic world view merging with behavior analysis. However, for this synthesis to be functional, a more careful research agenda concerning the development of people with disabilities will be necessary (Holvoet, 1989). In many past applications of the organicismic world views and behavior analysis, normal child development was taken as the template for planning instruction. However, neither the validity nor the necessity of normal sequences of development is well established. A closer study of the development of children with severe and profound disabilities will aid the field in the identification of alternative sequences of development.

There have been some important efforts in this direction. Stillman and Battle (1985), for instance, have conducted a consistent program of research that documents the developmental sequences of students with profound disabilities. From this analysis they have produced the Callier–Azuza Scales, which are a sequenced series of activities and responses that persons with profound disabilities can display. The Callier–Azuza Scales offer a validated sequence to use for assessment and planning of instruction, based on atypical child development, not on responses that are typical for developing children.

A similar research strategy was employed by N. G. Haring, White, Edgar, Affleck, and Hayden (1981) in the development of another assessment instrument, the Uniform Performance Assessment System (UPAS). The UPAS consists of ordered sequences of responses that were determined from analyzing the development of disabled children as well as normally developing children. Sequences are provided for the development of communication, social, self-help, gross motor, and preacademic skills. The development of the UPAS represents a better synthesis of a behavior model with the organicismic model than with many other applications because, in the UPAS, Skinner's (1935) functional definition of responses classes is explicitly retained (White, 1980). In this analysis, it is sufficient that a child show a form of a response to accomplish a certain goal or function, even if that form is atypical. Thus, the ability to perform a *function* is stressed over the specific *form* (topography) of responses used to accomplish that function. For example, in gross motor development, an increased ability to walk and run is an important component of all developmental sequences. In the UPAS, students with disabilities who use a wheelchair for mobility get credit for development of higher level mobility skills, even though their means of mobility is atypical.

In summary, although organicism is the least compatible of the four world views with the basic tenets of behavior analysis, there have been several attempts to integrate these theories and procedures. Recent changes in extending intervention to young children and infants should promote further research in this area. Thus, as with mechanism and formism, there is potential for important future contributions from an organicismic behavior analysis.

A Contextualistic Behavior Analysis

The root metaphor for contextualism is an event within history. For this world view, an event can only be understood in relationship to the meaning and sequence of events that precede and follow it. However, contextualism is concerned not with past events as implied by the historical metaphor, but rather with the unfolding of events in the here and now. An example of an event within contextualism is making a trip downtown to buy a loaf of bread. This trip entails the unfolding of specific actions (e.g., getting into a car and taking certain roads) whose purpose and meaning are understood in reference to the context—a trip to buy bread. The meaning, significance, or relevance of any one component in the process of taking this trip is best understood in reference to the *function* of the whole sequence. Ethnographic interviews and observations that attempt to construct the meaning of social events or institutions from the perspective of people participating in these systems are examples of contextual research processes.

Contextualism, among the four world views, is perhaps the most compatible with behavior analysis and has been advocated as a direction for its future growth (Hayes et al., 1988; Baer, Wolf, & Risley, 1987). The similarities between tenets of contextualism and behavior analysis will be discussed as the contextualistic world view is defined. These similarities have specific implications for how behavioral analyses are conducted for people with developmental disabilities.

Contextualism as a Basis for Behavior Analysis

Both contextualism and behavior analysis view events as part of the context in which they occur. It is from the complete event within a context that the contextualist derives meaning. For Pepper (1942), "contextualism denies that there are absolute elements . . . that a whole is nothing but the sum of its parts" (p. 238). Similarly, behavior analysis views events as being composed of a dynamic unit that cannot be understood by breaking the event down into its constituent elements (unlike mechanism). For behavior analysts, this manifests itself in the basic unit of analysis: the interrelation between behavior and environment (Skinner, 1935; 1953). These two elements are not separable within a behavioral analysis. The response stripped of the environment and the environment without the organism acting upon it have no independent meaning to a behavior analyst (Barnes, 1989; Sidman, 1986; Zeiler, 1986). It is the dynamic interaction between behavior and environment, or more precisely, the functional relations that are derived from the interaction, that constitute a behavioral analysis.

Another feature of contextualism that is compatible with behavior analysis is that both systems view the world as understandable at multiple levels. Within behavior analysis, behavior–environment interactions can be studied at varying levels of complexity (cf. Thompson & Zeiler, 1986). For example, on a fine-grained level, conversational behavior might be analyzed in terms of the stimulus control relations between two members of a conversational dyad. On a broader level, complex and interacting patterns of behavior over an extended duration might be the focus of analysis.

An example of this multilevel approach comes from research sponsored by NASA to study how astronauts spend time in space (e.g., during space shuttle missions). These experiments (e.g., Brady, Bigelow, Emurian, & Williams, 1975; Emurian, Emurian, & Brady, 1985) analyze how individuals living in a self-contained environment spend their time (eating, sleeping, exercising, using a computer, etc.) and how specific task requirements and sequences of tasks affect the allocation of behavior. The information from these studies is analyzed and integrated at various levels. For instance, at the broadest level, the percentage of time a person spends with particular activities across several days is analyzed (e.g., computer use versus interpersonal communication). At a narrower level, the behavior–environment interrelations are examined to see how juxtaposing and interspersing task sequences affects the allocation of an individual's time across a single day (e.g., the effects of conducting a certain procedure on the duration of the lunch break that follows). At an even more refined level, the behavior of participants (e.g., rate of responding) during specific tasks can be compared. Thus, research in this area can span multiple levels (i.e., "molar" to "molecular") while still holding the behavior–environment interaction as the basic unit.

An additional feature of contextualism and behavior analysis that appears consistent is the criterion for judging the adequacy of an analysis (i.e., the truth criterion employed). A primary means of judging whether something is true or not for contextualism focuses on *successful functioning*. "The successful action is the true one, the unsuccessful actions are false" (Pepper, 1942, p. 270). This is similar to behavior analysts' adherence to the control of behavior as the ultimate goal of analysis. The degree to which behavior can be successfully changed (e.g., learning a new skill) is the degree to which we understand it (Skinner, 1974).

Implications for Instruction

Task Analysis

Contextualism analyzes or describes events using an "action-based," instead of a "thing-based," language (Hayes et al., 1988). The actions of life are described using verbs such as shopping, buying lunch, and communicating with others. This action-based language fits well with the idea of task analysis in the sense that task analyses deal with sequences of action. However, a contextualistic behavior analysis places the response sequence within the larger social context in which it occurs. The quality of an event is not necessarily comprised solely of a specific skill taught to a learner (e.g., paying for an item in a store). The skill itself has to be understood in relation to the person's life-style, quality of life, and goals.

A contextualistic approach to task analysis includes a recognition of the broader (multilevel) context within which response sequences are taught. For example, Wilcox and Bellamy (1987) have presented a system for individualized plan development that emphasizes the activities within which specific skills can be taught. Particular goals are identified and embedded within activities. Specific skills are subgoals that can be taught within the framework of the larger activity or context. Thus, if the goal of instruction is to have the student learn a specific skill such as more fluent expansion of conversational responses, this skill is taught within multiple naturally occurring contexts, such as talking to peers while lifting weights in a gym or talking to a barber while getting a haircut. This type of approach stresses the broader context in which instruction occurs, so that skills are imparted within socially meaningful situations. This avoids teaching the skill in isolation and stripping it of its context by using massed practice and other artificial instructional strategies.

Incidental teaching (e.g., Goetz et al., 1985; Hart & Risley, 1975; Haring, T.G., et al., 1987; Warren & Kaiser, 1988), mentioned previously in this chapter, is another example of contextualized skill training because it embeds instruction within the flow of events across a student's day. A contextualistic behavior analyst, aware of the social context in which actions occur, should emphasize the social/interactive elements that are part of sequences, activities, and the school day. Teaching and facilitating social interactions within task analyses, even though these responses may not be "critical" to completing the task, are integral parts of events that participate in the overall meaning of social integration and community participation.

Problem Behavior

As we move toward a more complete integration of all students and adults with developmental disabilities into local communities, the challenge of successfully coping with problem behaviors previously not present in these settings must be addressed. Problem behaviors—such as self-injury, property destruction, and injury to others—have in the past led to individuals' removal from the community and placement in more restrictive settings. A purely mechanistic behavioral analysis may have difficulty meeting the challenges presented by these recent changes in policy. Although a mechanistic behavioral analysis has been effective in dealing with discrete antecedent, response, and consequence units in a fairly isolated manner, new approaches are having to deal with the broader physical and social contexts in which these behaviors occur (Horner et al., 1990).

One means of contextualizing the analysis of problem behavior has focused on the communicative function of some problem behaviors (Carr & Durand, 1985) or the functions that the behavior seems to serve for the student within a context (Iwata, Dorsey, Slifer, Bauman, & Richman, 1982). Within this approach, variables that control a student's problem behavior are identified (e.g., obtaining teacher attention through having a tantrum) and incorporated into an intervention that establishes alternative responses that operate as effectively or more effectively within the context (e.g., signing "Play with me"). However, instead of treating the occurrence of a problem behavior as having fixed properties (as a mechanistic or formistic approach does), contextually bound behavioral analyses assess the function and forms of behavior across settings (Iwata et al., 1982; White, 1980). For example, Haring and Kennedy (1990) demonstrated that problematic stereotypic behavior (e.g., body rocking), although topographically the same across contexts, can serve different functions depending on the context in which it occurs (e.g., escaping from instruction or providing pleasurable self-stimulation during leisure). This type of relationship is not inherently obvious from a mechanistic or formistic analysis because these approaches assume fixed operations or consistent physical classifications, respectively. That is, because context is viewed as not relevant to function, the differential functions of behavior or the differential effects of intervention across context could not be anticipated.

Another approach to understanding why problem behaviors occur has focused on an expanded analysis of the stimulus situations across settings and times that occasion problem behavior. J.R. Kantor's (1958) concept of the "interbehavioral field" and Michael's (1982) "establishing operations" are consistent with an expanded analysis of antecedent contextual conditions. Within Kantor's theory, discrete stimulus–behavior units occur within a more complex field of events that influence their occurrence and nonoccurrence. Setting factors are one major set of variables identified by Kantor. Essentially, setting factors are social (e.g., the tone of voice used when talking); environmental (e.g., ambient noise level); and biological events (e.g., hunger) that affect or influence the more discrete units typically dealt with by a mechanistic behavioral analysis.

Recent strategies for identifying why problem behaviors occur have used scatterplots that identify the times and contexts during the day when problems occur and do not occur (Touchette, MacDonald, & Langer, 1985) and specific variables, similar to setting factors, that coincide with the occurrence and nonoccurrence of problem behaviors (O'Neill,

Horner, Albin, Storey, & Sprague, 1989). An example of this more contextualized approach is a high school student who intermittently attacks and injures other students in the classroom. From a discrete antecedent → response → consequence analysis, no clear antecedent appeared to regularly occasion the problem behavior (e.g., teacher demands, being ignored by others). However, by using a scatterplot strategy for documenting occurrences of the problem behaviors, it was revealed that certain types of activities or contexts do not occasion problem behaviors, whereas other contexts coincide with the student's aggression. This conclusion would have been difficult to arrive at from more mechanistic analyses that considered only specific discriminatory stimuli that preceded a response. A contextually based approach, by expanding the qualities and textures of events assessed, reveals more-difficult-to-identify controlling variables.

Friendships and Social Networks

A focal challenge for support technologies in the 1990s will be the development of technologies for building and maintaining social relationships among people with and without disabilities. The previous reliance on a mechanistically based analysis, although providing an extremely effective set of strategies for teaching social skills, has not dealt with social relationships within a broader social framework. For example, the study of social skills that facilitate social interactions is a rich area of research; however, if a contextually based behavioral analysis is adopted, research will need to deal with the larger social context in which such skills are embedded.

Several possible strategies are available (cf. Haring, T.G., & Breen, 1989). A multilevel approach is one strategy that could be adopted for studying the social lives of students with disabilities. This approach views people's social relationships as existing across several distinct levels, each of which has meaning and specific aspects that are not captured when analyses are conducted at the other levels. The initial, most molecular focus, centers on the *social interactions* and response patterns that occur between individuals. This area of research already represents a substantial body of literature (e.g., Goldstein & Wickstrom, 1986; Haring, T.G., et al., 1987; Kohler & Fowler, 1985; Sasso & Rude, 1987) that has sought to understand the behavior of students with and without disabilities at the level of social interactions and moment-to-moment changes that occur. Broadening the analysis changes the focus to the *contact patterns* among people and the *meaning of the contacts* to the interactants. At this level, the development, maintenance, and dissolution of social relationships are studied over several months or years, providing analyses such as how often individuals have opportunities for contact, how often contacts occur, how rates change over time, and what variables influence contact patterns (Haring, T.G., Breen, Weiner, Pitts-Conway, & N.G. Haring, 1989; Kennedy, Horner, & Newton, 1989). At another level, analyses focus on the *social networks* of people (e.g., Bruininks & Abery, 1989; Kennedy, Horner & Newton, 1990). Social networks, or the individuals who are identified as socially important to a person (cf. Barrera, 1986; Gottlieb, 1981, 1988), have been studied to better understand who the individuals are that enter and become significant individuals in a person's life.

Strengths and Limitations

A contextualistic behavior analysis is an appealing means of extending the philosophic foundations on which our technological efforts are based. When compared, for example, to a mechanistic or formistic behavioral analysis, a contextual approach offers alternatives and solutions for curricular areas that have proven difficult to address in the past (e.g., problem behaviors, social relationships). However, there are potential reasons for concern if a contextually derived behavior analysis is adopted by researchers. The dispersive nature of contextualism is potentially problematic. By *dispersive* what is meant is that contextualism does not inherently seek to group facts into a systematic and orderly structure. Instead, it views facts and how they are structured as imposed upon nature, not as part of nature. An implication of this may be to resort to implicit use of other world views to structure our knowledge, thus confusing contextualism with other world views. For example, contextualism may not be well suited for identifying sequences of development that are necessary for the occurrence of more complex repertoires (e.g., language development). However, another world view, such as organicism, which is well suited for this purpose, could be implicitly used without one necessarily being aware of its adoption. It is possible, then, that a contextual behavioral analysis could foster an eclecticism that obfuscates the distinct qualities of each world view and leads to approaches to analysis that are not internally consistent. The tendency for contextualism to revert to mechanism is a frequent example of this.

A clear strength of a contextualistic behavior analysis is the potential that this world view offers to expand the variables considered as viable for technological development. In some aspects, contextually based analyses appear to focus on variables that have sometimes been referred to as *ecological* (e.g., Rogers-Warren & Warren, 1977). Contextualism provides a framework for reassessing theoretical systems that posit a broader set of controls than the stimulus → response → consequence model (e.g., Kantor, 1958; Michael, 1982).

Understanding behavior in natural social contexts and how it is changed in those contexts is the purpose of applied behavior analysis. We should assess how intervention affects the student and other people within the context over time (Kazdin, 1977; Wolf, 1978). If behavior analysis is to continue to help improve the lives of people with disabilities, the social meaningfulness and acceptability of behavior-analytic efforts deserve a more primary focus (Baer, 1986). For contextually based behavior analysis, successful functioning means more than changing discrete behaviors. Most important, behavior change must endure across time, or maintain. Maintenance can be viewed as the primary criterion for successful functioning because for behavior change to endure, it must succeed at multiple levels (e.g., change people's attitudes, not demand too much effort) in addition to suppressing or increasing particular responses.

In summary, emerging research in the areas of task analysis, problem behaviors, social relationships, and the social validity of behavior is highly contextualistic. A contextualistic behavior analysis warrants further development and analysis as a future foundation upon which to develop support technologies.

Conclusions

We have attempted to show the potential for syntheses between behavior analysis and the four world views as outlined by Pepper (1942). The review indicates that there are examples of research programs that have been conducted and future research questions that could be productively asked within the context of each of these four world views. From a theoretical perspective, as well as an applied perspective, how successful have these integrations been?

In the case of mechanism, there is an excellent fit between the major components of the mechanistic world view and the tenets of behaviorism. We have argued that the majority of instructional research and behavior change interventions to date have been conducted from the framework of mechanism. Indeed, from our initial review, a question might be raised as to what inconsistencies exist between these world views. There is one very critical difference between mechanism and behavior analysis: The truth criteria of these two theories are opposed.

In mechanism, the truth criterion is hypothetico-deductive. In hypothetico-deductive research, the investigators predict that an operation will be successful, and the success or failure of the data to conform to the prediction constitutes the truth test. After the principles and laws that control the operation of the parts of the machine are discovered, truth is determined by predicting the outcomes of the law under new situations. The ability to predict successful application provides the truth of the mechanistic understanding. In behavior analysis, the truth criterion is both inductive and pragmatic. The truth criterion is inductive in that when the researcher is solving a problem or designing instruction, the behavior of the student is first studied to identify existing response systems, contexts, and direct antecedent and consequent events that might control the behavior. Potential hypotheses are generated from this basic level of observation. The success of an intervention is ultimately judged against a criterion of successful operation within natural contexts. The investigation proceeds on a dynamic basis to test potential interventions and modify them until the criterion of successful operation is met.

The history of special education and applied behavior analysis has been largely a history of a mechanistic behavior analysis. Because the truth criteria for applied behavior analysis and contextualism stress successful working and pragmatic solutions, this does not pose a major theoretical concern or threat to the integrity of either model. However, if mechanistic analysis is insufficient, it is an indication that a return to the fundamental tenets of a more contextualistic behavior analysis is necessary. We have argued that many of the current problems facing researchers and practitioners cannot be solved through mechanistic analysis. Foremost among these problems are the analysis and support of friendships; the analysis of developmentally complex tasks; the social perceptions of interventions; and the development of procedures to ensure that people within a student's social environment value, support, and maintain the results of an intervention.

Formism, too, has been integrated into a program of behavior-analytic research, most notably in the theories of direct instruction and general case programming. Although definitions of classes constitute the major analytic tool across both theories, there is a fundamental incompatibility between how a response class is defined within formism (structurally), and how it is defined within behavior analysis (functionally). Formism and behavior analysis share, at least in part, the same truth criterion: inductive reasoning. Formism can be expected to contribute important research in the areas of generalization of skills. In addition, formism provides a model through which one can study and classify the characteristics of the natural environment. As has been demonstrated within the research conducted by Horner et al. (1985), this can be an important means to create behavior change that is sensitive to the variation of stimulus characteristics within natural contexts. Formism is, however, severely limited in its ability to understand and promote more dynamic social interactions and relationships between people.

Organicism is theoretically the world view least compatible with behavior analysis. In particular, organicism assumes that development is directed from internal structures and that these internal structures are a means of understanding the stagelike course of development. Basic tenets of behavior analysis reject the internal organization and direction of development and instead concentrate on the observable accomplishments of the child and how the structure of the social environment creates the structure of behavior. The truth criteria for these two theories are also incompatible. Behavior analysis stresses successful problem solving with no necessity for an integration of all solutions into an ultimate understanding. Organicism assumes that all facts must interrelate and that truth is the ability to interrelate all facts into an understanding of the entire system. Most syntheses of behavior analysis and organicism have employed the stagelike progression of development inherent in organicism, with behavioral technology to teach students skills that are needed to better integrate their responses within one stage or teach responses that might promote progress to higher stages. Although the theories are basically incompatible, the future expansion of programming under Public Law 99–457 to young children and infants with disabilities should continue to provide a fertile basis for research of this type. In particular, research into prelinguistic development in terms of necessary developmental milestones needed for more complex linguistic development is an important area for research. However, for older learners, models based on organicism have little to offer in solving emerging problems, such as friendship and the contextualization of instruction within natural environments and social interaction contexts.

We have argued that contextualism is a world view closely related to behavior analysis. There are several important points of similarity between these two theories. They share a pragmatic criterion of successful working as the truth criterion. In addition, both theories share the ability to analyze events across multiple levels from the most fine-grained, individual responses to progressively larger aggregates of responses that comprise events. The contextualistic world view offers an important means to extend applied behavior analysis from its overly mechanistic applications. As Hayes et al. (1988) have pointed out from a contextual perspective, there is nothing inherently wrong with employing a mechanistic world view as long as that world view leads to the successful solving of problems. Contextualism is the most flexible of the world views because it allows the adoption of procedures and analyses from other systems if these are successful. However, contextualism is itself a comprehensive theory, not merely an eclectic adoption of multiple viewpoints.

From the perspective of the development of special education, the contextualistic world view would appear to be the best suited for solving the major problems currently confronting the field. In the area of friendship and integration into social support systems, adopting a more contextualistic viewpoint may prove essential. As this becomes a major goal for special education, it is critical to assess the contexts within which students behave. An important part of context is the social context and the support that people within a student's environment can give to newly emerging skills and the maintenance of behaviors. In addition, in understanding problem behaviors, it is important to realize that the functional control of behavior, and hence the interventions that will be effective in changing that behavior, can be mediated by contextual variables (Haring, T.G., & Kennedy, 1990).

A critical factor in training and in promoting social interaction is the context for interaction (Haring, T.G., in press). Contexts can be analyzed as to both physical parameters and social parameters. Physical parameters vary as to the richness in opportunities for interaction and the degree of support for interaction provided by the setting or materials. For example, an important physical contextual characteristic is providing students with access to integrated school, classroom, and community experiences. In addition, the activities that are within settings can vary greatly in the degree to which they set the occasion for behavior. For example, when playing on a seesaw, in order for the activity to proceed, two children must coordinate their behavior in a socially reciprocal fashion. Other toys, or more passive activities such as watching TV, do not occasion high levels of social interchange or may encourage more isolate play. These contextual characteristics are important to analyze in the design of programs, activities, and environments.

In addition to physical parameters such as types of activity or toys, or the characteristics of the physical setting that influence behavior, aspects of the *social* context can also affect the amount of responding. For example, from a contextualistic viewpoint, all instruction is conducted within a context that includes not only the aspects of the physical environment that determine context but also the social context of the teacher–learner relationship. Teachers who have established a history of positive interactions with a student, whose social interaction can serve as a generalized reinforcer for a child, establish increased attention and responsiveness from a child under instruction. Clearly, these are key problems for many people with disabilities and their teachers.

As our interventions become more contextualized, it will be increasingly important to include all individuals who participate in a student's life into the planning and implementation of interventions. Increasingly, the identification of problem behaviors, as well as behaviors for instruction, must come directly from the perspectives of the learner and the people with whom the learner is interacting, not *solely* from developmental checklists or analyses from the perspective of the teacher, psychologist, or even the parent. When people within a student's social context participate in identifying targets for change, their perspectives must also form the criteria for the ongoing assessment of the success or failure of intervention. Finally, people within the student's natural social contexts should be included in the intervention process as well as in the planning process.

In summary, our review has indicated that all four world hypotheses can be expected to contribute important means of designing interventions. From our analysis, contextualism would appear to be the most productive approach for many of the emerging challenges facing special education. Progressive growth and evolution of a scientific paradigm is a hallmark of its health and adequacy (Hull, 1989). Given the potential of behavior analysis to grow in these diverse and largely orthogonal directions, it must be considered a healthy and important paradigm for the future development of special education.

References

Albin, R.W., & Horner, R.H. (1988). Generalization with precision. In R.H. Horner, G. Dunlap, & R.L. Koegel (Eds.), *Generalization and maintenance: Lifestyle changes in applied settings* (pp. 99–120). Baltimore: Paul H. Brookes.

Baer, D.M. (1986). In application, frequency is not the only estimate of the probability of behavior units. In T. Thompson & M.D. Zeiler (Eds.), *Analysis and integration of behavioral units* (pp. 117–136). Hillsdale, NJ: Erlbaum.

Baer, D.M., Wolf, M.M., & Risley, T.R. (1987). Some still current dimensions of applied behavior analysis. *Journal of Applied Behavior Analysis*, *20*, 313–327.

Baldwin, J.D. (1988). Mead and Skinner: Agency and determinism. *Behaviorism*, *16*, 109–127.

Barnes, D. (1989). Behavior-behavior analysis, human schedule performance, and radical behaviorism. *Psychological Record*, *39*, 339–350.

Barrera, M. (1986). Distinctions between social support concepts, measures, and models. *American Journal of Community Psychology*, *14*, 413–445.

Becker, W.C., Engelmann, S., & Thomas, D. (1975). Systems for basic instruction: Theory and applications. In A.C. Catania & T. Brigham (Eds.), *Handbook of applied behavior analysis: Social and instructional processes* (pp. 325–378). New York: Irvington.

Bellamy, G.T., Horner, R.H., & Inman, D.P. (1979). *Vocational habilitation of severely retarded adults: A direct service technology*. Baltimore: University Park Press.

Brady, J.V., Bigelow, G.E., Emurian, H.H., & Williams, D.M. (1975). Design of a programmed environment for the experimental analysis of individual and small group behavior. In C.G. Miles (Ed.), *Experimentation in controlled environments: Its implications for economic behavior and social policy making* (pp. 134–144). Toronto: Addictive Research Foundation.

Bricker, W., & Bricker, D. (1970). A program of training language for the severely language handicapped child. *Exceptional Children*, *37*, 101–111.

Brown, F., Evans, I.M., Weed, K.A., & Owen, V. (1987). Delineating functional competencies: A component model. *Journal of The Association for Persons With Severe Handicaps*, *12*, 117–123.

Bruininks, R.H., & Abery, B. (1989, December). *Social networks of youth with disabilities*. Session presented at the Annual Meeting of the Association for Persons With Severe Handicaps, San Francisco, CA.

Carr, E.G., & Durand, V.M. (1985). Reducing problem behaviors through functional communication training. *Journal of Applied Behavior Analysis*, *18*, 111–126.

Chomsky, N. (1959). Review of Skinner's *Verbal Behavior*. *Language*, *35*, 26–58.

Cohen, M., & Haring, N.G. (1979). Developmental Pinpoints. In N.G. Haring & L. Brown (Eds.), *Teaching the severely handicapped* (Vol. 1, pp. 35–110). Seattle, WA: American Association for Education of the Severely and Profoundly Handicapped.

Cuvo, A.J., & Davis, P.K. (1983). Behavior therapy and community living skills. In M. Hersen, R.M. Eisler, & D.M. Miller (Eds.), *Progress in behavior modification* (Vol. 14, pp. 125–172). New York: Academic.
Engelmann, S., & Carnine, D. (1982). *Theory of instruction: Principles and applications*. New York: Irvington.
Emurian, H.H., Emurian, L.S., & Brady, D.V. (1985). Positive and negative reinforcement effects on behavior in a three-person microsociety. *Journal of the Experimental Analysis of Behavior*, *44*, 157–174.
Gardner, H. (1985). *The mind's new science: A history of the cognitive revolution*. New York: Basic Books.
Goetz, L., Gee, K., & Sailor, W. (1985). Using a behavior chain interrupted strategy to teach communication skills to students with severe disabilities. *Journal of The Association for Persons With Severe Handicaps*, *10*, 21–30.
Goldstein, H., & Wickstrom, S. (1986). Peer intervention effects on communicative interaction among handicapped and nonhandicapped preschoolers. *Journal of Applied Behavior Analysis*, *19*, 209–214.
Gould, S.J. (1981). *The mismeasure of man*. New York: W.W. Norton.
Gottlieb, B.H. (1981). *Social networks and social support*. Beverly Hills, CA: Sage.
Gottlieb, B.H. (1988). *Marshalling social support: Formats, processes, and effects*. Newbury Park, CA: Sage.
Guess, D., Sailor, W., Rutherford, G., & Baer, D.M. (1968). An experimental analysis of linguistic development: The productive use of the plural phoneme. *Journal of Applied Behavior Analysis*, *1*, 297–306.
Haring, N.G., White, O.R., Edgar, E.B., Affleck, J.Q., & Hayden, A.H. (1981). *UPAS: Uniform Performance Assessment System criterion tests*. Columbus, OH: Charles E. Merrill.
Haring, T.G. (1985). Teaching between-class generalization of toy play behavior to handicapped children. *Journal of Applied Behavior Analysis*, *18*, 127–139.
Haring, T.G. (in press). Research basis of instructional procedures to promote social interactions and integration. In S. Warren (Ed.), *Advances in mental retardation and developmental disabilities, Vol. 5: Research basis of instruction*.
Haring, T.G., & Breen, C. (1989). Units of analysis in social interaction outcomes in special education. *Journal of The Association for Persons With Severe Handicaps*, *14*, 255–262.
Haring, T.G., Breen, C., Weiner, J., Pitts-Conway, V., & Haring, N.G. (1989, December). *Intervention and technology to promote social integration*. Session presented at the Annual Meeting of the Association for Persons With Severe Handicaps, San Francisco, CA.
Haring, T.G., & Kennedy, C.H. (1988). Units of analysis in task-analytic research. *Journal of Applied Behavior Analysis*, *20*, 207–215.
Haring, T.G., & Kennedy, C.H. (1990). Contextual control of problem behavior in students with severe disabilities. *Journal of Applied Behavior Analysis*, *23*, 235–243.
Haring, T.G., Neetz, J.A., Lovinger, L., Peck, C.A., & Semmel, M.I. (1987). Effects of four modified incidental teaching procedures to create opportunities for communication. *Journal of The Association for Persons With Severe Handicaps*, *12*, 218–225.

Hart, B.M., & Risley, T.R. (1975). Incidental teaching of language in a preschool. *Journal of Applied Behavior Analysis*, *8*, 411–420.

Hayes, S.C., Hayes, L.J., & Reese, H.W. (1988). Finding the philosophical core: A review of Stephen C. Pepper's *World Hypotheses: A study in evidence. Journal of the Experimental Analysis of Behavior*, *50*, 97–111.

Holvoet, J.F. (1989). Research on persons labeled profoundly retarded: Issues and ideas. In F. Brown & D. Lehr (Eds.), *Persons with profound disabilities: Issues and practices* (pp. 61–82). Baltimore: Paul H. Brookes.

Horner, R.H., Dunlap, G., Koegel, R.L., Carr, E.G., Sailor, W., Anderson, J., Albin, R.W., & O'Neill, R.E. (1990). Toward a technology of "nonaversive" behavioral support. *Journal of The Association for Persons with Severe Handicaps*, *15*, 215–132.

Horner, R.H., Williams, J.A., & Knobbe, C.A. (1985). The effect of "opportunity to perform" on the maintenance of skills learned by high school students with severe handicaps. *Journal of The Association for Persons With Severe Handicaps*, *10*, 172–175.

Iwata, B.A., Dorsey, M.F., Slifer, K.J., Bauman, K.E., & Richman, G.S. (1982). Toward a functional analysis of self-injury. *Analysis and Intervention in Developmental Disabilities*, *5*, 357–372.

Kantor, J.R. (1958). *Interbehavioral psychology*. Chicago: Principia.

Kazdin, A.E. (1977). Assessing the clinical or applied significance of behavior change through social validation. *Behavior Modification*, *1*, 427–453.

Hull, D.L. (1989). *Science as a process*. Chicago: University of Chicago Press.

Kennedy, C.H., Horner, R.H., & Newton, J.S. (1989). Social contacts of adults with severe disabilities living in the community: A descriptive analysis of relationships patterns. *Journal of The Association for Persons with Severe Handicaps*, *14*, 190–196.

Kennedy, C.H., Horner, R.H., & Newton, J.S. (1990). The social networks and activity patterns of adults with severe disabilities: A correlational analysis. Journal of The Association for Persons With Severe Handicaps, *15*, 86–90.

Kohler, F.W., & Fowler, S.A. (1985). Training prosocial behaviors to young children: An analysis of reciprocity with untrained peers. *Journal of Applied Behavior Analysis*, *18*, 187–200.

Lerner, R.M., Hultsch, D.F., & Dixon, R.A. (1983). Contextualism and the character of developmental psychology in the 1970s. *Annals of the New York Academy of Sciences*, *412*, 101–128.

Macpherson F., & Butterfield G. (1988). Sensorimotor intelligence in severely handicapped children. *Journal of Mental Deficiency Research*, *32*, 465–478.

Michael, J. (1982). Distinguishing between the discriminative and motivational properties of stimuli. *Journal of the Experimental Analysis of Behavior*, *37*, 149–155.

Morris, E.K. (1988). Contextualism: The world view of behavior analysis. *Journal of Experimental Child Psychology*, *46*, 289–323.

O'Neill, R.E., Horner, R.H., Albin, R.W., Storey, K., & Sprague, J. (1989). *Functional analysis: A practical assessment guide*. Urbana, IL: Sycamore Press.

Peck, C.A., & Furman, G.C. (1990). Qualitative research in special education: An illustrative review. In R. Gaylord-Ross & J. Campoine (Eds.), *Research issues in special education*. (pp. 151–173). San Diego, CA: College Hill.

Peck, C.A., Schuler, A.C., Tomlinson, C., Theimer, R.K., & Haring, T. (1984). *The social competence curriculum project: A guide to instructional programming for social interactions* (Contract No. 300–83–0353). Washington, DC: U.S. Office of Special Education.

Pepper, S.C. (1942). *World hypotheses: A study in evidence*. Berkeley, CA: University of California Press.

Piaget, J. (1952). *The origins of intelligence in children*. (M. Cook, Trans.). New York: International University Press.

Ravish, N. (1987). *The relationship between cognitive concepts developed during the sensorimotor period, language, and adaptive behavior in autistic and mentally retarded children*. Unpublished doctoral dissertation, University of California, Santa Barbara, CA.

Rogers-Warren, A., & Warren, S.F. (1977). *Ecological perspectives in applied behavior analysis*. Baltimore: University Park Press.

Rosnow, R.L., & Georgoudi, M. (1986). *Contextualism and understanding in behavioral science: Implications for research and theory*. New York: Praeger.

Sasso, G.M., & Rude, H.A. (1987). Unprogrammed effects of training high-status peers to interact with severely handicapped children. *Journal of Applied Behavior Analysis*, *20*, 35–43.

Saunders, R.R., & Sailor, W. (1979). A comparison of three strategies of reinforcement on two-choice learning problems with severely retarded children. *Journal of The Association for Persons With Severe Handicaps*, *4*, 323–332.

Schoenfeld, N., & Farmer, J. (1970). Reinforcement schedules and the "behavior stream." In W.N. Schoenfeld (Ed.), *The theory of reinforcement schedules* (pp. 215–245). New York: Appleton-Century-Crofts.

Shimp, C.P. (1989). Contemporary behaviorism versus the old behavioral straw man in Gardner's *The Mind's New Science: A History of the Cognitive Revolution*. *Journal of the Experimental Analysis of Behavior*, *51*, 163–171.

Sidman, M. (1986). Analysis of emergent verbal classes. In T. Thompson & M.E. Zeiler (Eds.), *Analysis and integration of behavioral units* (pp. 213–245). Hillsdale, NJ: Earlbaum.

Skinner, B.F. (1935). The generic nature of the concepts of stimulus and response. *Journal of General Psychology*, *12*, 40–65.

Skinner, B.F. (1953). *Science and human behavior*, New York: Macmillan.

Skinner, B.F. (1974). *About behaviorism*. New York: Vintage.

Skrtic, T. (1988). *Establishing causality and generality*. Proceedings of the Project Directors Meeting, Office of Special Education Programs, U.S. Department of Education. Reston, VA: The Council for Exceptional Children.

Stillman, R., & Battle, C. (1985). *Callier Azusa Scale (H): Scales for the assessment of communicative abilities*. Dallas, TX: University of Texas, Callier Center for Communication Disorders.

Thompson, T., & Zeiler, M.D. (1986). *Analysis and integration of behavioral units*. Hillsdale, NJ: Erlbaum.

Touchette, P.E., MacDonald, R.F., & Langer, S.N. (1985). A scatter plot for identifying stimulus control of problem behavior. *Journal of Applied Behavior Analysis*, *18*, 343–351.

Vincent, L., Bricker, D.D., & Bricker, W.A. (1973). Receptive vocabulary: Performances and selection strategies of delayed and nondelayed toddlers. *American Journal of Mental Deficiency*, *77*, 576–584.

Warren, S., & Kaiser, A. (1988). Research in early language intervention. In S.L. Odom & M.B. Karnes (Eds.), *Early intervention for infants and children with handicaps: An empirical base*. Baltimore: Paul H. Brookes.

White, O.R. (1980). Adaptive performance objectives: Form versus function. In W. Sailor, B. Wilcox, & L. Brown. (Eds.), *Methods of instruction for severely handicapped students* (pp. 47–69). Baltimore: Paul H. Brookes.

Wilcox, B., & Bellamy, G.T. (1987). *A comprehensive guide to The Activities Catalog: An alternative curriculum for youth and adults with severe disabilities*. Baltimore: Paul H. Brookes.

Williams, J.A., Koegel, R.L., & Egel, A.L. (1981). Response-reinforcer relationships and improved learning in autistic children. *Journal of Applied Behavior Analysis, 14*, 53–60.

Wolf, M.M. (1978). Social validity: The case for subjective measurement, or how applied behavior analysis is finding its heart. *Journal of Applied Behavior Analysis, 11*, 203–214.

Wolfensberger, W. (1983). Social role valorization: A proposed new term for the principle of normalization. *Mental Retardation, 21*, 254–259.

Zeiler, M.D. (1986). Behavior units and optimality. In T. Thompson & M.D. Zeiler (Eds.), *Analysis and integration of behavioral units* (pp. 81–116). Hillsdale, NJ: Erlbaum.

4
Behavior Analysis in Supported Education

CATHERINE G. BREEN

Introduction

The Least Restrictive Environment (LRE)

Perhaps the most significant change in the lives of individuals with disabilities over the past two decades has been in the structure of education within the school environment. Since the passage of Public Law 94–142 (the Education for All Handicapped Children Act of 1975), and the development of the least restrictive environment (LRE) concept, researchers, policymakers, and teachers have made numerous attempts to find the best educational solutions for children with disabilities. Not very long ago, these children experienced complete exclusion not only from state-of-the-art practices but also from public educational services in general. Arguments continue as to what constitutes the least restrictive environment, both in terms of the educational placement of students and the curriculum to be adopted. What is agreed upon is that children with disabilities must have contact with their nondisabled peers. There is disagreement, however, concerning the conditions under which this contact should occur.

Continuum of Placement Options

Taylor (1988) analyzed LRE as it has come to be interpreted, in terms of the continuum of services that should be offered to individuals with disabilities, both from a traditional analysis of LRE (e.g., Zettel & Ballard, 1982) and from a current analysis of the law (e.g., Brown et al., 1983). Within a traditional continuum, special education placement options range from residential school or homebound instruction (as the most restrictive option) to full inclusion in a regular class on a regular public school campus (as the least restrictive option). Falling between these two extremes are options that include placement in a special school, placement in a self-contained class in a regular school, placement in a self-contained class with regular class services provided, and placement in a regular class with special class services provided. In contrast, in current interpretations of the LRE continuum, the most restrictive option is the placement of students in a self-contained class in a regular school with no regular class services provided. Sailor et al. (1989) argue that the continuum should be "best conceived as an array of potential service placements that are available if needed" (p. 17). Regardless of the LRE model advocated, placement choices should be decided only according to the needs and best interests of each individual.

Definition of Supported Education

The term *supported education*, which reflects the most current analysis of LRE, structures both the placement and curricular choices for individuals with special needs. Within supported education students are, to the maximum extent possible, integrated into regular classes, school activities, and critical community environments. Supported education is defined, not solely by regular class placement but also by integration into non-classroom-based activities, such as breaks between classes, lunch, school assemblies, school clubs, after-school sports, other recreational activities, and school jobs; and integration into non-school-based activities, such as community employment, accessing public transportation, the use of community shops, and participation in community recreational activities. The concept of supported education is also defined by the amount, type, and source of support needed for an individual to successfully participate in typical school and community settings. The most critical factor to the concept of supported education is that students are provided with opportunities for participation in the mainstream and with the support needed to participate with nondisabled peers in activities throughout the day. Placement and activity decisions must remain flexible and responsive to the specific needs of the individual.

Behavior Analysis and Supported Education

Although placement issues remain critical to the success of supported education within a school context, placement alone will probably not ensure successful integration (e.g., Gresham, 1983; Hamre-Nietupski & Nietupski, 1981). Direct intervention (which includes student, peer, and teacher training) and environmental manipulations and contextual interventions are necessary components of a program designed to promote successful integration. Behavior analysis has made significant contributions over the past two decades to the development and implementation of integrated school services, and remains key to the evaluation of current processes being applied in supported education. This chapter will include (a) a review of the behavioral research that has been conducted within the areas of social interaction and social integration since the early 1970s, (b) a review of research in the area of instructional integration, and (c) a review of validated techniques for assessing and evaluating the social validity of efforts to teach social interaction skills and to promote integration within school contexts.

Methods to Affect Social Interaction

Empirical efforts to examine social interaction can be generally organized according to three overall strategies: direct instruction, contextual interventions, and environmental manipulations. Research from each of these approaches has aided substantially in creating a validated system for systematically implementing and evaluating integration of students into supported educational contexts. Within direct instruction, the research has validated specific procedures to teach social interaction skills within a dyadic or multiple peer context. Within contextual interventions, the research focuses on processes that change social or relational events as a means to affect social interaction. Finally, within environmental manipulations, the research examines the effects of modifying physical variables within a context of social interaction.

Direct Instruction

Table 4.1 provides an overview of the direct instruction strategies that have been demonstrated to positively affect the social interaction between individuals with and without disabilities.

Adult-Mediated Instruction

Much research has been done that targets behavior change through adult mediation, in which the training of specific social interaction skills (including prompting, modeling, correcting, and reinforcing) is conducted by a teacher or other adult (e.g., Bates, 1980; Ford, Evans, & Dworkin, 1982; Haring, Roger, Lee, Breen, & Gaylord-Ross, 1986; McEvoy et al., 1988). For example, in Haring et al. (1986) social initiations and conversational expansions were taught by an adult to three elementary-school-age children with moderate disabilities within the natural environment in the absence of peers. Training consisted of delay procedures, indirect verbal prompts, and modeled prompts followed by contingent reinforcement of appropriate responding in the context of teaching socially scripted initiations and expansions. Social scripts were based on a list of conventionally appropriate conversational initiations (which were referenced to conversational topics of interest to same-age peers who attended the school), followed by a class of appropriate

TABLE 4.1. Direct instructional strategies.

- Adult-mediated instruction
    - Antecedent prompting
        - Modeling
        - Time delay
        - Prompt-fade
    - Shaping
    - Social script training
- Peer-mediated instruction
    - Peer initiation training
        - Antecedent prompting
            - Modeling
        - Time delay
            - Prompt-fade
        - Shaping
        - Social script training
    - Student initiation training
        - Antecedent prompting
            - Modeling
            - Time delay
            - Prompt-fade
        - Shaping
        - Social script training
- Peer- + Student-initiation training
    - Antecedent prompting
        - Modeling
        - Time delay
        - Prompt-fade
    - Shaping
    - Social Script training
- Adult + peer-mediated instruction

reponses, which were in turn followed by a class of appropriate conversational expansions. During training, the student with disabilities was assigned one part of the social script (initiator) and the teacher was assigned the second part (respondent). Probes were conducted within two natural contexts, with results indicating generalization of trained and novel responses to natural contexts.

Procedures that involve teacher attention or teacher-delivered reinforcement contingent on the production of appropriate social behavior as a procedure to shape responding have also been documented (e.g., Apolloni & Cooke, 1975; Russo & Koegel, 1977; Strain & Timm, 1974). In Russo and Koegel, token and social reinforcers were delivered to a 5-year-old girl with autism whenever she displayed appropriate social behaviors toward her peers without disabilities. The results showed that the social interactional behaviors of the student increased as a result of adult reinforcement. Adult-mediated interventions have been used effectively to teach specific social behaviors; however, they have also been criticized for their cost in terms of teacher time (e.g., Allen, Hart, Buell, Harris, & Wolf, 1964); lack of maintenance over time in the absence of teacher reinforcement (e.g., Walker, Greenwood, Hops, & Todd, 1979); failure to generalize to more natural contexts in the presence of same-age peers (e.g., Bates, 1980; Berler, Gross, & Drabman, 1982); and disruptiveness to the ongoing social interaction (e.g., Strain & Odom, 1986). Bates (1980), for example, introduced an interpersonal skills training program to eight adults with moderate to mild retardation. The instructional package included verbal instruction, modeling, role playing, feedback, contingent incentives, and homework. Although the program resulted in the acquisition of new social skills within role-play situations, there was not a substantial improvement in interactions within more natural settings. Finally, with more students with disabilities being educated within regular classrooms, in the absence of a special education teacher, the feasibility of implementing systematic adult-mediated interventions is in doubt.

Peer-Mediated Instruction

Peer-mediated strategies were developed in response to the problems found within adult-mediated training procedures (e.g., Egel, Richman, & Koegel, 1981; Gaylord-Ross, Haring, Breen, & Pitts-Conway, 1984; Goldstein & Wickstrom, 1986; Hunt, Alwell, & Goetz, 1988; Lancioni, 1982; Strain, Shores, & Timm, 1977). Within peer-mediated strategies peers are taught to initiate toward, respond to, prompt, and/or reinforce their peer with disabilities. For example, Goldstein and Wickstrom taught specific social interaction strategies to two peer confederates to be used with three preschool-age children with disabilities. The results showed that teaching the nonhandicapped peers to use specific strategies led to increases in the frequency of social responding by the peers with disabilities during free-play activities.

Within peer-mediated strategies, the role of the peer generally takes one of three forms. The peer can be used as a direct change agent, someone who directly prompts and reinforces social responding in the peer with disabilities (e.g., Apolloni & Cooke, 1979; Goldstein & Wickstrom, 1986; Lancioni, 1982); the peer can act as the initiator of social interaction, in "peer-initiation strategies" (e.g., Odom, Hoyson, Jamieson, & Strain, 1985; Ragland, Kerr, & Strain, 1978; Shafer, Egel, & Neef, 1984; Strain, Kerr, & Ragland, 1979); or the peer can be used as a confederate within a training context as a respondent to the initiations of the peer with disabilities, in "student-initiation strategies" (e.g., Brady et al., 1984; Gaylord-Ross et al., 1984; Haring et al., 1988; Hunt & Lovinger, 1989; Kohler & Fowler, 1985). Results from each of these efforts indicate that through systematic peer-mediated interventions, increased levels of appropriate social responding occur by the student with disabilities for the duration of the intervention in settings where intervention was targeted. For example, Ragland et al. (1978) trained a peer without disabilities to initiate scoial interactions with three children with autism, resulting in increases in positive social behavior by the children with disabilities. In a study by Hunt et al. (1988), students with severe disabilities initiated and participated in 10-minute conversations with peers without disabilities as a result of prompt-fade teaching strategies and of using conversational books. These results were not systematically extended to nonexperimental settings or peers, although anecdotal reports from parents, teachers, and peers suggested that gains from the training settings were being observed in other contexts.

In *peer-initiation strategies*, the peer acts as the initiator of a social interaction. The student with disabilities is then taught by either the teacher or the peer to respond appropriately to the peer initiation. Social responding is a very important social skill, in that individuals who do not respond to social attempts will eventually (if not immediately) extinguish any future social initiations made by their peers (e.g., Strain, Odom, & McConnell, 1984). Additionally, Strain (1983) found a relationship between student social responding to peer initiations and peer social acceptance in mainstream classes. A critical feature of peer-initiation strategies (particularly with young children), however, is that in order for peers to successfully implement and maintain programming, they must receive at least intermittent prompts and reinforcement (Odom et al., 1985). Trained effects are typically not maintained after teacher prompting and reinforcement are removed, although some researchers report the maintenance of levels of social responding above baseline levels (e.g., Goldstein & Wickstrom, 1986). An additional criticism of peer-initiation strategies has been that the individual with disabilities may become artificially dependent on another person for social interaction (Gaylord-Ross et al., 1984). By programming for social initiations from one group of people only, a second group of people is denied the choice to initiate and engage in an interaction. These effects are particularly noticeable when interactions are examined within contexts where the peer confederates are not present, or where trained peers are present but do not choose to initiate. Within both contexts, the frequency of interaction between individuals with and without disabilities is extremely low. Therefore, although the instruction of appropriate social responding through peer-initiation training is critical to social reciprocity, it is not alone sufficient for producing fully competent social participants.

Student-initiation strategies attempt to address the problem of creating social dependencies by teaching students with disabilities to initiate interactions toward their peers without disabilities. Through skill training, student-initiation strategies are designed to allow all individuals more social control. Social control is not only critical in terms of allowing individuals with disabilities more opportunities for social participation, but it is also a critical variable in determining how individuals are perceived. Persons without social control, or persons who depend on others for social participation are generally perceived as deviant and are devalued. As soon as individuals are perceived as deviant, the expectations for deviant behavior become greater, and the frequency of greater deviant behavior concomitantly rises (Wolfensberger, 1972, 1983). Student-initiation strategies have been found to be successful in increasing the frequency of interactions within nontrained contexts between individuals with and without disabilities. For example, in Gaylord-Ross et al. (1986), three high school students with autism were successfully taught, through the use of social scripts and peer confederates, to initiate and extend social conversations about attractive leisure items to untrained peers during school breaks.

Adult- and Peer-Mediated Instruction

Research has been conducted recently that attempts to bring together direct instructional strategies to intervene more extensively in the interaction between persons with and without disabilities. Odom and Strain (1986) compared two procedures for improving social interactions of three preschool-age children with autism. In one condition, peer confederates were taught to initiate interaction with their peers with disabilities. In a second condition, teachers prompted the targeted students to initiate toward peers who had been taught to respond. The results showed that the peer-initiation strategy was successful in increasing the social responses of the children with autism, whereas the student-initiation strategy was successful in increasing the social initiations *and* responses of the targeted children. Additionally, when the students with autism were prompted to begin an interaction, the interaction was typically of a longer duration than an interaction that was begun by the nondisabled peer. Finally, the study showed that an equal number of prompts were needed for all children to begin an interaction, but fewer prompts were needed for the children without disabilities to respond to student initiations than for the children with disabilities to respond to peer initiations. Although the research supports the use of teacher-antecedent, student-initiated interventions, the study also argues for intervention targeted at the social initiations and social responses of individuals both with and without disabilities to best achieve reciprocal interaction.

In Haring and Lovinger (1989), a research program was conducted that combined an awareness activity, peer-initiation training, student-initiation training, and appropriate play strategies. The program was designed to affect the frequency of peer and student initiations and peer and student responding. Training included the use of attractive, desirable materials and procedures for teaching strategies to use in the event that social initiations are rejected by another (i.e., What do you do if you ask someone to play and they say no? Go ask someone else). The results showed that the awareness activity and peer-initiation training alone increased the frequency of peer initiations, but did not affect peer responding. After students with disabilities were taught to initiate interactions and to play appropriately, the frequency of student initiation and the level of peer responding to student initiations increased. The authors discuss the importance of maintaining or increasing peer responding to levels that will maintain and encourage future social bids made by students with disabilities.

In recent work by Haring and Breen (1990), instruction of social skills occurred within multiple contexts to increase the frequency and quality of social interaction between two junior-high-school-age students with severe disabilities and two groups of four or five peers without disabilities across a school day. Within this investigation, four to five peers were taught during a weekly group meeting (and through intermittent problem solving with a teacher) strategies to prompt, reinforce, and correct the social behavior of a peer with disabilities, as well as strategies for responding to and extending initiations. Simultaneously, the student with disabilities was taught by a teacher, through social script training, appropriate initiations and responses to peer initiations that could be used across multiple contexts and peers. Opportunities for interaction were increased by mapping student and peer schedules across a school day and assigning peers at least one time per day to "hang out" with the targeted student, so that during all integrated activities (mainstream classes, breaks between classes, lunch, and nonacademic school activities) the student with disabilities hung out with at least one of the peers from his social network. Interactions were maintained through scheduling, weekly peer feedback, and the self-monitoring of the student with disabilities. Interactions were evaluated for the occurrence and appropriateness of targeted behaviors through written peer assessments of each interaction and through intermittent teacher probes. The results showed an increase in (a) opportunities for interaction, (b) frequency of interaction, (c) frequency of appropriate responding by the student with disabilities, and (d) duration of interaction. Additionally, satisfaction measures indicated positive ratings by all of the peers. Anecdotal reports indicated "spillover" effects within two domains. Friends of peers included within the social network expressed satisfaction with the program and with their interactions with the student with disabilities and reported more frequent and more positive contacts with the student following the intervention. Second, for one student, the frequency of peer-arranged contacts between members of the network away from school increased following intervention. Therefore, in this investigation adult- and peer-mediated strategies (in addition to environmental and contextual interventions) were used in combination to positively affect the reciprocal social interaction of individuals with and without disabilities.

Contextual Interventions

Contextual variables are those variables that define multiple stimulus conditions that "surround" a social interaction and that are oftentimes not physically observable, but that can be systematically measured through more complex quantitative and qualitative measurement systems. Contextual variables can include such things as disability awareness activities, manipulating the status and role of a participant, and activities that target group behaviors.

Disability Awareness

An important component of integration efforts is to provide information about disabilities and about the process that will be used to best achieve integration to the administrators, teachers, and students. Anderson (1984) involved a group of students who had had no structured contact with their peers with disabilities in a disability awareness program and measured the effects of the program on duration and quality of interactions between students with and without disabilities during recess. Simulation activities and information regarding individual students with disabilities resulted in increases in amount and quality of interaction. As reviewed previously, Haring and Lovinger (1989) included disability awareness activities within a more complex experimental design as a means to increase the frequency of initiations among preschool-age children. They found that disability awareness activities, in combination with direct instruction and inclusion of preferred activities, resulted in improved reciprocal interactions.

Manipulating the Responding of Individuals Through Altering the Status of a Participant in an Interaction

By modifying how someone is perceived, in terms of his or her abilities, ties to peers, associated reinforcing behaviors, or power, it is possible to significantly affect the degree of acceptance and resulting levels of social interaction (e.g., Breen & Haring, 1991; Dougherty, Fowler, & Paine, 1985; Kirby & Toler, 1970; Sainato, Maheady, & Shook, 1986; Sasso & Rude, 1987). Sainato et al. (1986) created the role of classroom manager for three young children who were socially withdrawn. The results showed that when the children were placed in the role of a manager, the following measures substantially increased: (a) the frequency of positive social initiations by the children who were socially withdrawn, (b) the frequency of positive social initiations by the classroom peers, (c) positive ratings by the classmates, and (d) the frequency of best-friend nominations by the classmates.

In a study by Sasso and Rude (1987), elementary-age nondisabled high- and low-status peers were taught to socially initiate interactions with students with severe disabilities during recess activities. Interactions from high-status peers led to higher levels of social initiations from untrained peers than did interactions from low-status peers.

In a manipulation of a social status variable, Breen and Haring (1991) investigated the effects of behavioral competence in playing computer games by junior-high-school-age students with moderate disabilities on the frequency of social initiations and participant satisfaction during dyadic interactions. The results indicated that there were greater frequencies of social initiations by participants both with and without disabilities. There were also greater degrees of overall satisfaction by both participants following interactions around computer games that had been trained to the student with disabilities than around computer games that had not been trained. This suggests that social reciprocity is enhanced when both members of a peer dyad are competent in the play activity.

Manipulating the Responding of Individuals Through Assignment of Participant Role

Two systematic programs that target social skills have emerged that specify a differential role of children without disabilities in relationships with peers with disabilities. In one program, peers act as peer tutors, who change instructional and social behavior through systematic teaching procedures (e.g., Kohl, Moses, & Stettner-Eaton, 1983; Lancioni, 1982; Maheady, Sacca, & Harper, 1988; McKenzie & Budd, 1981). In an alternative program, peers act as "buddies," or friends who change instructional and social behavior through incidental modeling, prompting, and feedback within the context of a supported friendship (Haring & Breen, 1990; Strain, Cooke, & Apolloni, 1976; Voeltz, 1980, 1982). Research has been conducted in both areas, with results indicating success in terms of increased levels of appropriate social and performance responding across school contexts by students with disabilities.

Peer Tutor Programs

Kohl et al. (1983) systematically taught fifth and sixth graders to act as instructional trainers with peers with severe disabilities in cafeteria jobs. The results indicated that through providing information sessions, direct instruction within the cafeteria, and feedback, the students were able to successfully teach job skills to their peers with disabilities. No measures were conducted of social interaction between peers. Lancioni (1982) used elementary- and junior-high-school-age children without disabilities within a structured classroom environment to systematically teach peers with moderate retardation delayed imitation, cooperative play, and two social verbalizations: "That's good" and "Thank you." As a result of peer tutoring, the levels of social responding by the students with disabilities increased within the training setting and across untrained contexts.

Friendship Programs

Strain et al. (1976) suggest pairing students with a buddy as a means to integrate the students with disabilities into peer groups. Haring and Breen (1990) increased positive social responding by two students with disabilities through assigning the students to "hang out" with members of an intact peer support group throughout the school day. Members of the group received informal training (consisting of teacher modeling of natural social behaviors, instruction of behavior management strategies, and delayed feedback regarding the naturalness and appropriateness of an interaction) as to how to most successfully interact and hang out with their friend with disabilities. An emphasis of the program was on establishing friendships and friendship-type interactions. All social skills training was conducted within a framework of what naturally occurs within peer groups during nonstructured times at a junior high school.

Peer Tutor Versus Friendship Programs

Voeltz (1981) discusses the importance of limiting tutorial-type relationships because peer tutoring programs promote hierarchical or vertical relationships where the peer assumes a higher status position as trainer and the student with disabilities assumes a lower status position as trainee. Programs that construct interventions around buddy-type relationships or friendships, in contrast, promote horizontal or more equal participation within a social relationship. Haring, Breen, Pitts-Conway, Lee, and Gaylord-Ross (1987) complared the levels of social interaction toward individuals with severe disabilities and attitudinal ratings of high-school-age students who had participated in a peer tutoring program to those who had participated in a "special friends" program. Statistical comparisons of the groups indicated that serving as a peer tutor was equivalent to serving as a special friend across the two measures, and both experiences resulted in greater degrees of interaction and willingness to interact than no experience. Thus, although there is some debate as to the types of roles that peers should assume, there is support for both types of relationships in terms of increasing the appropriateness of social responding of peers with disabilities and affecting the attitudes of peers without disabilities.

Manipulating the Responding of Individuals Through Classroom Structure

Within traditional academically competitive classroom structures, students with disabilities are often targets of negative comments and are often rejected by their more academically competent peers (Slavin, 1990). By manipulating the classroom structure so that students work within cooperative groups, where each member is able to contribute to the overall success of the group and where interdependent participation of individual members is critical, it is likely that the frequency of negative nominations by peers will decline (e.g., Madden & Slavin, 1983). Research has been conducted that supports the use of cooperative over competitive or individual learning situations in terms of its effects on achievement (Johnson, D. W., Maruyama, Johnson, R. Nelson, & Skon, 1981) and its positive effects on the quality of relationships between students (e.g., Altman, 1971; Johnson, D.W., & Johnson, R. 1984; Johnson, D.W., Johnson, R. & Maruyama, 1983; Rynders, Johnson, R. Johnson, D.W. & Schmidt, 1980).

Manipulating the Responding of Individuals Through Group Contingencies

The manipulation of group contingencies in social and academic responding has received some experimental attention (e.g., Dougherty et al., 1985; Greenwood & Hops, 1981; Kohler & Fowler, 1985; Speltz, Shimamura, & McReynolds, 1982). Within group contingencies, "the behavior of one or more group members determines the consequences received by at least one other member of the group" (Speltz et al., 1982, p. 533). As with cooperative group structuring, this procedure can have very powerful effects on responding because it involves multiple interdependent social controls. As part of a larger study investigating the training and maintenance of prosocial behaviors, Kohler and Fowler (1985) implemented two group contingencies to increase play invitations from three peers to a target child. During Group Contingency 1, the four children each received a sticker if they met their predetermined criterion of three to six positive invitations from the target student and one invitation from each of the three peers. Additionally, the whole class received a large-group award if the target group met the criterion for 3 consecutive days. During Group Contingency 2, awards were given for peer invitations only. The contingency phase resulted in an increase in positive invitations from all members of the group. The rate of positive invitations from the peers increased slightly and remained high for the target student during Group Contingency 2. After the contingency was removed, the levels of interaction returned to baseline levels.

In Speltz et al. (1982), various individual and group contingencies were applied to the performance on arithmetic problems of two students with learning disabilities. The results were analyzed in terms of effects on academic performance and social interaction. Each of the imposed contingencies was effective in improving arithmetic worksheet performance. Group rewards that were based on the number of correct problems completed during the work period by an identified target student and an unidentified group member resulted in the greatest percent of social interaction among group members, suggesting more frequent instances of helping behavior and encouragement when one individual in a group was responsible for the reward outcomes of the group. Student ratings of group contingencies also gave support for the use of a identified responder group over individual contingencies.

Manipulating the Responding of Individuals Through Group Size

An extension of group management techniques is the use of group of peers rather than single peers as a way to facilitate social inclusion into peer networks. Most of the research, aside from that which targets group contingencies or cooperative learning, has been conducted within dyadic interactions. That is, instruction to criterion is conducted using one peer confederate or targeting initiations toward one peer at a time. Programs that include multiple (albeit independent) peer training have found greater success in generalization of social responding to novel contexts than programs which include single peer confederates (Brady et al., 1984; Gaylord-Ross et al., 1984); however, the interventions tend to be lengthy and costly in terms of teacher time. Haring and Breen (1990) have recently investigated the effects of an intervention that was designed around a small group of nondisabled peers who, prior to the investigation, were members of one social network. The results were analyzed in terms of acquisition of responses, generalization of responses, maintenance of effects, and spillover effects with nontrained peers. Through structuring interventions around a peer social support network, in combination with a structured training package, positive results were found across all dependent variables.

In Breen, Lovinger, and Haring (1989), a large group of peers with and without disabilities participated in a lunchtime recreational club (PAL Club) where peers "hung out" in small groups during lunch periods and in a large group one lunch period per week. Social interaction skills were taught incidentally, embedded within natural interactions during lunch and within systematic training periods after lunch. Attitudinal measures and measures of frequency and duration of interaction were gathered across a 1-year period, indicating positive attitudinal and behavioral effects for both students with and without disabilities.

Environmental Manipulations

One of the most efficient ways to encourage, elicit, and maintain social interaction is to manipulate physical aspects of the environment in which interaction is desired. This can include altering the materials or activities within the environment in terms of (a) the number and variety of materials, which can allow for greater choice; (b) student preference; (c) attractiveness; and (d) interactiveness of activies and materials. Manipulation of seating arrangements and use of space in a classroom can also lead to substantial increases in social interaction.

Amount and Variety of Materials and Activities

In an early study by M.W. Johnson (1935), increases in the frequency of social contacts between classmates was seen as a function of reducing the amount of playground equipment. In contrast, Horner (1980) increased the frequency of appropriate adaptive behaviors by increasing the number of toys in an institutional environment. Spangler and Johnson (1983) similarly increased the purposeful play activity of boys with severe and profound disabilities by increasing the availability of toys. The presence of placemats illustrated with conversational topics and games led to increases in social conversation among family members in a study by Green, Harbison, and Greene (1984).

Student-Preferred Materials and Activities

In a study by Koegel, Dyer, and Bell (1987), 10 students with mental retardation and autism engaged in decreased levels of social avoidance behavior and increased levels of social initiation when provided access to child-preferred activities than to activities selected arbitrarily by an adult. Wong et al. (1987) similarly decreased the rate of stereotypic vocalizations in adults with schizophrenia during preferred recreational activities with or without contingent reinforcement for on-task behavior.

Attractiveness of Materials and Activities

In order for interactions to maintain across time and context, each participant in the interaction must in some way be reinforced. Objects or activities which are valued or appealing to the potential interactants can serve as the reinforcement needed to extend the duration of the interaction and lead to predicted future exchanges. In the study by Gaylord-Ross et al. (1984), attractive, age-appropriate leisure materials were selected as stimuli around which social conversations and social interactions would be likely to occur within a high school environment. The authors discussed the need for the teaching of social skills in addition to the availability of attractive materials in order to positively affect the rates of social interaction. Haring and Lovinger (1989) also found that the presence of attractive materials in combination with direct skill training facilitated the interaction between young children with and without disabilities and increased the likelihood of interactions within nontrained contexts.

Interactiveness of Materials and Activities

Similar to the effects found with providing access to attractive materials, materials and activities that require the participation of more than one individual can also lead to higher levels of interaction. Quilitch and Risley (1973) found that the type of play, social or isolate, differed according to the type of toy available for play; they encouraged the use of interactive play materials to promote social interaction. Hand-held video games that required the participation of two individuals were used in the study by Gaylord-Ross et al. (1984). Hunt et al. (1988) used picture communication books to structure conversations between students with and without disabilities.

Summary of Methods to Affect Social Interaction and Integration

A synthesis of the vast research in the area of social interaction and integration indicates a number of instructional, contextual, and environmental procedures that have been successfully validated:

1. Procedures that are adult-mediated, that is, strategies that include both adult shaping of social behavior and the antecedent prompting of behavior, have been used effectively to teach specific social responses; however, they are limited in terms of their generalized and maintained effects and pose logistical concerns in integrated contexts.
2. Procedures that are peer-mediated, are similarly effective in promoting the acquisition of social responses, but have found somewhat greater generalized effects, because the change agents are more closely aligned with the natural population.
3. Within peer-mediated programs, strategies that target student-initiated interactions are generally more effective than peer-initiated interactions in terms of the frequency and duration of interactions between students with and without disabilities.
4. The participation of both members of a dyad as initiators and respondents in order to promote reciprocity within interactions is found to be more successful in leading to maintenance and generalization of trained effects.
5. By manipulating the status of a participant in an interaction, whether he or she is a participant with disabilities or a nondisabled peer, the

social acceptance and resulting levels of interaction with participants with disabilities can be significantly affected within natural contexts.

6. The role of peers with disabilities (peer tutor relationships and friendship relationships) can facilitate the social integration and teaching of social responses of individuals with disabilities across multiple contexts.
7. Manipulation of group contingencies and group interaction patterns can improve the performance and social responding of students, resulting in more positive attitudes toward persons with disabilities.
8. Preliminary investigations show that the inclusion of peer networks to facilitate integration can be effective in promoting the maintenance and generalization of trained social responding.
9. Altering physical aspects of a social context, including providing access to highly attractive materials, interactive materials, and more choices of materials and social activities can facilitate the occurrence of interactions.
10. Manipulation of seating arrangements and use of space in a classroom can affect the level of social interaction.
11. Experimental programs that combine the above strategies lead to the greatest success in terms of levels of social responding, generalization of trained responses, maintenance of trained responses, and satisfaction by members of the school population.

Methods to Affect Instructional Integration

Supported education is intended to increase the opportunities and systems for social responding and social interaction, and also to increase performance of nonsocial responses within integrated contexts. Behavioral research that has been conducted in the area of instructional integration in many ways parallels that being done in the area of social integration, with research efforts that include direct instruction through adult mediation (e.g., Bryant & Budd, 1982; Guevremont, Osnes, & Stokes, 1988; Knapczyk, 1989; Rhode, Morgan, & Young, 1983; Singh & Singh, 1984) and peer mediation (e.g., Dineen, Clark, & Risley, 1977; Egel et al., 1981; Greenwood et al., 1984; Greenwood, Sloane, & Baskin, 1974; McKenzie & Budd, 1981), and contextual interventions that include manipulation of group contingencies (e.g., McCarty, Griffen, Apolloni, & Shores, 1977; Pigott, Fantuzzo, & Clement, 1986; Pigott, Fantuzzo, Heggie, & Clement, 1984; Speltz et al., 1982); manipulation of the role of the student within a group (e.g., Pigott et al., 1986; Stern, Fowler, & Kohler, 1988); individual self-management (e.g., Ayllon & Roberts, 1974; Dunlap & Dunlap, 1989; Harris, 1986; Lloyd, Bateman, Lundrum, & Hallahan, 1989; Stevenson & Fantuzzo, 1986); and procedures to infuse individual performance objectives into a regular education curriculum (Peck, Killen, & Baumgart, 1989). To date, the greatest number of behavior analytic research efforts have targeted inclusion of students with learning disabilities, underachievers, and students with behavior disorders into mainstream classes. Few efforts (beyond analyses of early education programs) have been made to target students with more severe disabilities. With the emergence of a strong philosophic movement toward integrating students with moderate, severe, and profound disabilities partially and fully into regular classes (e.g., Sailor et al., 1989; Stainback & Stainback, 1987), there exists a critical need for data-based behavior analytic research to determine the best practices to use in transitioning, implementing, and evaluating programs that are being supported within the mainstream for students with more severe disabilities.

Direct Instruction

Adult-Mediated Instruction

Adult-mediated instruction strategies have been used to help students make a transition from a more to a less restrictive classroom placement and to teach skills that will allow students to perform at levels similar to those of their classmates. Knapczyk (1989), for example, taught question asking to three 4th-grade students with mild disabilities using videotape modeling, rehearsal, and feedback strategies within a resource room. Measures of the frequency of question asking and percentage of accuracy on assignments were gathered in the regular classroom, indicating greater levels across both measures following intervention. The use of videotapes of regular class activities (as exemplars of the regular education program) is discussed as a strategy to facilitate generalization.

Singh and Singh (1984) taught students with moderate disabilities to decrease reading errors and increase self-corrections by manipulating the student's familiarity with the targeted text through teacher previewing of the material. In previewing, the teacher and the students discussed the story that was to be read and new words that would be found in the story prior to the students' reading of the material. Previewing resulted in increased rate of self-corrections and a reduction in the number of errors for all students.

Guevremont et al. (1988), as a follow-up to work done by Bryant and Budd (1982), taught preschool-age children who demonstrated poor independent work performance to self-instruct overtly (i.e., audibly) during classroom work periods. Self-instruction followed steps outlined by Meichenbaum and Goodman (1971), which included the following: (a) Define task (e.g., What do I have to do first?); (b) define required responses (e.g., I have to circle the words that have the same letters); (c) guide correct responding (e.g., This one, so I will circle it); and (d) acknowledge task completion (e.g., Good job). The authors found that through overt self-instruction, students were able to increase their accuracy in performance of tasks that were similar to those used during training and for two out of three children in tasks that were dissimilar. Children generalized their use of self-instructional strategies from the training setting to the classroom only after given instruction to use self-verbalizations in the classroom. Efforts to train covert (silent) self-instruction following training of overt (audible) self-instruction found inconsistent results. The authors discussed a need for caution when proceeding from overt to covert instructional strategies, particularly with students who show limited or transient success with overt self-instruction.

Peer-Mediated Instruction

Because of large class sizes and the heterogeneity of classroom populations, adult-mediated instructional strategies that differ from those strategies that are used with the class as a whole may be less feasible after students are placed within the regular class. Using peer-mediated instruction strategies has been described (Jenkins & Jenkins, 1985) as a way to increase academic engaged time, defined as the time a student spends in academically relevant tasks that are moderately difficult (Berliner, Fisher, Filby, & Marlieve, 1976). McKenzie and Budd (1981) used a peer tutor to improve the accuracy of mathematics performance of two students with learning and behavioral disabilities. In Egel et al. (1981), peers modeled correct responses on five discrimination tasks to four students with autism, resulting in increased correct responding across tasks by the targeted students. Criterion performance maintained after the peer models were removed.

Teacher- Versus Peer-Mediated Instruction

In a study by Jenkins, Mayhall, Peschka, and Jenkins (1974), teacher-mediated small-group instruction was compared with one-to-one peer-mediated instruction on the academic performance of students with mild disabilities. Performance measures were found to be higher when the student received one-to-one instruction from a peer than when instruction was delivered by the teacher in a small group context. Similarly, Greenwood et al. (1984) as part of a larger investigation compared the effects of teacher-mediated to peer-mediated instruction on academic responding, finding greater weekly achievement effects and a greater diversity of academic responding under peer-mediated conditions.

Although peer-mediated instruction has been validated as being an effective strategy for increasing the academic performance of students with special needs, some concerns arise as to the effects and the benefits to the tutor. Within peer-tutoring programs, positive effects (both attitudinal and performance) have been demonstrated for both the tutor and tutee. For example, Dineen et al. (1977) enlisted a peer treatment program targeted to improve spelling performance. The results showed increased spelling performance for both the targeted students and the tutors, indicating mutually beneficial effects. Maheady et al. (1988) found that classwide peer tutoring (Delquadri, Greenwood, Whorton, Carta, & Hall, 1986) resulted in increased academic performance by high school students with disabilities and their nondisabled peers. Additionally, anecdotal measures reported high degrees of satisfaction from both the teacher and the students with the tutoring procedures and outcomes.

Contextual Interventions

As with social integration, educational integration can be strongly affected by such variables as manipulation of group contingencies within the classroom structure, manipulation of the role of the student within the classroom, transfer of control from the teacher to the student in self-determining goals and outcomes of daily and weekly performance, and transfer of performance objectives from a self-contained classroom to a regular classroom curriculum. Some of the research that will be reviewed within this section is work that was conducted within a self-contained classroom; however, because the processes used are those that could be applied within a regular classroom, the work is viewed as relevant to an analysis of performance-enhancing procedures that can be used to successfully integrate students with different needs.

Manipulating the Responding of Individuals Through Group Contingencies

McCarty et al. (1977) increased the arithmetic performance of behavior-disordered adolescents through manipulation of group contingencies. Similarly, Pigott et al. (1986) increased the arithmetic performance of 12 underachieving fifth-grade students to levels indistinguishable from those of their nondisabled classmates by applying a group contingency to groups of four targeted students who were assigned different roles within the group. Both studies discuss the positive effects of group contingencies on promoting cooperative behavior in students. Additionally, Pigott et al. found an increased amount of peer affiliation outside of the work period among members who participated together in the treatment group.

Manipulating the Responding of Individuals Through Assignment of Participant Role

Within Pigott et al. (1986), students selected one of four rotating roles within the group ("coach," "scorekeeper," "referee," and "manager"). The roles were designed to provide peer instruction, peer observation, peer evaluation, and peer reinforcement. As discussed, the participation of students within a group with applied group contingencies resulted in increased arithmetic performance. Further research is needed to assess more systematically the contribution of each role in the group on the resulting performance increase and satisfaction.

Stern et al. (1988) examined the effects of assigned roles on arithmetic performance and off-task behavior of two 5th-grade students with high rates of disruptive behavior. Within this research students were appointed within an alternating treatments design as a peer monitor or a point earner within a dyad. The results indicated that both roles led to a similar decrease in off-task behavior and an increase in the rate of math performance. Additional measures of consumer satisfaction indicated positive ratings by both students for both roles, with a slight preference for the point-earner role.

Manipulating the Responding of Individuals Through Altering Student Control Within a Classroom

Self-management has been used as a means to transfer learned social and performance responses from training settings to criterion environments, to decrease the amount of direct teacher-to-student time, and to increase student motivation through the provision of more self-controlled learning.

In a study by Rhode et al. (1983), self-evaluation procedures were taught to six elementary students with behavior disorders by the teacher within a resource room. As soon as the students demonstrated appropriate behavior using self-evaluation and minimal external reinforcement, the self-evaluation strategy was transferred to the regular classroom. The results indicated that the students transferred and maintained high levels of appropriate classroom behavior with the use of self-evaluation in the regular classrooms.

Dunlap and Dunlap (1989) introduced a self-monitoring checklist to improve the subtraction skills of students with learning disabilities within a resource room. The self-monitoring checklist resulted in an increased percentage of correct responses for all students. When the self-monitoring checklist was withdrawn, the students continued to perform at improved levels and maintained their performance for the duration of the maintenance period (4–16 consecutive days).

In an early study by Lovitt and Curtiss (1969), the academic responding of one student with behavioral disorders was compared when contingency requirements were made by the teachers and when they were determined by the student. The results indicated that self-imposed contingencies were associated with greater academic response rates than were teacher-imposed contingencies.

In Stevenson and Fantuzzo (1986), underachieving students, through the use of self-score cards, self-selected daily goals, and reinforcers recorded and charted correct arithmetic problems. The results demonstrated that self-management led to increased arithmetic performance across multiple settings and times to levels comparable to those found with untreated students. Additionally, measures were conducted that positively evaluated the appropriateness and acceptability of the procedure to the classroom teachers.

Lloyd et al. (1989) applied self-recording to attentive behavior and to arithmetic productivity with students with learning and behavioral disabilities within a self-contained classroom. During the first intervention phase of the study, the students recorded (at the sound of a tape-recorded tone) whether they were paying attention to their assignments. During the subsequent phase, the students recorded how many problems they had completed at the sound of the tone. The results indicated that self-recording of both attentiveness and productivity resulted in increased levels of performance (with neither procedure producing superior levels of performance) and increased attention to task.

Transfer of Performance Objectives

In order for partial or full inclusion into the regular class to be warranted, it must be clear that the individual needs as specified by the student's individualized educational plan (IEP) are being addressed within the mainstream context. Although the successful transfer of performance objectives is one of the most critical components of integration efforts, it has rarely been experimentally validated. Extensive experimental research is needed in this area in order to make specific recommendations regarding critical amount of time in the mainstream classroom, and effectiveness of integrated programming on social and performance objectives.

Peck et al. (1989) conducted two investigations that assessed procedures for increasing the implementation of IEP-related instruction for children with mild to moderate disabilities in regular preschool and day-care programs. In one study, a nondirective consultation intervention was implemented. Through consultation, the regular teacher observed videotapes of teacher/student activities and provided suggestions for techniques to be used to include a specific IEP objective into the regular program. The intervention resulted in increased implementation of instruction related to IEP objectives within instructional settings that were trained as well as untrained. The second study replicated the findings of the first study without the use of videotape observations. The results are discussed in terms of the strength of nondirective consultations between regular and special education teachers in increasing implementation of IEP objectives within the regular class program.

Summary of Methods to Affect Instructional Integration

A limited amount of experimental research has been conducted that directly targets the education of students with disabilities within regular education classrooms. Much of the behavior analytic research that has been done targets students with mild to moderate disabilities and examines the remediation of academic skills. Based on this work some preliminary instructional procedures can be summarized, although caution should be taken when applying these procedures to individuals with more severe disabilities:

1. Adult-mediated instruction has been shown to be successful in teaching specific learning strategies, such as oral self-instruction of identified tasks, question-asking strategies, or previewing work to be completed; with increasing classroom size and diversity of student need, adult-mediated instruction (as it would be used with an individual or small group of students) may be inefficient or may require that teacher time be pulled away from the needs of the group.
2. One-to-one peer-mediated instruction may result in greater rates of academic performance than adult-mediated small-group instruction.
3. Peer-mediated instruction can be effective in improving the academic performance of classmates with disabilities with no deleterious effects to the peers.
4. Instruction within groups is an alternative to instruction within a one-to-one context, allowing for more efficient use of teacher time.
5. By manipulating group contingencies, the academic performance of students can be improved with concomitant improvements in cooperative behavior.
6. Manipulation of the role of a student within a group can improve the academic performance of students, with concomitant increases in peer ratings.
7. Procedures that incorporate self-management techniques have been shown to be effective in reducing the need for individual teacher attention, in facilitating the transfer of learned skills to nontrained contexts, and in improving the academic performance of students.
8. Through nondirective consultation between regular and special education staff, the number of IEP objectives infused into the regular education curriculum can be increased.

Measures of Social Validity

Traditionally, social validation research has provided data that indicate that application of specific research methods result in behavior occurring at a normative rate (e.g., Stevenson & Fantuzzo, 1986) or that the effects of intervention are discriminable to people removed from the research (e.g., Haring et al., 1986). Measures typically reflect frequency counts or rates of social behavior. More recently, social validation research has examined the effects of treatment programs on those individuals within the student's immediate social environment (e.g., Breen & Haring, 1991; Haring & Breen, 1990). Efforts are being made to assess whether the behavior change is valued by persons not directly targeted by the intervention but who are in contact with those directly targeted. Measures have gone beyond simple frequency counts of individual behaviors and now include more qualitative assessments of behavior change. One goal of integration is to affect "relationships" (indicating reciprocal satisfaction). Social validation measures must be included that assess the true impact of behavioral interventions on individuals who are directly and indirectly involved in programming. Those interventions that positively affect a person's social and instructional ecology—in terms of the resultant behavior change being perceived, valued, and needed—should be enlisted and maintained within a school curriculum. Those interventions that result in behavior that is proven to hold no value or that does not positively affect the context in which it occurs should be removed from current practice.

Various measurement systems are currently being used to assess the social validity of programs designed to promote social and instructional integration.

Questionnaires

Within a questionnaire format, students without disabilities, students with disabilities, and/or teachers respond to a list of questions that may (a) assess satisfaction with the processes and the results of systematic programming; (b) solicit specific feedback regarding elements of the program; and/or (c) assess the willingness of peers to engage in the same, related, or different activities with a person with disabilities (e.g., Breen et al., 1989; Haring & Breen, 1990; Haring et al., 1987; Hiroshige, 1989). Questionnaires can be delivered after each treatment session to evaluate ongoing satisfaction with the program (e.g., Breen & Haring, 1991), intermittently to assess changes (or stability) over time in consumer satisfaction (e.g., Haring & Breen, 1990); or as single pre/post measures to assess changes in attitudes regarding people with disabilities and/or programs designed to serve people with disabilities (e.g., Haring et al., 1987).

Student/Teacher Ratings

Related to measures gathered within a questionnaire, are measures that are assessed through a single question format, which rates the overall satisfaction with a program or a preference for one aspect of the program over another (Speltz et al., 1982; Stern et al., 1988). Ratings are gathered through written assessments or through individual interviews. Teacher ratings of the appropriateness of specific interventions, in terms of the usability within a classroom and perceived impact on classroom population, have also been conducted as a means to socially validate research efforts (e.g., Stevenson & Fantuzzo, 1986).

Observation of Behavioral Interactions

Frequency counts, or assessments of rate of interaction when conducted within natural contexts that are not targeted for intervention, can serve as validity measures of the generalized impact of intervention efforts. These measures can be evaluated in terms of a student's willingness to participate in unrelated contexts or activities as a result of systematic programming (e.g., Haring et al., 1987; Pigott et al., 1986).

Future Directions for Behavior Analysis in Supported Education

Behavior analytic research has been successful in developing and evaluating specific social and educational processes for use with students with disabilities. Research efforts have validated procedures that will produce behavior change within trained and untrained settings, in the presence of trained and untrained peers, and behavior change that is likely to maintain in the absence of programming. Behavior analysts have specified the effects of manipulating antecedent and consequent events on responding. In general, research to date has been highly responsive to the need for fine-grained analyses of specific learning processes both in terms of simple stimulus–response–consequence (S–R–C) learning and of more complex multidimensional analyses. Behavior analysis has not been as responsive, however, to the need for analyses that examine broader contextual variables and the development of human relationships, which are the goals of supported education.

Friendship Relationships

One of the most important arguments for increasing the amount of contact between students through supported education is that more frequent contacts within natural contexts will lead to (a) increased acceptance of persons with different abilities, and (b) the development of friendship relationships. Although the validity of this argument has been supported by emotional and subjective assessments, very few systematic, data-based analyses have been conducted that empirically validate and warrant the degree of change that educational systems are currently undertaking. We do not know empirically that increasing contacts will increase friendship relationships. We do know that by increasing opportunities for interaction and introducing systematic behavior change program variables, the frequency of initiations, the duration of interaction, or the rate of initiations can be increased. However, it is not clear that these variables are actual indicators of friendships. Friendships must be defined by multiple interrelated factors that define the topography of an interaction across contexts (e.g., school–nonschool, dyadic–group, presence of friends–presence of acquaintances, structured–nonstructured, in class–out of class). Friendship relationships can differ in quality and intensity. Some (but not all) of the relationships that friendships can include are (a) acquaintance-type relationships, in which peers may have a class together and will exchange a greeting in passing; (b) membership in a same social clique, in which peers eat lunch together and attend common large-group activities outside of school; (c) good-friend relationships, in which peers from the same social clique hang out during nonstructured times at school and after school in small-group and occasionally dyadic interaction; and (d) best-friend relationships, in which two or three peers hand out during all nonstructured times at school, after school, and on weekends, and call each other on the telephone at least once per day.

In addition to the frequency and location of contact that peers can have at different friendship levels, there also exist different types of interactions, including the makeup of conversational exchanges and differential exclusionary or exceptance behavior toward other peers. In total, assessing and intervening on friendship relationships goes far beyond measuring single variables within sampled contexts. Behavior analysis can and must successfully affect this area with a broadening of measures to include multicomponent contextual variables. (See chapter 3 for a more inclusive discussion of contextualism and a contextual behavior analysis.)

Mainstreaming

Two major questions that emerge when we discuss mainstreaming, that is, the placement of students with disabilities into one or more regular education classes, are, (a) Given our initial argument that increasing contacts will affect friendship relationships and attitudes, what systematic manipulations must be conducted to ensure these goals? and (b) How can the nonsocial instructional needs of individual students be met within a regular class placement? Behavior analysis again has provided us with a basis for teaching or influencing social interaction and instruction. What is still largely unknown within behavior analytic research is how to integrate these processes into the mainstream. Empirical investigations must seek answers to the following questions:

1. What types of classes or classroom structures best facilitate or allow opportunities for interaction (partial responses include classes with cooperative learning groups and nonacademic classes)?
2. What duration is optimal for mainstreaming within classes to result in stronger friendship relationships and attitudes compared to placement within a self-contained classroom with integration into all nonclassroom-based activities?

3. Are students who are fully mainstreamed meeting instructional objectives that facilitate future participation in community activities (i.e., independent living and work), and if not, how can this be achieved without a total restructuring of the regular education curriculum?
4. Are students who are mainstreamed perceived more positively by their nondisabled peers?
5. How are students best supported within a regular education classroom?
6. What systems are effective in evaluating social and instructional integration outcomes?
7. What are the effects of a pull-out model to teach critical skills on the attitudes of peers without disabilities?

Supported Education and Systematic Interventions for Students With Profound Disabilities

Much of the research in the area of social interaction targets students with mild to severe disabilities. Virtually all empirical research in the area of instructional integration is relevant to persons with mild disabilities. Caution should be taken in applying instructional strategies validated with students with more independent critical skills and intact communication systems to persons who have fewer skills. In great need of expansion is the development and analysis of social and instructional interventions involving students with profound disabilities. Pilot procedures developed by Haring and Kennedy (1990) teach students with profound disabilities to signal (through manipulating a tape recorder via an electronic switch) a change in social activity with nondisabled peers. The procedure allows students more independent control over their social environment and demonstrates to the peers levels of competent social responding that prior to the intervention were absent. Further research of this type would be critical to the extent data base.

Administrative Issues Surrounding the Achievement of Supported Education Goals

A significant amount of change is currently under way within special education. In many areas across the United States, regular education and special education are converging in terms of available monies and resources, administrative powers, and education of children. Students with mild, moderate, severe, and profound disabilities of all ages are being served to a greater extent than ever before within mainstream settings. Some students are currently attending their neighborhood school within the age-matched regular classroom with consultative or direct support from special education resource personnel. These administrative changes are currently being undertaken in the absence of strong empirical data to support fuller inclusion of students with disabilities into the mainstream. We do not know empirically what the short-term or long-term effects of increased mainstreaming will be on the targeted individual and on the mainstream population. Most important, there is a paucity of research that details the administrative and educational processes that can lead to positive outcomes. The following questions are in extreme need of examination:

1. Given the standard allotment of state and federal monies per student, what administrative processes can be used to place students individually within mainstream contexts with enough educational support so that there are no negative effects on the individual, the regular education teacher, or the classmates?
2. What administrative processes are most successful in negotiating with regular education teachers about the inclusion of students with disabilities in their classrooms?
3. What are the best procedures for shifting a school district to a full inclusion model?
4. What systems are effective in developing team approaches to curricular infusion.
5. How can school systems establish a continuum of services throughout a student's public educations?
6. What systems are effective in evaluating social and instructional integration process variables and outcomes?

Overall, behavior analytic research has provided us with a strong instructional and conceptual framework from which to develop systematic programs for the education of students with disabilities. Educators should continue to create and analyze new methods for promoting behavior change. In addition, however, behavior analysis must be extended to include (a) analyses of broader, contextual variables, and within these analyses more systematic assessment of the social validity of integration efforts; (b) analyses of procedures that can be utilized to more fully include persons with profound disabilities in the mainstream; and (c) analyses and determination of administrative strategies to facilitate supported education.

Conclusion

This chapter has reviewed the behavior analytic research in the areas of social and instructional integration over the past two decades. Research efforts have moved from an emphasis on the teaching of single, isolated skills within a controlled, adult-mediated context to the teaching of a more comprehensive class of responses within natural contexts using peers as trainers, peers as confederates, and peers as support. Interventions are beginning to shift from teacher-determined objectives and criteria to student- and peer-determined variables. In addition, behavior analysts are placing a greater emphasis on measures of social validity within their research. It is critical that the procedures that are the most experimentally sound are also the most socially relevant. As a result of these transitions, experimental research is demonstrating greater generalized and maintained effects, and greater levels of satisfaction from students, peers, and teachers. Continued expansion of the process and outcome variables (e.g., Haring, & Breen, 1989) within behavior analysis is critical as the values and practices within the educational community continue to change. As researchers, we must be committed to developing, validating, and evaluating systems that will inevitably improve the quality of life of individuals.

References

Allen, K.E., Hart, B., Buell, J.S., Harris, F.R., & Wolf, M.M. (1964). Effects of social reinforcement on isolate behavior of a nursery-school child. *Child Development*, *35*, 511–518.

Altman, K. (1971). Effects of cooperative response acquisition on social behavior during free-play. *Journal of Experimental Child Psychology*, *12*, 387–395.

Anderson, J. (1984). San Francisco school district evaluation report: Jose Ortega School study (1982–83). Unpublished manuscript, San Francisco State University, California Research Institute.

Apolloni, T., & Cooke, T.P. (1975). Peer behavior conceptualized as a variable influencing infant and toddler development. *American Journal of Orthopsychiatry*, *45*, 4–17.

Apolloni, T., & Cooke, T.P. (1979). Integrated programming at the infant, toddler, and preschool levels. In M. Guralnick (Ed.), *Early intervention and the integration of handicapped and nonhandicapped children (pp. 147–165)*. Baltimore: University Park Press.

Ayllon, T., & Roberts, M.D. (1974). Eliminating discipline problems by strengthening academic performance. *Journal of Applied Behavior Analysis*, *7*, 71–76.

Bates, P. (1980). The effectiveness of interpersonal skills training on the social skill acquisition of moderately and mildly retarded adults. *Journal of Applied Behavior Analysis*, *13*, 237–248.

Berler, E.S., Gross, A.M., & Drabman, R.S. (1982). Social skills training with children: Proceed with caution. *Journal of Applied Behavior Analysis*, *15*, 41–54.

Berliner, D.C., Fisher, C.W., Filby, N., & Marlieve, R. (1976). Proposal for Phase 3 of beginning teacher evaluation study. San Francisco: Far West Laboratory for Educational Research and Development.

Brady, M.P., Shores, R.E., Gunter, P., McEvoy, M.A., Fox, J.J., & White, C. (1984). Generalization of an adolescent's social interaction behavior via multiple peers in a classroom setting. *Journal of the Association for Persons With Severe Handicaps*, *9*, 278–286.

Breen, C.G., & Haring, T.G. (1991). Effects of contextual competence on social initiations. *Journal of Applied Behavior Analysis*, *24*, 337–347.

Breen, C.G., Lovinger, L., & Haring, T.G. (1989, December). *PAL (Partners at Lunch) Club: Evaluation of a program to support social relationships in a junior high school.* Paper presented at the 16th Annual TASH Conference, San Francisco, CA.

Brown, L., Nisbet, J., Ford, A., Sweet, M., Shirage, B., York, J., & Loomis, R. (1983). The critical need for nonschool instruction in educational programs for severely handicapped students. *Journal of the Association for Persons With Severe Handicaps*, *8*, 71–77.

Bryant, L.E., & Budd, K.S. (1982). Self-instructional training to increase independent work performance in preschoolers. *Journal of Applied Behavior Analysis*, *15*, 259–271.

Delquadri, J., Greenwood, C.R., Whorton, D., Carta, J.J., & Hall, R.V. (1986). Classwide peer tutoring. *Exceptional Children*, *52*, 535–542.

Dineen, J.P., Clark, H.B., & Risley, T.R. (1977). Peer tutoring among elementary students: Educational benefits to the tutor. *Journal of Applied Behavior Analysis*, *10*, 231–238.

Dougherty, B.S., Fowler, S.A., & Paine, S.C. (1985). The use of peer monitors to reduce negative interaction during recess. *Journal of Applied Behavior Analysis*, *18*, 141–153.

Dunlap, L.K., & Dunlap, G. (1989). A self-monitoring package for teaching subtraction with regrouping to students with learning disabilities. *Journal of Applied Behavior Analysis*, *22*, 309–314.

Egel, A., Richman, G., & Koegel, R. (1981). Normal peer models and autistic children's learning. *Journal of Applied Behavior Analysis*, *14*, 3–12.

Ford, D., Evans, J.H., & Dworkin, L.K. (1982). Teaching interaction procedures: Effects upon the learning of social skills by an emotionally disturbed child. *Education and Treatment of Children*, *5*, 1–11.

Gaylord-Ross, R.J., Haring, T.G., Breen, C., & Pitts-Conway, V. (1984). The training and generalization of social interaction skills with autistic youth. *Journal of Applied Behavior Analysis*, *7*, 611–621.

Goldstein, H., & Wickstrom, S. (1986). Peer intervention effects on communicative interaction among handicapped and nonhandicapped preschoolers. *Journal of Applied Behavior Analysis*, *19*, 209–214.

Green, R.B., Harbison, W.L., & Greene, B.F. (1984). Turning the table on advice programs for parents: Using placemats to enhance family interaction at restaurants. *Journal of Applied Behavior Analysis*, *17*, 497–508.

Greenwood, C.R., Dinwiddie, G., Bailey, V., Carta, J.J., Dorsey, D., Kohler, F.W., Nelson, C., Rotholz, D., & Schulte, D. (1987). Field replication of classwide peer tutoring. *Journal of Applied Behavior Analysis*, *20*, 151–160.

Greenwood, C.R., Dinwiddie, G., Terry, B., Wade, L., Stanley, S., Thibadeau, S., & Delquadri, J. (1984). Teacher- versus peer-mediated instruction: An ecobehavioral analysis of achievement outcomes. *Journal of Applied Behavior Analysis*, *17*, 521–538.

Greenwood, C.R., & Hops, H. (1981). Group-oriented contingencies and peer behavior change. In P.S. Strain (Ed.), *The utilization of classroom peers as behavior change agents*. pp. 189–259 New York: Plenum.

Greenwood, C.R., Sloane, H.N., & Baskin, A. (1974). Training elementary aged peer behavior managers to control small group programmed mathematics. *Journal of Applied Behavior Analysis*, *7*, 103–114.

Gresham, F.M. (1983). Misguided mainstreaming: The case for social skills training with handicapped children. *Exceptional Children*, *48*, 321–328.

Guevremont, D.C., Osnes, P.G., & Stokes, T.F. (1988). The functional role of preschoolers' verbalizations in the generalization of self-instructional training. *Journal of Applied Behavior Analysis*, *21*, 45–56.

Hamre-Nietupski, S., & Nietupski, J. (1981). Integral involvement of severely handicapped students within regular public schools. *Journal of the Association for the Severely Handicapped*, *6*, 30–39.

Haring, T.G., & Breen, C.G. (1989). Units of analysis of social interaction outcomes in supported education. *Journal of the Association for Persons With Severe Handicaps*, *14*, 255–262.

Haring, T.G., & Breen, C.G. (1990 May). *A peer-mediated social network intervention to enhance social integration for persons with severe disabilities*. Paper presented at the National Conference for Applied Behavior Analysis, Nashville, TN.

Haring, T.G., Breen, C., Pitts-Conway, V., Lee, M., & Gaylord-Ross, R. (1987). Adolescent peer tutoring and special friend experiences. *Journal of the Association for Persons With Severe Handicaps*, *12*, 280–286.

Haring, T.G., & Kennedy, C.H. (1990). *The training and generalization of social control procedures to students with profound disabilities*. Unpublished manuscript, University of California, Santa Barbara, Social Context Research Project.

Haring, T.G., & Lovinger, L. (1989). Promoting social interaction through teaching generalized play initiation responses to preschool children with autism. *Journal of the Association for Persons With Severe Handicaps*, *14*, 58–67.

Haring, T.G., Roger, B. Lee, M., Breen, C., & Gaylord-Ross, R. (1986). Teaching social language to moderately handicapped students. *Journal of Applied Behavior Analysis*, *19*, 159–171.

Harris, K.R. (1986). Self-monitoring of attentional behavior versus self-monitoring of productivity: Effects on on-task behavior and academic response rate among learning disabled children. *Journal of Applied Behavior Analysis*, *19*, 417–423.

Hiroshige, J.A. (1989). *Effects of direct instruction of social skills and peer facilitation on free play at recess of students with physical disabilities*. Unpublished doctoral dissertation, University of California, Santa Barbara.

Horner, R.D. (1980). The effects of an environment "enrichment" program on the behavior of institutionalized profoundly retarded children. *Journal of Applied Behavior Analysis*, *13*, 159–171.

Hunt, P., Alwell, M., & Goetz, L. (1988). Acquisition of conversation skills and the reduction of inappropriate social interaction behaviors. *Journal of the Association for Persons With Severe Handicaps*, *13*, 20–27.

Jenkins, J.R., & Jenkins, L. (1985). Peer tutoring in elementary and secondary programs. *Focus on Exceptional Children*, *17*, 1–12.

Jenkins, J.R., Mayhall, W.F., Peschka, C.M., & Jenkins, L.M. (1974). Comparing small-group and traditional instructon in resource rooms. *Exceptional Children*, *40*, 245–251.

Johnson, D.W., & Johnson, R. (1984). The effects of intergroup cooperation and intergroup competition on ingroup and out-group cross-handicap relationships. *Journal of Social Psychology*, *124*, 85–94.

Johnson, D.W., Johnson, R., & Maruyama, G. (1983). Interdependence and interpersonal attraction among heterogeneous and homogeneous individuals: A theoretical formulation and meta-analysis of the research. *Review of Educational Research*, *53*, 5–54.

Johnson, D.W., Maruyama, G., Johnson, R., Nelson, D., & Skon, L. (1981). The effects of cooperative, competitive, and individualistic goal structures on achievement: A meta-analysis. *Psychological Bulletin*, *89*, 47–62.

Johnson, M.W. (1935). The effect on behavior of variation in amount of play equipment. *Child Development*, *6*, 56–68.

Kirby, F.D., & Toler, H.C. (1970). Modification of preschool isolate behavior: A case study. *Journal of Applied Behavior Analysis*, *3*, 309–314.

Knapczyk, D.R. (1989). Generalization of student question asking from special class to regular class settings. *Journal of Applied Behavior Analysis*, *22*, 77–83.

Koegel, R.L., Dyer, K., & Bell, L.K. (1987). The influence of child-preferred activities on autistic childrens social behavior. *Journal of Applied Behavior Analysis*, *20*, 243–252.

Kohl, F.L., Moses, L.G., & Stettner-Eaton, B.A. (1983). The results of teaching fifth and sixth graders to be instructional trainers with students who are severely handicapped. *Journal of the Association for Persons With Severe Handicaps*, *8*, 32–40.

Kohler, F.W., & Fowler, S.A. (1985). Training prosocial behaviors to young children: An analysis of reciprocity with untrained peers. *Journal of Applied Behavior Analysis*, *18*, 187–200.

Lancioni, G.E. (1982). Normal children as tutors to teach social responses to withdrawn mentally retarded schoolmates: Training, maintenance, and generalization. *Journal of Applied Behavior Analysis*, *15*, 17–40.

Lloyd, J.W., Bateman, D.F., Landrum, T.J., & Hallahan, D.P. (1989). Self-recording of attention versus productivity. *Journal of Applied Behavior Analysis*, *22*, 315–324.

Lovitt, T.C., & Curtiss, K.A. (1969). Academic response rate as a function of teacher- and self-imposed contingencies. *Journal of Applied Behavior Analysis*, *2*, 49–53.

Madden, N.A., & Slavin, R.E. (1983). Effects of cooperative learning on the social acceptance of mainstreamed academically handicapped students. *Journal of Special Education*, *17*, 171–182.

Maheady, L., Sacca, M.K., & Harper, G.F. (1988). Classwide peer tutoring with mildly handicapped high school students. *Exceptional Children*, *55*, 52–59.

McCarty, T., Griffin, S., Apolloni, T., & Shores, R.E. (1977). Increased peer-teaching with group-oriented contingencies for arithmetic performance in behavior-disordered adolescents. *Journal of Applied Behavior Analysis*, *10*, 313–320.

McEvoy, M.A., Nordquist, V.M., Twardosz, S., Heckman, K.A., Wehby, J.H., & Denny, R.K. (1988). Promoting autistic children's peer interaction in an integrated early childhood setting using affection activities. *Journal of Applied Behavior Analysis*, *21*, 193–200.

McKenzie, M.L., & Budd, K.S. (1981). A peer tutoring package to increase mathematics performance: Examination of generalized changes in classroom behavior. *Education and Treatment of Children*, *4*, 1–15.

Meichenbaum, D.J., & Goodman, J. (1971). Training impulsive children to talk to themselves: A means of developing self-control. *Journal of Abnormal Psychology*, *77*, 115–126.

Odom, S.L., Hoyson, M., Jamieson, B., & Strain, P.S. (1985). Increasing handicapped preschoolers' peer social interactions: Cross-setting and component analysis. *Journal of Applied Behavior Analysis*, *18*, 3–16.

Odom, S.L., & Strain, P.S. (1986). A comparison of peer-initiation and teacher-antecedent interventions for promoting reciprocal social interaction of autistic preschoolers. *Journal of Applied Behavior Analysis*, *19*, 59–71.

Peck, C.A., Killen, C.C., & Baumgart, D. (1989). Increasing implementation of special education instruction in mainstream preschools: Direct and generalized effects of nondirective consultation. *Journal of Applied Behavior Analysis*, *22*, 197–210.

Pigott, H.E., Fantuzzo, J.W., & Clement, P.W. (1986). The effects of reciprocal peer tutoring and group contingencies on the academic performance of elementary school children. *Journal of Applied Behavior Analysis*, *19*, 93–98.

Pigott, H.E., Fantuzzo, J.W., Heggie, D.L., & Clement, P.W. (1984). A student-administered group-oriented contingency intervention: Its efficacy in a regular classroom. *Child and Family Behavior Therapy*, *6*, 41–55.

Quilitch, H.R., & Risley, T.R. (1973). The effects of play materials on social play. *Journal of Applied Behavior Analysis*, *6*, 573–578.

Ragland, E.U., Kerr, M.M., & Strain, P.S. (1978). Effects of peer social initiation on the behavior of withdrawn autistic children. *Behavior Modification*, *2*, 565–578.

Rhode, G., Morgan, D.P., & Young, K.R. (1983). Generalization and maintenance of treatment gains of behaviorally handicapped students from resource rooms to regular classrooms using self-evaluation procedures. *Journal of Applied Behavior Analysis*, *16*, 171–188.

Russo, S., & Koegel, R. (1977). A method for integrating the autistic child into a normal public school classroom. *Journal of Applied Behavior Analysis*, *10*, 579–590.

Rynders, J., Johnson, R., Johnson, D., & Schmidt, B. (1980). Producing positive interaction among Down's syndrome and nonhandicapped teenagers through cooperative goal structuring. *American Journal of Mental Deficiency*, *85*, 268–273.

Sailor, W., Anderson, J.L., Halvorsen, A.T., Doering, K., Filler, J., & Goetz, L. (1989). *The comprehensive local school*. Baltimore: Paul H. Brookes.

Sainato, D.M., Maheady, L., & Shook, G.L. (1986). The effects of a classroom manager role on the social interaction patterns and social status of withdrawn kindergarten students. *Journal of Applied Behavior Analysis*, *19*, 187–196.

Sasso, G.M., & Rude, H.A. (1987). Unprogrammed effects of training high-status peers to interact with severely handicapped children. *Journal of Applied Behavior Analysis*, *20*, 35–44.

Shafer, M.S., Egel, A.L., & Neef, N.A. (1984). Training mildly handicapped peers to facilitate changes in the social interaction skills of autistic children. *Journal of Applied Behavior Analysis*, *17*, 461–476.

Singh, N.N., & Singh, J. (1984). Antecedent control of oral reading errors and self-corrections by mentally retarded children. *Journal of Applied Behavior Analysis*, *17*, 111–119.

Slavin, R.E. (1990). *Cooperative learning: Theory, research, and practice*. Englewood Cliffs, NJ: Prentica-Hall.

Spangler, P.F., & Marshall, A.M. (1983). The unit play manager as facilitator of purposeful activities among institutionalized profoundly and severely retarded boys. *Journal of Applied Behavior Analysis*, *16*, 345–349.

Speltz, M.L., Shimamura, J.W., & McReynolds, W.T. (1982). Procedural variations in group contingencies: Effects on children's academic and social behaviors. *Journal of Applied Behavior Analysis*, *15*, 533–544.

Stainback, W., & Stainback, S. (1987). Facilitating friendships. *Education and Training in Mental Retardation*, *51*, 18–25.

Stern, G.W., Fowler, S.A., & Kohler, F.W. (1988). A comparison of two intervention roles: Peer monitor and point earner. *Journal of Applied Behavior Analysis*, *21*, 103–109.

Stevenson, H.C., & Fantuzzo, J.W. (1986). The generality and social validity of a competency-based self-control training intervention for underachieving students. *Journal of Applied Behavior Analysis*, *19*, 269–276.

Strain, P.S. (1983). Identification of peer social skills for preschool mentally retarded children in mainstreamed classes. *Applied Research in Mental Retardation*, *4*, 369–382.

Strain, P.S., Cooke, T.P., & Apolloni, T. (1976). *Teaching exceptional children: Assessing and modifying social behavior*. New York: Academic.

Strain, P.S., Kerr, M.M., & Ragland, E.U. (1979). Effects of peer-mediated social initiations and prompting/reinforcement procedures on social behavior of autistic children. *Journal of Autism and Developmental Disorders*, *9*, 41–54.

Strain, P.S., & Odom, S.L. (1986). Peer social initiations: Effective intervention for social skills development of exceptional children. *Exceptional Children*, *52*, 543–551.

Strain, P.S., Odom, S.L., & McConnell, S. (1984). Promoting social reciprocity of exceptional children: Identification, target behavior selection, and intervention. *Remedial and Special Education*, *5*, 21–28.

Strain, P.S., Shores, R.E., & Timm, M.A. (1977). Effects of peer social initiations on the behavior of withdrawn preschool children. *Journal of Applied Behavior Analysis*, *10*, 289–298.

Strain, P.S., & Timm, M.A. (1974). An experimental analysis of social interactions between a behaviorally disordered preschool child and her classroom peers. *Journal of Applied Behavior Analysis*, *7*, 583–590.

Taylor, S.J. (1988). Caught in the continuum: A critical analysis of the principle of the least restrictive environment. *Journal of the Association for Persons With Severe Handicaps*, *13*, 41–53.

Voeltz, L.M. (1980). Children's attitudes toward handicapped peers. *American Journal of Mental Deficiency*, *84*, 455–464.

Voeltz, L.M. (1982). Effects of structured interactions with severely handicapped peers on children's attitudes. *American Journal of Mental Deficiency*, *86*, 380–390.

Walker, H.M., Greenwood, C., Hops, H., & Todd, N. (1979). Differential effects of reinforcing topographic components of social interaction. *Behavior Modification*, *3*, 291–321.

Wolfensberger, W. (1972). *Normalization*. Toronto: National Institute on Mental Retardation.
Wolfensberger, W. (1983). Social role valorization: A proposed new term for the principle of normalization. *Mental Retardation*, *21*, 254–259.
Wong, S.E., Terranova, M.D. Bowen, L., Zarate, R., Massel, H.K., & Liberman, R.P. (1987). Providing independent recreational activities to reduce stereotypic vocalizations in chronic schizophrenics. *Journal of Applied Behavior Analysis*, *20*, 77–81.
Zettel, J.J., & Ballard, J. (1982). The Education for All Handicapped Children Act of 1985 (P.L. 94–142): Its history, origins, and concepts. In J. Ballard, B.A. Ramirez, & F.J. Weintraub (Eds.), *Special education in America: Its Legal and governmental foundations (pp. 11–22)*. Reston, VA: Council for Exceptional Children.

5
Achieving Schooling Success for All Students

Margaret C. Wang

Building an educated citizenry has been a persistent goal of educational reform efforts in this country. Indeed, by stressing the value of education and seeing it as a way of achieving social and economic equity, we have made great progress in ensuring equal opportunity to a free public education for all children in this country. We have increased the percentage of the population in school; the diversity in student characteristics (with respect to the learning needs of the students, as well as the ethnic, cultural, and socioeconomic backgrounds of their families); and the kinds of educational programs we offer.

However, these accomplishments fall far short of our vision of schooling success for every child. The statistics clearly point to a trend of increasing numbers of students who drop out of school or graduate without attaining the basic literacy skills necessary to function effectively in an increasingly technological world. Based on the projected demographic changes in student populations (cf. Hodges et al., 1980), the failure to provide for the schooling success of all students in our educational system will become even more alarming in the coming decade. A major school improvement goal of the 1990s is for the schools to achieve schooling success of all students with diverse learning characteristics and educational and related service support needs. Educational equity in this context is defined in terms of learning outcomes for every student—a conception of educational equity that goes beyond the current practice of only providing access to educational opportunities.

Achieving the goal of educational equity in the context of outcomes will require a major conceptual shift in the way we think about differences among students, how we view the purpose of elementary and secondary education, and the way we choose to organize schools. If schooling success is recognized as possible for everyone through effective intervention and related service support, then a major task of the schools is clearly the creation of learning environments that uphold a standard of educational equity in terms of schooling outcomes for all students. The central focus in efforts to improve educational equity, therefore, is the identification of practices that deny equal access to schooling success, as well as practices that promote it.

The overall purpose of this chapter is to discuss the prospect of utilizing well-confirmed knowledge to enhance the chances for the schooling success of every student in today's schools. The chapter begins with a brief discussion of the state of practice. It is followed by an illustration of how to apply research and practical wisdom toward the design and implementation of innovative practices aiming to improve the schools' capabilities to achieve equity in schooling outcomes for all students, including and especially those requiring greater-than-usual educational support—students whose learning success depends on educational interventions that are of high quality and effectiveness.

The State of the Practice

Advances in theory and research during the past two decades have provided substantial conceptual changes in the type of information available on individual students and their learning. Among the significant developments is an increased recognition that certain personal and learning characteristics are alterable (Bloom, 1976). Some prime examples of variables that are no longer considered to be static are family characteristics, such as parental expectations and family involvement (Walberg, 1984); cognition and processes of learning (Chipman, Segal, & Glaser, 1985; Segal, Chipman, & Glaser, 1985); and student motivation and the roles students play in their own learning (Wang & Palincsar, 1989; Zimmerman, 1986).

The recognition of the alterability of these learner characteristics leads researchers to study ways to modify the psychological processes and cognitive operations used by individual students, as well as to modify learning environments and instructional strategies to accommodate learner differences (Wang & Walberg, 1985). It is the responsibility of the schools to structure educational programs to account for these alterable differences and ensure educational outcomes for every student while still maintaining the standard of mastering a common curriculum of elementary and secondary education in this country (Fenstermacher & Goodlad, 1983).

Schools' Response to Student Diversity

Despite the advances in theory and research on individual differences in learning and effective teaching, the knowledge base has had very little impact on how schools respond to these issues in practice. For example, although we provide opportunities for students requiring greater-than-usual educational support through well-intentioned "special" programs (e.g., special education, Chapter 1, and other compensatory and remedial programs), implementation of these programs for the most part has not measured up to the outcome standards that are considered to be critical indicators of educational equity (cf. Brandt, 1989). Many students have difficulty in achieving learning success, and they need better help than they are now receiving.

There are serious problems in how individual differences are characterized and in the way information is generated and used for instructional decision making. In current practice, diversity in processes of learning and instructional support needs among students is typically handled by classifying or labeling the perceived differences in terms of macro-level characteristics (i.e., children at risk, low-achieving children from poor families, children with learning disabilities, or socially/emotionally disturbed children). Then, the "identified" or "certified" students with these spuriously defined labels are placed homogeneously in narrowly framed categorical or special education programs.

Although well intentioned, implementation of these programs has become a major problem source in schools. In too many cases, this practice of classifying students for instruction based on certain perceived differences involves the delivery of radically altered and not always appropriate curriculum to selected students. There is a tendency to seriously neglect fundamental content (Oakes, 1985), and there is substantial evidence to suggest that students may actually receive *less* instruction when schools provide them with specially designed programs to meet their particular learning needs (Allington & Johnston, 1986; Haynes & Jenkins, 1986).

Current approaches to provide for student diversity often contribute to children's learning problems. One such problem is characterized by the "Matthew Effect" (Stanovich, 1984). Students who show limited progress in early phases of instruction in basic subjects, such as reading, tend to show progressive retardation over succeeding years. It has been estimated, for example, that the lowest achieving students in the middle elementary grades may be reading only one tenth as many words per day in school as students in a highly skilled reading group (Reynolds, 1989). The Matthew Effect is also reflected in teacher expectancy research. For example, teachers tend to give less feedback to students with special learning needs, calling on them less often or waiting less time for them to answer (Cooper, 1983). Such differences in educational practices that work to the disadvantage of selected groups of students have contributed to, rather than ameliorated, the problem of school failure among an alarming number of students.

Providing educational opportunities without ensuring educational outcomes only perpetuates inequity in a more subtle form. Schools cannot address the equity issue to simply provide educational opportunities for students through establishing special programs. Educational outcomes must apply for every student. The practice of compensating for learner differences by making school success easier for selected students through differential standards cannot be accepted as an indicator of educational equity.

Prospects for Improvement

If all students are to successfully complete a "basic" education or common curriculum, today's schools must undergo major conceptual and restructural changes. Some students require more time and extraordinary instructional support to achieve mastery of the common curriculum, and others require less time and little direct instruction. Thus, achieving equity in educational outcomes requires a shift from a fixed to a flexible system for effective implementation of the common curriculum.

Findings from recent research, along with the practical wisdom culled from implementing innovative programs in schools, significantly contribute to our current understanding of what constitutes effective teaching and how student learning can be enhanced. These findings suggest alternate approaches to delivering instruction and related service supports that are substantially superior to widespread traditional practices (cf. U.S. Department of Education, 1986, 1987; Wang, Reynolds, & Walberg, 1987, 1988; Wittrock, 1986). Based on the wealth of findings from the past two decades of "effectiveness" research, many varieties of experimental programs can be envisioned to enhance the capabilities of schools to more effectively address student diversity and equity in student learning outcomes.

However, although a number of innovative programs are in operation and can be replicated or extended, there is very little evidence of systematic application of advances from the past two decades of research on effective teaching and school effectiveness. If widespread systematic implementation of knowledge from the past decade of research and innovative program development efforts is to occur in schools with a high level of precision and credibility, significant efforts need to be made in building a knowledge base on the "how to" aspects of program implementation in school settings.

We need to build a data base on implementation requirements of a variety of demonstrably effective alternative programs/practices, as well as information delivery systems in forms that are usable by school personnel. Local schools and related social service agencies are presently faced with two demanding tasks: first, surmounting the difficulty of obtaining information on the design, implementation requirements, and efficacy of innovative programs/practices; and second, specifying criteria for making informed decisions on the feasibility and the site-specific compatibility of program(s)/practices that will best serve the program development and implementation objectives of a particular school district/school.

The need for systematic information that addresses program design and implementation-related concerns has been widely expressed by school personnel and policymakers. Presently, there is little available information (in forms that are usable) to assist local schools/school districts in selecting programs/practices for meeting their specific program improvement and implementation needs. Systematically organized information is needed on what constitutes school effectiveness and the conditions that influence effective implementation. Information is also needed on critical program features, implementation and training requirements, program cost, program delivery systems, program impacts, and a host of other relevant factors critical to enable schools to make informed choices—to identify demonstrably effective programs/practices for adoption or adaptation that are aligned with their respective program improvement goals, resources, and needs.

A Framework for Building an Information Base for Making Programming Decisions

Research on effective teaching and implementation of innovative school improvement programs has identified a large number of variables that are important to learning (cf. Wittrock, 1986; Wang, Reynolds, & Walberg, 1987–1989; Williams, Richmond, & Mason, 1986). However, researchers, policymakers, and practitioners find the research base on the multiplicity of learning influences perplexing and are in need of clearer guidance concerning the relative importance of the particular variables most likely to maximize school learning. To address this need, the following section provides an illustration of how to draw upon well-confirmed knowledge on effective practices to make informed decisions on educational programming.

Based on findings from a recently completed synthesis of the research base and an analysis of the consensus from the field on variables that are important to learning (Temple University Center for Research in Human Development and Education, 1989), a framework was developed for systematic description of program features and assessment of implementation requirements and outcomes of approaches and practices. This framework, the Consensus Marker-Outcome Variable System (CMOVS), incorporates variables that are considered by professionals to be "important" and "alterable" so as to improve chances for students' learning success. A major design goal of the CMOVS is the development of a common language that can be used to improve communication about program features and implementation requirements among educational professionals (i.e., principals, regular education teachers, special education teachers, school psychologists, counselors, subject matter specialists, etc.).

The Development of the CMOVS

There have been several notable theoretical developments attempting to synthesize and explicate the interactive effects of the many variables identified by research as related to school learning. The 1960s and 1970s were marked by the introduction of several important models of learning, including those of Carroll (1963), Bruner (1966), Bloom (1976), Harnischfeger and Wiley (1976), Glaser (1975), and Bennett (1978). All of these models recognize the primary importance of student ability and include constructs such as aptitude, prior knowledge, and other learning and personal characteristics of the individual students. Most of them also address the importance of motivation by employing such constructs as perseverance, self-concept of the learner, and attitude toward school subject matter. This acknowledgement of individual difference variables among learners stood in contrast to more narrow psychological studies of influences on learning, which generally treated individual differences as a source of error and focused on instructional-treatment variables (Hilgard, 1964).

Although these models brought some refinement in the ways in which individual difference variables and instructional variables were defined and the ways in which they were related to one another, the primary contributions of more recent models have been in extending the range of variables considered. Findings from a study by Haertel, Walberg, and Weinstein (1983), for example, showed that previous models of school learning neglect extramural and social-psychological influences. The evolution of models of school learning was further advanced with the introduction of models of adaptive instruction (Glaser, 1975; Wang & Walberg, 1985). School-based implementation of models of adaptive instruction are designed to help schools create learning environments that maximize each student's opportunities for success in school. These models pay particular attention to new variables associated with instructional delivery systems, program design, and implementation.

Another contribution to contemporary models of school learning came from sociologists concerned with the identification of effective schools. Ronald Edmonds (1979a, 1979b, 1979c) is most strongly associated with this identification of variables associated with exceptionally effective schools, especially for the urban poor. Significant contributions to effective school models were also made by Brookover (1979); Brookover and Lezotte (1977); and Rutter, Maughan, Mortimore, and Ouston (1979). Illustrations of the types of variables characterizing effective schools include degree of curriculum articulation and organization, schoolwide staff development, parental involvement and support, schoolwide recognition of academic success, maximized learning time, district support, clear goals and high expectations, orderly and disciplined school environment, and leadership of the principal characterized by attention to quality of instruction (Purkey & Smith, 1983).

There is a substantial research base on what makes learning more productive. Indeed, a pressing task for policymakers and practitioners interested in improving teaching and learning in school is delineation of variables most likely to maximize school learning. The CMOVS which will be discussed in this section, aims to provide a systematic framework for addressing the variables that are important to consider in designing educational programs for achieving educational equity in student outcomes.

The CMOVS was developed based on a synthesis of professional literature and expert opinions to answer the following questions: What aspects of school and instruction enhance student learning? What kinds of social relationships are important to enhance student learning in regular classroom settings? What learner characteristics are important and alterable in improving the learning of students with special needs? Answers to these questions were then analyzed and summarized as the basis for the development of the CMOVS. (For a detailed discussion of the development and the research base of the CMOVS, see Wang, Haertel, & Walberg, 1990).

Briefly, the development of the CMOVS involved a detailed reading of the literature to make a "first approximation" list of variables important to learning using a conceptual model of influential variables (Wang, 1986) shown in Figure 5.1. The model is a schematic representation of the multidimensional variables and hypothesized interactive effects on classroom learning (Wang, 1986). This interactive view of school learning is supported by findings in the contemporary literature on cognitive-social-psychological research on learning, research on effective teaching and school effectiveness, and studies of school change from a sociological perspective.

For example, distinct patterns of interaction among program features, student and teacher behaviors, and student outcomes have been noted in studies of the differential effects among instructional approaches (e.g., Berliner, 1983; Hedges, Giaconia, & Gage, 1981; Walberg, 1984; Wang & Walberg, 1986; Webb, 1982a; Webb, 1982b; Webb, 1983c). Findings from a study of program implementation and effects recently completed by Wang and Walberg (1986) suggest that programs that feature student choice, task flexibility, teacher monitoring, peer tutoring, student-initiated requests for teacher help, a variety of curriculum materials, and task-specific instructions are associated with student self-management, personal interactions between students and teachers, student work in small groups, and substantive interactions between teachers and students.

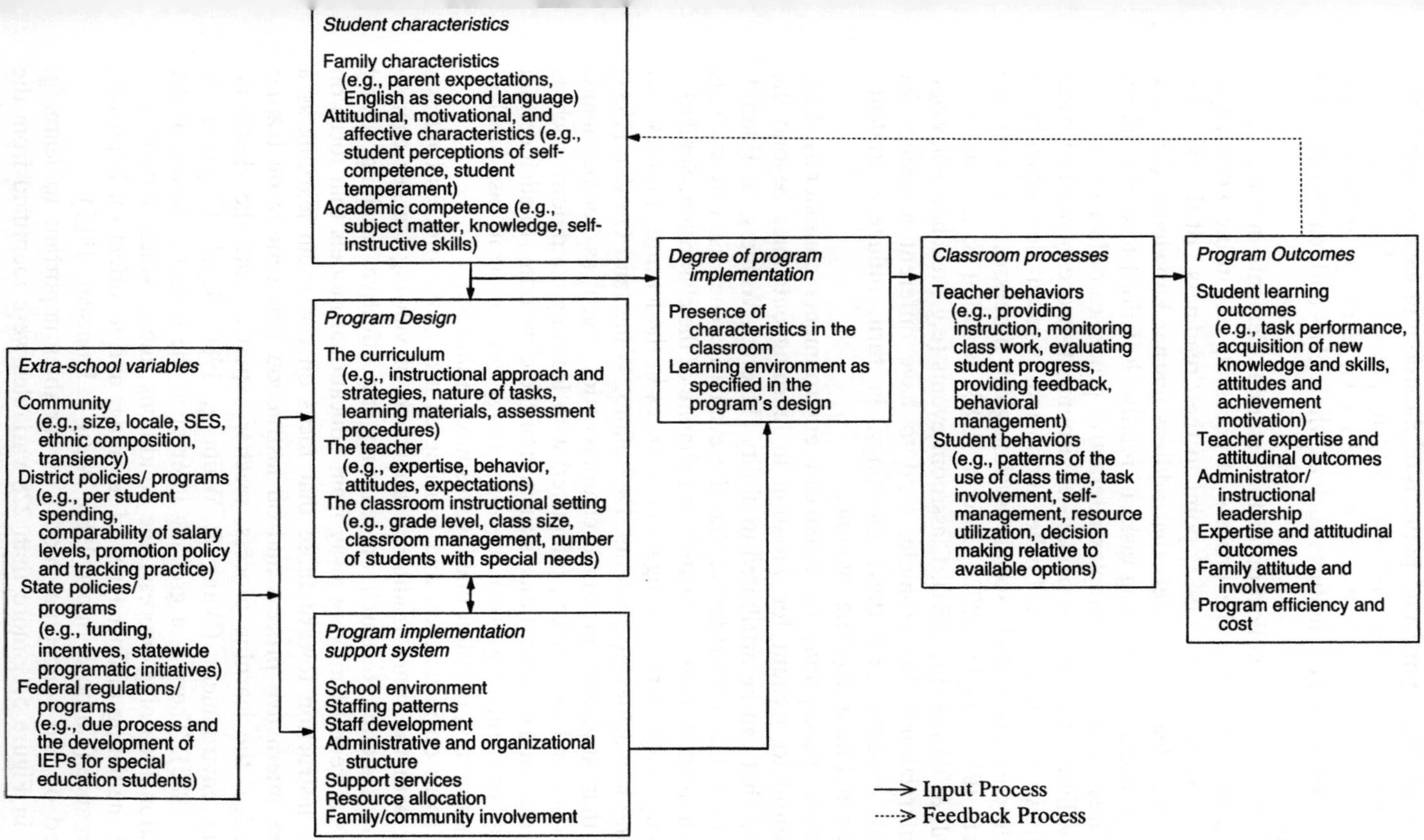

FIGURE 5.1. Conceptual model of variables that are important to learning.

Note: Variables listed are intended to be illustrative only. They are not intended to reflect a comprehensive analysis

From Wang et al. (1990). Reprinted with permission of the Helen Dwight Reid Educational Foundation. Published by Heldref Publications, 4000 Albemarle St., N.W., Washington, D.C. 20016. Copyright© 1990.

Furthermore, these particular patterns of classroom processes were found to be positively associated with instructional approaches that recognize an active role for students in mediating their own learning, and negatively associated with program features such as whole-class and teacher-directed instruction.

Similarly, in their explication of the essential elements in the acquisition of information and the process of accessing and using knowledge, Brown, Day, and Jones (1983) point to the "readiness" of the field for moving from learning models that address learner knowledge (i.e., the learning process and learning tasks in relative isolation) toward a model that addresses the more complex interactive processes of learning.

The validity of using the person–environment–process–product paradigm shown in Figure 5.1 is further supported by recent developments in research concerned with social psychological processes and attitudes (Bossert, 1979; Doyle, 1977; Gordon, 1983; Madden & Slavin, 1982; Marshall & Weinstein, 1984). Classroom events (e.g., teacher behaviors, peer interactions), for example, tend to have different meanings for different students, and these meanings, in turn, influence students' behavior and their learning outcomes.

Students' perceptions of classroom environments consistently have been found to account for variation in learning outcomes beyond the variation that can be attributed to ability (Haertel, Walberg, & Haertel, 1981). Weinstein (1984) found that the evaluative cues used by students vary as a function of the structure and climate of the classroom. Similarly, in a study designed to investigate differences in the learning processes of high- and low-achieving students, DeStefano, Wang, and Gordon (1984) found that students' personal characteristics, such as temperament, knowledge, and motivation, interacted with learning conditions, such as the physical and organizational structure of the classroom, to elicit certain learning behaviors (e.g., time on-task, energy development, task involvement, autonomy, decision making, resource utilization).

This focus on instruction and learning as a dynamic process contrasts sharply with the more traditional approach of viewing learner characteristics as static. Research on learning and effective teaching clearly suggests a trend of moving away from educational models that focus on teacher instruction toward those that focus on classroom learning as a complex interactive process and on instruction that centers on learner knowledge, the learning process, teacher expertise, and the classroom learning environment (Wang & Walberg, 1986; Segal, Chipman, & Glaser, 1985). There is a growing interest in the dynamic nature of the instructional-learning process, the conditions under which it occurs, its role in mediating distinct types of learning, and its effect on improving performance (Corno & Snow, 1986; Wang & Palinscar, 1989).

Based on the conceptual model of variables important to learning, shown in Figure 5.1, more than 228 variables were identified from the literature as important to school learning. A list of these variables is presented in the appendix to this chapter (Wang, Haertel, & Walberg, 1990). The literature review focused on a synthesis of authoritative reviews and handbook chapters, especially those sponsored by the American Educational Research Association and other organizations, and selected additional syntheses in government documents and other sources. A preliminary list of sources was reviewed by the Scientific Advisory Panel and revised following the panel's recommendations. Following this review, specific sources were chosen. They included 86 chapters from special reviews such as the American Educational Research Association's *Handbook of Research on Teaching* (Wittrock, 1986); 45 handbook chapters from the *Handbook of Special Education: Research and Practice* (Wang, Reynolds, & Walberg, 1987–1989); 11 major review articles from the past decade or more of the *Review of Research in Education*, the *Annual Review of Psychology*, and the *Annual Review of Sociology*; 18 book chapters, such as Brophy's chapter in *Designs for Compensatory Education* (Williams, Richmond, & Mason, 1986); and a number of journal articles chosen to assure coverage of all of the areas addressed in the conceptual model (Figure 5.1). (For a complete bibliography of the literature included in the review, see Wang, Haertel, & Walberg, 1990.)

Using the CMOVS for Making Programming Decisions

In this section an illustration is provided of the use of the CMOVS as a guiding framework for analyzing and describing program features and, perhaps more important, for making systematic programming decisions that facilitate and improve articulation and coordinate innovative efforts by special and regular education professionals to improve instructional effectiveness in student learning. The CMOVS can be used as a systematic guideline for making informed decisions on design, identification, and selection of innovative practices for adoption and adaptation, and for describing and documenting program implementation and outcomes.

Table 5.1 provides an illustration of how the CMOVS can be used to analyze the critical design features and outcomes of extant programs or discuss features of an innovative program being implemented or considered for implementation by a group of teachers, a school, or school district. Column 1 of Table 5.1 shows a list of 30 categories of variables included in the CMOVS that are considered important to learning, as well as the anticipated program outcomes. The second column shows the average weightings of each variable category based on the consensus from the field (Temple University Center for Research in Human Development and Education, 1989). A rating of 3 for a given variable category (as listed in column 2 of Table 5.1) means that, based on the consensus from the field, that particular variable category received a mean rating of 3,

TABLE 5.1 Decision-making framework: A preliminary analysis of the programmatic emphases of selected programs.

Variable categories	Variable weighting (based on consensus from the field)*	Program A: A peer collaboration approach	Program B: A teacher collaboration approach	Program C: A classroom approach	Program D: A curriculum modification approach	Program E: A comprehensive, integrated, education and related service delivery approach
I. Variables considered important to learning						
A. State and district variables						
1. District level demographics and marker variables	(2)		x	x		x
2. State level policy variables	(2)		x			x
B. Out of school contextual variables						
1. Community variables	(2)					x
2. Peer Group variables	(2)	x				x
3. Home environment and parental support variables	(3)				x	x
4. Student use of out of school time variables	(2)	x		x		x
C. School level variables						
1. Demographic and marker variables	(1)					x
2. Teacher/administrator decision making variables	(3)		x	x		x
3. School culture variables (ethos conducive to teaching and learning)	(3)	x	x	x		x
4. Schoolwide policy and organizational variables	(2)		x	x		x
5. Accessibility variables	(2)			x		x
6. Parental involvement policy variables	(2)					x

D. Student variables						
1. Demographic and marker variables	(1)			x		x
2. History of educational placements	(2)			x	x	x
3. Social and behavioral variables	(3)	x		x	x	x
4. Motivational and affective variables	(3)	x	x	x	x	x
5. Cognitive variables	(2)	x	x	x	x	x
6. Metacognitive variables	(3)	x	x	x	x	x
7. Psychomotor variables	(2)	x	x	x	x	x
E. Program design variables						
1. Demographic and marker variables	(2)			x		x
2. Curriculum and instructional variables	(2)	x	x	x		x
3. Curriculum design variables	(2)	x		x		x
F. Implementation, classroom instruction, and climate variables						
1. Classroom implementation support variables	(2)			x		x
2. Classroom instructional variables	(3)	x	x	x	x	x
3. Quantity of instruction variables	(2)			x	x	x
4. Classroom assessment variables	(2)			x	x	x
5. Classroom management variables	(3)	x		x		x
6. Student and teacher interactions: social variables	(3)	x		x		x
7. Student and teacher interactions: academic variables	(2)	x		x		x
8. Classroom climate variables	(3)	x		x		x
II. Expected program outcomes						
A. Student learning outcomes		x	x	x	x	x
B. Teacher expertise and attitudes		x	x	x	x	x
C. Administrator/instructional leader expertise and attitudes			x	x		x
D. Family expectation-attitudes						x
E. Program cost effectiveness		x	x	x	x	x

* Abstracted from Temple University Center for Research in Human Development and Education (1989). "Effective Educational Practices: A Consensus on Learning."

indicating high importance (on a 3-point scale) in arranging learning environments. A rating of 1 for a given variable category, on the other hand, indicates that the particular variable category was of low importance based on the consensus from the field.

The Xs listed under each program column indicate that the particular variables were explicitly considered in the design of a specific program. For example, for Program B, a hypothetical program based on a teacher collaboration approach, variable categories that were explicitly considered under the heading of State and District Variables include district level demographics and marker variables and state level policy variables; while variable categories under the heading of School Level Variables include teacher/administrator decision making variables, school culture variables, and schoolwide policy and organizational variables. It is important to note, the listing of program approaches and the specific programs under each approach are hypothetical, and they are included here for illustrative purposes.

Regular and special educators, for example, can work together using the CMOVS to identify, describe, and evaluate the program features that best meet their implementation needs and the needs of their students. The CMOVS, in this context, serves as a systematic mechanism that enhances communication and implementation of demonstrably effective research-based practices. One major expected outcome of utilizing the CMOVS is improved communication and coordination of work among regular educators and specialists through a common knowledge base on effective practices.

Calculating Indices Based on the CMOVS

Several simple indices can be generated to provide a data base for identifying program development needs and/or selecting a particular approach or practice for adoption or adaptation in order to meet the improvement needs of a particular school.

One such index is the Program Effectiveness Index. Using the variable weightings based on findings from the consensus from the field (Temple University Center for Research in Human Development and Education, 1989), as well as information on features explicitly considered in the design of the various programs as shown in Table 5.1, potential adopters of specific programs or practices can develop an effectiveness index that serves as an indication of site-specific needs.

The first step in developing a Program Effectiveness Index is to calculate the "importance rating" by the user (e.g., potential adopter of the program/approach). This is done by asking the users to rate the importance of the CMOVS variable categories according to their own judgments about the program improvement needs of their respective situations, using a 3-point scale. A rating of 3 indicates that a particular variable category is considered of high importance in terms of the user's site-specific needs; a rating of 2 indicates that a particular variable category is of moderate importance; and a rating of 1 indicates that a particular variable category is of low importance. The ratings may be based on a variety of user-specific information (e.g., their own experiences, current programs implemented in their respective schools, knowledge on a particular set of research findings, philosophical alliances or differences on a specific instructional approach, the importance of the variables from their own perspective or those of particular stakeholder groups).

In essence, the importance ratings represent the users' ratings of each variable category included in the CMOVS based on multiple information sources that suggest the relative importance of selected variable categories according to their site-specific perspectives. The quantitative index derived from the potential users' importance ratings will enable them to make decisions on the extent to which the various educational approaches and program specific practices of the various extant programs being considered meet the program improvement and implementation support needs of their respective schools/school districts.

For example, if a particular hypothetical user were interested in adopting either Program A, which uses the peer collaboration approach, or Program B, which uses a teacher collaboration approach, he or she can use the Program Effectiveness Index for each of the programs being considered as one of the criteria for making selection decisions.

Table 5.2 is an example of how a hypothetical user calculates a Program Effectiveness Index based on the CMOVS. The second column of Table 5.2 shows the variable weighting scores (based on findings from the Temple University Center for Research in Human Development and Education, 1989 study on the consensus from the field for variables considered important to learning) of each of the variable categories included in the CMOVS. The hypothetical user's importance ratings of each of the variables included in the CMOVS are listed in Column 3 of Table 5.2. The number listed in the last row of column 3 is 79, which represents the total possible importance rating. The Program Effectiveness Index is calculated based on the user's own assessment of the relative importance of the variables included in the CMOVS (column 3), the variable weighting of the variables based on the consensus from the field (column 2), and whether a given variable in the CMOVS is emphasized in the design of a given program (columns 4 and 6 for Programs A and B, respectively).

Thus, the Program Effectiveness Index is the sum of the Effectiveness Ratings (calculated by using the importance rating multiplied by the variable weighting score for each of the variables considered in a given program design). For example, the effectiveness rating for variable category B.2 (peer group variables) for Program A is 4. The Program Effectiveness Index for variable category B.2 is derived by multiplying a

TABLE 5.2 An illustration of using the decision-making framework to calculate effectiveness index.

Variable categories	Variable weighting (based on consensus from the field)*	Importance rating by the potential user	Program A: A peer collaboration approach — Variables emphasized in program design	Program A: A peer collaboration approach — Effectiveness rating**	Program B: A teacher collaboration approach — Variables emphasized in program design	Program B: A teacher collaboration approach — Effectiveness rating**
I. Variables considered important to learning						
A. State and district variables						
1. District level demographics and marker variables	(2)	1	0	0	x	2
2. State level policy variables	(2)	2	0	0	x	4
B. Out of school contextual variables						
1. Community variables	(2)	1		0	0	0
2. Peer Group variables	(2)	2	x	4	0	0
3. Home environment and parental support variables	(3)	3		0	0	0
4. Student use of out of school time variables	(2)	1	x	2	0	0
C. School level variables						
1. Demographic and marker variables	(1)	2	0	0	0	0
2. Teacher/administrator decision making variables	(3)	3	0	0	x	9
3. School culture variables (ethos conducive to teaching and learning)	(3)	3	0	0	0	0
4. Schoolwide policy and organizational variables	(2)	3	x	6	x	6
5. Accessibility variables	(2)	3	0	0	x	6
6. Parental involvement policy variables	(2)	3	0	0	0	0

D. Student variables						
1. Demographic and marker variables	(1)	1	0	0	0	0
2. History of educational placements	(2)	1	0	0	0	0
3. Social and behavioral variables	(3)	3	x	9	0	0
4. Motivational and affective variables	(2)	2	x	4	x	4
5. Cognitive variables	(2)	1	x	3	x	3
6. Metacognitive variables	(3)	1	x	3	x	3
7. Psychomotor variables	(2)	1	x	2	x	2
E. Program design variables						
1. Demographic and marker variables	(2)	2	0	0	0	0
2. Curriculum and instructional variables	(2)	2	x	4	x	4
3. Curriculum design variables	(2)	2	x	4	0	0
F. Implementation, classroom instruction, and climate variables						
1. Classroom implementation support variables	(2)	3	0	0	0	0
2. Classroom instructional variables	(3)	3	x	9	0	0
3. Quantity of instruction variables	(2)	3	0	0	x	6
4. Classroom assessment variables	(2)	3	0	0	0	0
5. Classroom management variables	(3)	3	x	9	0	0
6. Student and teacher interactions: social variables	(3)	3	x	9	0	0
7. Student and teacher interactions: academic variables	(2)	3	x	6	0	0
8. Classroom climate variables	(3)	3	x	9	0	0
II. Expected program outcomes						
A. Student learning outcomes		3	x	3	x	3
B. Teacher expertise and attitudes		3	x	3	x	3
C. Administrator/instructional leader expertise and attitudes		2	0	0	x	0
D. Family expectation-attitudes		2	0	0	0	0
E. Program cost effectiveness		2	x	2	x	2
Program effectiveness index		79		91		57

Note: * Importance rating scale: 3 (high importance); 2 (moderate importance); 1 (low importance).
** Effectiveness rating: variable weighting × importance rating for variables emphasized in a given program.

variable weighting of 2 by an importance rating of 2 × 1 (1 indicates that this variable is emphasized in the design of Program A, as indicated by an X; a 0 is used for variable categories that are not emphasized in the design of the program).

Columns 5 and 7 list the effectiveness ratings for each variable category in Program A and Program B. The Program Effectiveness Index for meeting the site-specific improvement needs for Program A and Program B are shown in the last row of columns 5 and 7, respectively. Based on the Program Effectiveness Indices (shown in Table 5.2), without considering other factors, Program A (with a score of 91) seems to match the particular hypothetical user's program improvement needs better than Program B (with a score of 57).

The Broader Implications for the Use of the CMOVS

Although the foregoing discussion emphasizes the application of the CMOVS by potential users (decision makers) of educational programs, it may also prove useful to curriculum designers and developers of innovative programs. The list of variables included in the CMOVS can serve as a checklist to determine which variables are critical to consider in program development and school implementation of innovative programs. The checklist ensures that the program design incorporates features that research suggests are important to learning. Thus, the CMOVS can provide a guiding framework for specific variables to be considered in program development and implementation in schools.

If all programmatic factors were equal, it could be anticipated that the fully implemented programs that included more significant variables (features) would improve learning the most. In actual practice, however, all the factors involved are unlikely to be equal. Programs with extensive features are likely to be more costly to implement and manage. Therefore, both program developers and users need to carefully analyze the site-specific constraints and needs and weigh the trade-offs between cost and effectiveness in identifying priorities and in making programmatic decisions.

Discussion

This chapter provides an illustration of the use of well-confirmed knowledge on effective practices to improve a school's capability to improve student learning. School implementation of innovative programs that work, together with the research base on effective programs and practices (cf. Wittrock, 1986; Wang & Walberg, 1985; Graden, Zins, & Curtis, 1988), has yielded a rich knowledge base regarding how schools can implement highly complex and sophisticated instructional procedures to meet the learning needs of their diverse student populations.

A premise underlying the concept and practice of educational equity is that schooling success can be nurtured through provision of effective educational intervention (i.e., incorporation of advances in theories and research on demonstrably effective practice and practical wisdom on school implementations of programs that aim to provide for the learning success of all students, including those with special learning needs). Rather than attempting to identify a general underlying deficit in students requiring greater-than-usual instructional support, effective practices are adaptively implemented to ensure equity in student learning outcomes. In the context of the CMOVS discussed in this chapter, for example, provision of equal opportunity for educational success is characterized in terms of the use of school time, the quality of instruction, the content of the instruction, and instructional grouping practices.

A useful application of the CMOVS is identification and evaluation of innovative programs that aim at achieving educational excellence for all students with a high level of precision and credibility. If widespread implementation of innovative programs/practices is to occur, information is needed to further the understanding and specification of what constitutes effectiveness, the conditions that influence effectiveness, and the features of cost-effective alternative programs and practices.

There is no doubt that we fail to provide for the schooling success of many students in our schools today. Little understood, however, is the fact that many schools faced with the challenge of achieving educational equity have adopted new pilot programs, refocused teacher training, engaged in school reform, and implemented many other interventions in efforts to do better. Many national, state, and local school improvement efforts have energized their most creative people to find ways to effectively provide for the diverse learning needs of every child in our schools. Among the examples of federal initiative include the national Head Start program and the national Follow Through program designed to improve schooling outcomes of students from economically disadvantaged homes. These programs were initiated in the late 1960s as part of the federal government's War on Poverty program, the Chapter 1 Program development effort to improve basic skills of students who have not achieved well and are from economically disadvantaged homes, and the recently implemented Regular Education Initiative (REI) designed to improve coordination and articulation of the work of special and regular educators to improve learning outcomes of students with special needs (Will, 1986). Such efforts have led to the implementation of innovative school programs to enhance instruction and learning that require major rethinking and restructuring—not an easy task for schools to accomplish (cf. Williams et al., 1986; Wang, Reynolds, & Walberg, 1987–1989).

In many cases the innovations are working, albeit for the small group of targeted children who participate in the new programs (Dawson, 1987; U.S. Department of Education, 1987). Now, the challenge for the 1990s is to put innovations that work in place everywhere, for all students. Dropping the poorly motivated or difficult-to-teach students, or segregating them in programs that make few demands and offer few opportunities to succeed in school learning, is not an option. There is not a lack of ideas about what to do to improve instruction. What is glaringly lacking is the knowledge base on systematic selection and implementation of programs that promote educational equity and accountability.

Experience with successful implementation of innovative approaches to instructional accommodation in the 1980s has demonstrated the possibility of achieving the vision of equity in educational outcomes in the 1990s. A central consideration is how to tie together resources (e.g., teacher expertise, curricular accommodations, and administrative and organizational support for program implementation) and outcomes in ways that simultaneously achieve equity goals and accountability. Achieving educational equity will require using the best of what we currently know about how to design and maintain educationally powerful school learning environments that provide coordinated and inclusive comprehensive services to meet the diverse needs of all of the students today's schools are challenged to serve. School improvement efforts for the 1990s must address the concerns of systematically utilizing school resources and facilitating the development of students who have the most difficulty, while providing *all* students with the best possible opportunities to succeed in learning.

Acknowledgments. The research reported herein was supported in part by the Temple University Center for Research in Human Development and Education and in part by a grant from the Office of Special Education Programs of the U.S. Department of Education. The opinions expressed do not necessarily reflect the position of the OSEP and no official endorsement should be inferred. The author would like to especially thank Kim Tihansky for her editorial assistance in the preparation of this manuscript.

References

Allington, R.L., & Johnston, P. (1986). The coordination among regular classroom reading programs and targeted support programs. In B.I. Williams, P.A. Richmond, & B.J. Mason (Eds.), *Designs for compensatory education: Conference proceedings and papers* (Vol. 6, pp. 3–40). Washington, DC: Research and Evaluation Associates, Inc.

Bennett, S.N. (1978). Recent research on teaching: A dream, a belief and a model. *British Journal of Educational Psychology*, *48*, 127–147.

Berliner, D.C. (1983). Developing conceptions of classroom environments: Some light on the T in classroom studies of ATI. *Educational Psychologist*, *18*, 1–13.

Bloom, B.S. (1976). *Human characteristics and school learning*. New York: McGraw-Hill.

Bossert, S.T. (1979). *Tasks and social relationships in classrooms*. New York: Cambridge University Press.

Brandt, R.S. (Ed.). (1989). Dealing with diversity: Ability, gender, and style differences. [Special issue]. *Educational Leadership*, *46*(6).

Brookover, W.B. (Ed.). (1979). *School social systems and student achievement: Schools can make a difference*. New York: Praeger.

Brookover, W.B., & Lezotte, L.W. (1977). *Changes in school characteristics coincident with changes in student achievement*. East Lansing, MI: Michigan State University, College of Urban Development.

Brown, A.L., Day, J.D., & Jones, R.S. (1983). The development of plans for summarizing texts. *Child Development*, *54*(4), 968–979.

Bruner, J.S. (1966). *Toward a theory of instruction*. New York: W.W. Norton.

Carroll, J.B. (1963). A model for school learning. *Teachers College Record*, *63*, 722–732.

Chipman, S.G., Segal, J.W., & Glaser, R. (Eds.). (1985). *Thinking and learning skills: Vol. 2. Research and open questions*. Hillsdale, NJ: Erlbaum.

Cooper, H.M. (1983). Communication of teacher expectations to students. In J.M. Levine & M.C. Wang (Eds.), *Teacher and student perceptions: Implications for learning* (pp. 193–211). Hillsdale, NJ: Erlbaum.

Corno, L., & Snow, R.E. (1986). Adapting teaching to individual differences among learners. In M.C. Wittrock (Ed.), *Handbook of research on teaching* (3rd ed., pp. 605–629). New York: Macmillan.

Dawson, P. (1987). Preface. In A. Canter, P. Dawson, J. Silverstein, L. Hale, & J. Zins (Eds.), *NASP Directory of Alternative Service Delivery Models*. Washington, DC: National Association of School Psychologists.

DeStefano, L., Wang, M.C., & Gordon, E.M. (1984, April). Differences in student temperament characteristics and their effects on classroom processes and outcomes. In M.C. Wang (Organizer), *Temperament characteristics and learning*. Symposium presented at the annual meeting of the American Educational Research Association, New Orleans, LA.

Doyle, W. (1977). Paradigms for research on teacher effectiveness. In L.S. Shulman (Ed.), *Review research in education* (Vol. 5, pp. 163–198). Itasca, IL: Peacock.

Edmonds, R.R. (1979a). Effective schools for the urban poor. *Educational Leadership*, *37*, 15–27.

Edmonds, R.R. (1979b). Some schools work and more can. *Social Policy*, *9*(5), 28–32.

Edmonds, R.R. (1979c). *A discussion of the literature and issues related to effective schooling (Vol. 6)*. St. Louis, MO: CEMREL.

Fenstermacher, G.D. & Goodlad, J.I. (Eds.). (1983). *Individual Differences and the Common Curriculum*. Chicago: University of Chicago Press.

Glaser, R. (1975). The school of the future: Adaptive environments for learning. In L. Rubin (Ed.), *The future of education: Perspectives on tomorrow's schooling*. Boston: Allyn & Bacon.

Gordon, E.W. (Ed.). (1983). *Human diversity and pedagogy*. Westport, CT: Mediax.

Graden, J.L., Zins, J.E., & Curtis, M.J. (1988). *Alternative educational delivery systems: Enhancing instructional options for all students*. Washington, DC: National Association of School Psychologists.

Haertel, G.D., Walberg, H.J., & Haertel, E.H. (1981). Socio-psychological environments and learning: A quantitative synthesis. *British Educational Research Journal*, *7*, 27–36.

Haertel, G.D., Walberg, H.J., & Weinstein, T. (1983). Psychological models of educational performance: A theoretical synthesis of constructs. *Review of Educational Research*, *53*(1), 75–91.

Harnischfeger, A., & Wiley, D.E. (1976). The teaching-learning process in elementary schools: A synoptic view. *Curriculum Inquiry*, *6*, 5–43.

Haynes, M.C., & Jenkins, J.R. (1986). Reading instruction in special education resource rooms. *American Educational Research Journal*, *23*(23), 161–190.

Hedges, L.V., Giaconia, R.M., & Gage, N.L. (1981). *Meta-analysis of the effects of open and traditional instruction*. Stanford, CA: Stanford University Program on Teaching Effectiveness.

Hilgard, E.R. (1964). A perspective of the relationship between learning theory and educational practices. In E.R. Hilgard (Ed.), *Theories of learning and instruction: 63rd yearbook of the National Society for the Study of Education* (pp. 402–415). Chicago: University of Chicago Press.

Hodges, W.L., Branden, A., Feldman, R., Follins, J., Love, J., Sheehan, R., Lumbley, J., Osborn, J., Rentfrow, J., Houston, J., & Lee, C. (1980). *Follow through: Forces for change in the primary schools*. Ypsilanti, MI: High/Scope Press.

Madden, N.A., & Slavin, R.E. (1982). *Count me in: Academic achievement and social outcomes of mainstreaming students with mild academic handicaps* (Report No. 329). Baltimore: The Johns Hopkins University, Center for the Social Organization of Schools.

Marshall, H.H., & Weinstein, R.S. (1984). Classroom factors affecting students' self-evaluations: An interactional model. *Review of Educational Research*, *54*(3), 301–325.

Oakes, J. (1985). *Keeping track: How schools structure inequality*. New Haven, CT: Yale University Press.

Purkey, S.C., & Smith, M.S. (1983). Effective schools: A review. *Elementary School Journal*, *83*, 427–452.

Reynolds, M.C. (Ed.). (1989). *Knowledge base for the beginning teacher*. Oxford, U.K.: Pergamon.

Rutter, M., Maughan, B., Mortimore, P., & Ouston, J. (1979). *Fifteen thousand hours: Secondary schools and their effects on children*. Cambridge, MA: Harvard University Press.

Segal, J.W., Chipman, S.G., & Glaser, R. (Eds.). (1985). *Thinking and learning skills: Vol. 1. Relating instruction to research*. Hillsdale, NJ: Erlbaum.

Stanovich, K.E. (1984). The interactive-compensatory model of reading: A confluence of developmental, experimental, and educational psychology. *Remedial and Special Eduation*, *5*(3), 11–19.

Temple University Center for Research in Human Development and Education. (1989). *Effective educational practices: A concensus on learning*. Philadelphia, PA: Author.

U.S. Department of Education. (1986). *What works: Research about teaching and learning*. Washington, DC: Author.

U.S. Department of Education. (1987). *Schools that work: Educating disadvantaged children*. Washington, DC: U.S. Government Printing Office.

Walberg, H.J. (1984). Families as partners in educational productivity. *Phi Delta Kappan*, *65*(6), 397–400.

Wang, M.C. (1986). *Enhancing the learning efficiency and outcomes of mainstreamed special education students* (Technical Proposal). Pittsburgh, PA: University of Pittsburgh, Learning Research and Development Center.

Wang, M.C., Haertel, G.D., & Walberg, H.J. (1990). What influences learning: A content analysis of review literature. *Journal of Educational Research*, *84*(1), 30–43.

Wang, M.C., & Palincsar, A.S. (1989). Teaching students to assume an active role in their learning. In M.C. Reynolds (Ed.), *Knowledge Base for the Beginning Teacher* (pp. 71–84). Oxford, U.K : Pergamon.

Wang, M.C., Reynolds, M.C., & Walberg, H.J. (Eds.). (1987–1989). *Handbook of special education: Research and practice* (Vols. 1–3). Oxford, U.K.: Pergamon.

Wang, M.C., Reynolds, M.C., & Walberg, H.J. (1988). Integrating the children of the second system. *Phi Delta Kappan*, *70*(3) 248–251.

Wang, M.C., & Walberg, H.J. (Eds.). (1985). *Adapting instruction to individual differences*. Berkeley, CA: McCutchan.

Wang, M.C., & Walberg, H.J. (1986). Classroom climate as mediator of educational inputs and outputs. In B.J. Fraser (Ed.), *The study of learning environments 1985* (pp. 47–58). Salem, OR: Assessment Research.

Webb, N.M. (1982a). Student interaction and learning in small groups. *Review of Educational Research*, *52*, 421–445.

Webb, N.M. (1982b). Peer interaction and learning in cooperative small groups. *Journal of Educational Psychology*, *74*, 642–655.

Webb, N.M. (1982c). Group composition, group interaction, and achievement in cooperative small groups. *Journal of Educational Psychology*, *74*(4), 475–484.

Weinstein, C. (1984). Spatial strategies: Implications for applied research. In C. Holley & D. Dansereau (Eds.), *Spatial learning strategies: Techniques, applications, and related issues* (pp. 293–300). New York: Academic.

Will, M.C. (1986). Educating children with learning problems: A shared responsibility. *Exceptional Children*, *51*, 11–16.

Williams, B.I., Richmond, P.A., & Mason, B.J. (1986). *Designs for compensatory education: Conference proceedings and papers*. Washington, DC: Research and Evaluation Associates, Inc.

Wittrock, M.C. (1986). Students' thought processes. In M.C. Wittrock (Ed.), *Handbook of research on teaching* (3rd ed., pp. 297–314). New York: Macmillan.

Zimmerman, B.J. (Ed.). (1986). Discussions of role subprocesses in student self-regulated learning. [Special Issue] *Contemporary Educational Psychology*, *11*(4).

Appendix

Master List of Variables and Definitions

Variables important to learning: A consensus from the field.

Variables	Number of effective practices (rated as important) in each variable category
Category I: State and district variables	
A. District level demographics and marker variables	3
B. State level policy variables	3
Category II: Out of school contextual variables	
A. Community variables	3
B. Peer group variables	5
C. Home environment and parental support variables	9
D. Student use of out of school time variables	3
Category III: School level variables	
A. Demographic and marker variables	3
B. Teacher/administrator decision-making variables	6
C. School culture variables (ethos conducive to teaching and learning)	8
D. Schoolwide policy and organizational variables	11
E. Accessibility variables	1
F. Parental involvement policy variables	2
Category IV: Student variables	
A. Demographic and marker variables	4
B. History of educational placements	3
C. Social and behavioral variables	5
D. Motivational and affective variables	9
E. Cognitive variables	12
F. Metacognitive variables	4
G. Psychomotor variables	1
Category V: Program design variables	
A. Demographic and marker variables	4
B. Curriculum and instructional variables	15
C. Curriculum design variables	13
Category VI: Implementation, classroom instruction and climate variables	
A. Classroom implementation support variables	4
B. Classroom instructional variables	26
C. Quantity of instruction variables	11
D. Classroom assessment variables	4
E. Classroom management variables	5
F. Student and teacher interactions: social variables	6
G. Student and teacher interactions: academic variables	5
H. Classroom climate variables	15

A summary of findings from a survey of consensus from the field.

Variables	Consensus rating
Category I: State and district variables	
These are variables associated with state and district level school governance and administration. They include state curriculum and textbook policies, testing and graduation requirements, and teacher licensure; as well as specific provisions in teacher contracts, and some district-level administrative and fiscal variables.	
I–A. District level demographics and marker variables	
1. School district size	
2. Degree of school district bureaucratization	
3. Degree of school district centralization	
4. Presence of contractual limits on after-school meetings	
5. Limits on class size	
6. Presence of contractual restrictions on activities performed by aides	
7. Degree of central office assistance and support for programs	*
8. Degree of board of education support for instructional programs	*
9. Per pupil expenditure	*
10. Efficiency of transportation system	
I–B. State level policy variables	
1. Teacher licensure requirements	*
2. Degree of state control over textbooks	
3. Degree of state control over curriculum	
4. Academic course and unit requirements	*
5. Minimum competency test requirements	
6. Adherence to least restrictive environment/mainstreaming	*
Category II: Out of school contextual variables	
These are variables associated with the home and community contexts within which schools function. They include community demographics, peer culture, parental support and involvement, and amount of time students spend out of school on such activities as television viewing, leisure reading, and homework.	
II–A. Community variables	
1. Socioeconomic level of community	**
2. Ethnic mix of community	*
3. Quality of social services for students	*
II–B. Peer group variables	
1. Level of peers' academic aspirations	**
2. Level of peers' occupational aspirations	**
3. Presence of well-defined clique structure	*
4. Degree of peers' substance abuse	**
5. Degree of peers' criminal activity	**
II–C. Home environment and parental support variables	
1. Educational environment (e.g., number of books and magazines at home)	**
2. Parental involvement in assuring completion of homework	**

(Continued)

Variables	Consensus rating
3. Parental involvement in assuring regular school attendance	**
4. Parental monitoring of student television viewing	**
5. Parental participation in school conferences and related activities	*
6. Parental application of appropriate, consistent discipline	**
7. Parental expression of attention to children	**
8. Parental interest in student's school work	**
9. Parental expectation for academic success	**
II–D. Student use of out of school time variables	
1. Student participation in clubs and extracurricular school activities	
2. Amount of time spent on homework	*
3. Amount of time spent on leisure reading	*
4. Amount of time spent viewing educational television	
5. Amount of time spent viewing noneducational television	*
Category III: School level variables	
These are variables associated with school-level demographics, culture, climate, policies, and practices. They include demographics of the student body, whether the school is public or private, levels of funding for specific categorical programs, school-level decision making variables, and specific school-level policies and practices, including policies on parental involvement in the school.	
III–A. Demographic and marker variables	
1. Public versus private school	
2. Size of school	
3. Level of Chapter 1 (compensatory education) funding	*
4. Level of Title VII (bilingual) funding	
5. Level of PL 94–142 (handicapped) funding	*
6. Mix of socioeconomic levels in the school	*
7. Mix of cultural/ethnic groups in the school	
8. Mix of student language backgrounds in the school	
III–B. Teacher/administrator decision making variables	
1. Teacher and administrator consensus on school values, norms, and roles	**
2. Principal actively concerned with instructional program	**
3. Teacher involvement in curricular decision making	**
4. Teacher involvement in instructional decision making	**
5. Teacher involvement in resource allocation decisions	*
6. Teacher involvement in finding ways to increase academic performance	**
III–C. School culture variables (ethos conducive to teaching and learning)	
1. Use of cooperative, not exclusively competitive, goal structures	*
2. Schoolwide emphasis on and recognition of academic achievement	**
3. Low staff absenteeism	*
4. Low staff turnover	*
5. Low staff alienation	**
6. Active collaboration between regular classroom teachers and special education teachers	**
7. Safe, orderly school climate	**
8. Degree of school personnel professional collaboration	**

Variables	Consensus rating
III–D. Schoolwide policy and organizational variables	
1. Presence of "effective schools program"	*
2. Explicit school grading and academic progress policies	*
3. Explicit schoolwide discipline policy	*
4. Explicit schoolwide attendance policy	*
5. Coordination of pullout programs for handicapped students with regular instructional programs	*
6. Use of multi-age grouping	
7. Use of instructional teaming	*
8. Use of cross-age tutoring	*
9. Use of peer tutoring	*
10. Use of academic tracking for specific school subject areas	*
11. Minimization of external classroom disruptions (e.g., broadcast announcements)	
12. Adherence to least restrictive environment/mainstreaming	*
13. Minimum use of suspension and expulsion as discipline tools	*
III–E. Accessibility variables	
1. Accessibility of educational program (overcoming architectural, communication, and environmental barriers	*
III–F. Parental involvement policy variables	
1. Parental involvement in improvement and operation of instructional programs	*
2. School-sponsored parenting skills workshops (e.g., behavior modification, parent effectiveness training)	*
Category IV: Student variables	
These are variables associated with individual students themselves, including demographics, academic history, and a variety of social, behavioral, motivational, cognitive, and affective characteristics.	
IV–A. Demographic and marker variables	
1. Chronological age	
2. Socioeconomic status	*
3. Gender	
4. Ethnicity	
5. First or native language	*
6. Physical and health status	*
7. Special education classifications (e.g., EMR, LD)	*
IV–B. History of educational placements	
1. Prior grade retentions	*
2. Prior special placements	*
3. Current placement in regular class versus self-contained special education class	*
IV–C. Social and behavorial variables	
1. Positive, nondisruptive behavior	**
2. Appropriate activity level	**
3. Cooperativeness with teacher	**
4. Cooperativeness with peers	**
5. Ability to make friends with peers	*

(Continued)

Variables	Consensus rating
IV–D. Motivational and affective variables	
1. Attitude toward school	**
2. Attitude toward teachers	**
3. Attitude toward subject matter instructed	**
4. Motivation for continual learning	**
5. Independence as a learner	**
6. Perseverance on learning tasks	**
7. Self-confidence	**
8. Academic self-competence concept in subject area instructed	**
9. Attributions for success and failure in subject area instructed	**
IV–E. Cognitive variables	
1. Piagetian stage of cognitive development	*
2. Level of reasoning (fluid ability)	**
3. Level of spatial ability	*
4. Memory	**
5. Level of general academic (crystallized) knowledge	**
6. Level of specific academic knowledge in subject area instructed	*
7. Level of reading comprehension ability	**
8. Level of writing ability	*
9. Level of computational ability	*
10. Level of oral fluency	*
11. Level of listening skills	**
12. Learning styles (e.g., field independent, visual/auditory learners, high cognitive complexity)	*
IV–F. Metacognitive variables	
1. Self-regulatory, self-control strategies (e.g., control of attention)	**
2. Comprehension monitoring (planning; monitoring effectiveness of attempted actions; monitoring outcomes of actions; testing, revising, and evaluating learning strategies)	**
3. Positive strategies for coping with failure	**
4. Positive strategies to facilitate generalization of concepts	**
IV–G. Psychomotor variables	
1. Psychomotor skills specific to area instructed	*
Category V: Program design variables	
These are variables associated with instruction as designed, and with the physical arrangements for its delivery. They include the instructional strategies specified by the curriculum, and characteristics of instructional materials.	
V–A. Demographic and marker variables	
1. Size of instructional group (whole-class, small-group, one-on-one instruction)	**
2. Proportion of students with special needs served in regular classes	*
3. Number of classroom aides required	*
4. Resources needed	*

Variables	Consensus rating
V–B. Curriculum and instructional variables	
1. Clearly presented academic, social, and attitudinal program goals/outcomes	**
2. Use of explicit goal/objective setting for instruction of individual student (e.g., individualized educational plans, IEPs)	*
3. Use of mastery learning techniques, including use of instructional cues, engagement, and corrective feedback	**
4. Use of cooperative learning strategies	*
5. Use of personalized instructional program	*
6. Use of prescriptive instruction combined with aspects of informal or open education	*
7. Use of diagnostic-prescriptive methods	*
8. Use of computer-assisted instruction	*
9. Use of crisis management techniques to control classroom disruptiveness	*
10. Use of program strategies for favorable affective climate	*
11. Alignment among goals, contents, instruction, assignments and evaluation	**
12. Curriculum units integrated around key discipline-based concepts	*
13. Use of multidisciplinary approaches to instructional planning (including diagnosis in educational planning)	*
14. Presence of information in the curriculum on individual differences and commonalities (including handicapping conditions)	*
15. Presence of culturally diverse materials in the curriculum	*
V–C. Curriculum Design Variables	
1. Materials employ alternative modes of representation	*
2. Material is presented in a cognitively efficient manner	**
3. Materials employ explicit and specific objectives	**
4. Materials employ advance organizers	*
5. Materials employ learning hierarchies	*
6. Materials are tied to assessment and diagnostic tests	*
7. Availability of materials and activities prepared specifically for use with whole classroom, small groups, or one-on-one instruction	*
8. Degree of structure in curriculum accommodates needs of different learners	**
9. Student interests guide selection of a significant portion of content	*
10. Availability of materials and activities for students with different abilities	**
11. Availability of materials and activities for students with different learning styles	**
12. Developmental issues considered	*
13. Student experiences considered	*
Category VI: Implementation, classroom instruction, and climate variables	
These are variables associated with the implementation of the curriculum and the instructional program. They include classroom routines and practices, characteristics of instruction as delivered, classroom	

(Continued)

Variables	Consensus rating
management, monitoring of student progress, and quality and quantity of instruction provided, as well as student–teacher interactions and classroom climate.	
VI–A. Classroom implementation support variables	
1. Creation and maintenance of necessary instructional materials	*
2. Adequacy in the configuration of classroom space	*
3. Availability of classroom aides	*
4. Use of written records to monitor student progress	
5. Establishing efficient classroom routines and communicating rules and procedures	
6. Developing student self-responsibility for independent study and planning of one's own learning activities	**
VI–B. Classroom instructional variables	
1. Prescribing individualized instruction based on perceived match of type of learning tasks to student characteristics (e.g., ability, learning style)	*
2. Use of procedures requiring rehearsal and elaboration of new concepts	*
3. Use of clear and organized direct instruction	**
4. Systematic sequencing of instructional events and activities	**
5. Explicit reliance on individualized educational plans (IEPs) in planning day-to-day instruction for individual students	*
6. Use of instruction to surface and confront student misconceptions	*
7. Use of advance organizers, overviews, and reviews of objectives to structure information	*
8. Clear signaling of transitions as the lesson progresses	*
9. Significant redundancy in presentation of content	*
10. Teacher conveys enthusiasm about the content	**
11. Directing students' attention to the content	**
12. Using reinforcement contingencies	**
13. Setting and maintaining clear expectations of content mastery	**
14. Providing frequent feedback to students about their performance	**
15. Explicitly promoting effective metacognitive learning strategies	*
16. Promoting learning through student collaboration (e.g., peer tutoring, group work)	*
17. Corrective feedback in event of student error	**
18. Flexible grouping that enables students to work to improve and change status/groups	**
19. Teaching for meaningful understanding	**
20. Degree to which student inquiry is fostered	**
21. Scaffolding and gradual transfer of responsibility from teacher to student	*
22. Degree to which assessment is linked with instruction	*
23. Skills taught within the context of meaningful application	**
24. Good examples and analogies to concretize the abstract and familiarize the storage	**
25. Consideration of the teacher's use of language in the instructional process	**
26. Explicitly promoting student self-monitoring of comprehension	**

Variables	Consensus rating
VI–C. Quantity of instruction variables	
1. Length of school year	
2. Length of school day	*
3. Time on task (amount of time students are actively engaged in learning)	**
4. Time spent in direct instruction on basic skills in reading	**
5. Time spent in direct instruction on basic skills in mathematics	**
6. Time allocated to basic skills instruction by regular classroom teacher	**
7. Time allocated to basic skills instruction by special education teacher	**
8. Difference between academic learning time and allocated learning time	*
9. Time spent out of school on homework	*
10. Time spent out of school viewing educational television	*
11. Time spent out of school in informal learning experiences (e.g., museum trips, scouts)	*
12. Nature of regular classroom content missed by students during participation in pullout programs	*
VI–D. Classroom assessment variables	
1. Use of assessments to create detailed learner profiles rather than simple classifications or unlaborated total scores	*
2. Use of assessment as a frequent, integral component of instruction	*
3. Accurate, frequent measurement of basic skills in reading	*
4. Accurate, frequent measurement of basic skills in mathematics	*
VI–E. Classroom management variables	
1. Minimal disruptiveness in classroom (e.g., no excessive noise, no students out of place during instructional activities, no destructive activities)	**
2. Group alerting (teaching uses questioning/recitation strategies that maintain active participation by all students)	**
3. Learner accountability (teacher maintains student awareness of learning goals and expectations)	**
4. Transitions (teacher avoids disruptions of learning activities, brings activities to a clear and natural close, and smoothly initiates new activity)	**
5. Teacher "withitness" (teacher is continually aware of events and activities and minimizes disruptiveness by timely and nonconfrontational actions)	**
VI–F. Student and teacher interactions: social variables	
1. Student initiates positive verbal interactions with other students and with teacher	*
2. Student responds positively to questions from other students and from teacher	**
3. Teacher reacts appropriately to correct and incorrect answers	**
4. Teacher reinforces positive social interactions with students rejected by peers	**
5. Teacher provides explicit coaching on appropriate social behaviors	**
6. Teacher provides explicit coaching to reduce aggression	**

(Continued)

Variables	Consensus rating
VI–G. Student and teacher interactions: academic variables	
1. Teacher asks academic questions frequently	**
2. Teacher asks questions predominantly low in difficulty	*
3. Teacher asks questions that are predominantly low in cognitive level	*
4. Teacher maintains high post-question wait time	*
5. Frequent calls for extended, substantive oral and written response (not one-word answers)	*
VI–H. Classroom climate variables	
1. Cohesiveness (members of class are friends sharing common interests and values and emphasizing cooperative goals)	*
2. Low friction (students and teacher interact in a considerate and cooperative way, with minimal abrasiveness)	**
3. Low cliqueness (students work with many different classmates, and not just with a few close friends)	*
4. Satisfaction (students are satisfied with class activities)	**
5. Speed (the pacing of instruction is appropriate for the majority of the students)	**
6. Task difficulty (students are continually and appropriately challenged)	**
7. Low apathy (class members are concerned and interested in what goes on in the class)	**
8. Low favoritism (all students are treated equally well in the class, and given equal opportunities to participate)	**
9. Formality (students are asked to follow explicitly stated rules concerning classroom conduct and activities)	*
10. Goal direction (objectives of learning activities are specific and explicit)	**
11. Democracy (all students are explicitly involved in making some types of classroom decisions)	*
12. Organization (class is well organized and well planned)	**
13. Diversity (the class divides its efforts among several different purposes)	*
14. Environment (needed or desired books and equipment are readily available to students in the classroom)	**
15. Competition (students compete to see who can do the best work)	*

Note: ** = highly important (mean rating of 2.6 and above, based on a 3-point scale).
* = moderately important (mean rating of 2.0–2.5, based on a 3-point scale).

6
Curricular Concerns in Educating Students With Disabilities

KATHLEEN A. LIBERTY

Introduction

Curriculum is the content of education, and instruction is the method by which the curriculum is taught to the students. The content of education for persons with disabilities is influenced by (a) the societal expectations for the role of people with disabilities, (b) the expectations and educational goals of the individual and his or her family, (c) the curriculum model or approach selected, and (d) practical considerations of educational situations.

Societal Expectations

Our expectations for our children shape the school curriculum within constraints of environment and history. If a child with disabilities is expected to live out her life with her parents or relatives, to be seen only by immediate family within the confines of the home, and to be cared for entirely within the family structure, school curriculum might be directed at improving skills to ease care. If, on the other hand, a child with disabilities is expected to become a self-supporting adult, school curriculum is directed at providing skills necessary to achieve that objective.

In the United States, curriculum foundations for students with disabilities are changing as a result of changing expectations about persons with disabilities and their role in society. At the beginning of the century, people with disabilities were expected to be cared for in institutional or private family settings, to be economically dependent, and to be essentially invisible to the community at large. As the end of the century approaches, people with disabilities are increasingly perceived to be capable of living in the community and becoming partly or completely economically self-supporting, if provided appropriate adaptive equipment and education.

Several factors contributed to changing expectations in the United States. At the turn of the century, education was reserved primarily for the children, usually boys, of the more affluent classes. Poor children worked at home or in factories. However, compulsory education laws and child labor laws were passed, although children from racial minorities and children with disabilities were often excluded from educational opportunities. Significant judicial decisions based on the U.S. Constitutional guarantees of equal opportunity provided the foundation for new laws that resulted in the desegregation of education for minorities (1950s), based on the idea that separate schools (for black and for white children) were not equal schools. This concept of equality of educational opportunity was followed by compensatory early education for poor children (1960s), an attempt to equalize each child's exposure to environmental stimulation and prerequisite "school" behaviors. Equal opportunity was extended to all children with disabilities in 1975.

The principle of normalization was one of the foundation stones of the drive to educate all students and to deinstitutionalize persons with disabilities in the United States. This concept originated in Scandinavia. The ideas of normalization were first published in the United States in a government monograph under the leadership of Kugel and Wolfensberger (1969). The chapter on normalization was written by one of the leaders of the Scandinavian movement, Bengt Nirje, who defined normalization as "making available to the mentally retarded patterns and conditions of everyday life which are as close as possible to the norms and patterns of the mainstream of society" (Nirje, 1969, p. 181). One of the results of the deinstitutionalization movement was the entry of thousands of students with disabilities into community schools, along with the decline in institution-based schools or other segregated facilities. Although often poorly prepared and hostile at first, communities began recognizing the needs and presence of people with disabilities. Franklin Roosevelt, president of the United States from 1933 to 1945, provided the public with the image of a leader in a wheelchair, and life stories of people with disabilities overcoming the effects of their disabilities became popularized through films such as *The Helen Keller Story*. Returning disabled veterans of four wars in the 1910s, 40s, 50s, 60s, and 70s created a sizable disabled population that could not be ignored, especially veterans of the Vietnam War, who joined with others to call publicly for rights for persons with disabilities in the 1980s.

One of the most striking results of the advocacy movement is the removal of architectural barriers to wheelchair access of public buildings and services and other special provisions in restaurants, shops, hotels, airports and airplanes, and public transportation. The "can do" attitude of Americans, an absolute faith that problems can and will be solved, has been fueled since the 1960s by research demonstrating rapid acquisition of new skills through specialized instruction by persons with even the most severe disabilities. Decades of advocacy and change have increased expectations for the adult lives of children with disabilities.

Individualized Goals

Within the overall change in general expectations, distinctions are still made according to the nature and severity of a person's disability. These differential expectations in turn influence educational goals. Thus, although overall expectations are rising, not all individuals are currently expected to become economically or domestically independent.

In the United States, individual educational goals are established for each student with disabilities. Goals are individualized on the basis of differential expectations for each learner with disabilities. Initial individualization of goals is based on diagnosis, prognosis, and treatment of disabling conditions. Diagnostic information from physicians regarding vision, hearing, motor development, neurological conditions, orthopedic functions, and other physical conditions; prognoses of changes in physiological or neurological functioning; and the availability and effect of treatments such as medication, physical therapy, occupational therapy, and prosthetic or adaptive equipment are all vital factors in the determination of individual education goals.

The second source of information used in planning educational programs is an evaluation of the individual's current level of functioning and achievement. This is usually accomplished in individual testing and assessment sessions, which might involve a variety of procedures ranging from the administration of intelligence tests to informal observations of play and mother–child interactions. Participants in establishing educational goals for the individual student reflect the multidisciplinary sources of information used to guide goal setting: communication specialist, language disorder specialist, speech therapist, physical therapist, nurse, occupational therapist, physician, psychologist, nutritionist, social worker, adaptive physical education specialist, rehabilitation counselor, dentist, and recreation specialist each might be called upon to assist the student, parents, teacher, and administrator in planning educational goals.

Educational goals define the content of the curriculum by stating general expectations for achievement within a specified period, which is usually one school year. For example, Larry R. will communicate verbally answers to yes/no questions and answers to personal identity questions (e.g., What's your name? and Where do you live?). After educational goals are established, instructional objectives and instructional plans are developed.

Models of Curriculum

Curricular models are the third factor influencing the content of educational programs for students with disabilities. A curriculum model provides a structure within which or through which the goals of education can be achieved by individual students. In general education, this core curriculum consists of basic academic skills (i.e., reading, writing, spelling, grammar, composition, computation), usually taught in the elementary grades, and basic knowledge in the domains of science, history, and literature, primarily taught at the secondary level. The core curriculum is used to achieve general educational goals, primarily the education of a person who will become a self-supporting, law-abiding citizen. However, in the United States, unlike in other countries such as New Zealand and Switzerland, the specific skills, objectives and content of the core curriculum are not standardized. Thus, one school's curriculum may include instruction in the parts of speech whereas another school's curriculum does not. One may teach set theory and another may not. Even within a single school and grade, content may vary across teachers. The absence of a standardized core curriculum is one of the current criticisms of schools (e.g., Hirsch, 1989). Instead of state-controlled curriculum, each local school determines curriculum content and selects textbooks, with community participation through school boards, parent groups, and business partnerships. Local-control produces a curriculum based on the shared values and perceived needs of the community for its children. This also is the basis for a curriculum for students with disabilities.

Instead of a standard set of skills for students with severe disabilities, teachers and parents have developed curricula to meet the needs of children in their communities. The general philosophy of curricula have paralleled changes in expectations for students with disabilities. Initially, curriculum development was based on the assumption that individuals with severe disabilities would be dependent on others throughout the lifecycle. Curriculum in such a "care-taking model" emphasized the provision of enjoyable experiences, and the maintenance of comfort and current levels of functioning. Next, curricula were based on the theory that children with severe disabilities would develop skills in the same order and sequence as Western children without disabilities, although more slowly. Curriculum in this "developmental model" emphasized provision of activities appropriate to the individuals assessed level of development. Alternatively, a theory that the disability is produced by a particular type of cognitive deficit produced curriculum based at teaching skills to overcome the deficit. An overview of some of the different models for curriculum is shown in Table 6.1.

Each model relies on different assessment procedures and instruments; thus, the assessments used to determine educational goals will differ according to the curricular model. For example, a caretaking model will involve assessing the current status of the individual's relative comfort and happiness and developing educational goals to improve or maintain current levels. A developmental model requires assessing which developmental milestones have been mastered and setting educational goals according to the subsequent stages of development. A deficit approach

TABLE 6.1. Curriculum models.

Model	Foundation	Description	Current application
Models with implicit assumption that intelligence is fixed			
Care-taking model	Care and service will improve life and comfort (learning may not be possible); Christian philosophy and teachings; implies that intelligence is not malleable.	Curriculum is determined by deciding what person with disabilities needs to improve his comfort and by providing that. No assessment instruments used, although expressions of like, dislike, anger, pain, and happiness (as interpreted by caregiver) may be considered. "Curriculum" may be divided into different activities (e.g., snack, music, free play, nap, movie).	For persons in large residential institutions; persons with multiple physical, sensory, and mental disabilities.
Adapted curriculum ("watered-down")	Typical academic curriculum found in public school programs represents basic knowledge and skill base required for adults to participate in this society; provide same curriculum to all, let each acquire as much as possible.	Curriculum is determined by identifying current grade level or mastery level in skills and knowledge. Assessment instruments include quarterly progress reports (grades), teacher-made tests; commercially available curriculum guides; achievement tests.	For persons with mild mental retardation, persons with sensory deficits, for persons predicted to be low achievers.
Models with implicit assumption that intelligence is malleable			
Developmental model	Developmental delay. Stages or milestones of development can be identified; everyone goes through stages, even if at different rates; development through stages may be expedited by instruction.	Curriculum is determined by identifying current developmental age or mental age, often broken down into different "domains" (e.g., communication, gross motor, fine motor, preacademic). Assessment instruments used: Denver Developmental Survey, Brigance.	For persons with developmental delays, mental retardation, infants and young children.
Remedial model	Skill deficit problems rest within specific skill performance. Specific nature of academic or learning problems can be identified; can remediate specific problems by instruction directed at	Curriculum is determined by identifying skill areas in which performance deficits are significant, often broken down into different academic areas (e.g., reading, math, spelling). Assessment instruments used: standardized	For persons with mild retardation, learning disabilities, behavior disorders, of school age.

(Continued)

TABLE 6.1. *Continued*

Model	Foundation	Description	Current application
	specific skill areas. Supported by research in discrimination and in how young children acquire basic academic and thinking skills, and by data on remediation effectiveness.	achievement and skill tests	
Compensatory model	Cognitive deficit specific or general deficits exist in cognitive and metacognitive functions; education aimed at correcting or ameliorating the deficit by teaching cognitive and metacognitive strategies. Supported by comparative research in learning and cognition. Curriculum may include finding alternative paths to achieve critical effect of skills inhibited by deficit.	Curriculum is determined by identifying deficits. Medical diagnosis, etiology, and special instruments such as Illinois Test of Psycholinguistic Abilities, Intelligence Test	For persons with minimal brain dysfunction, dyslexia, learning disabilities.
Enrichment model	Environmental deficits at early age (prenatal, infancy, early childhood) will affect learning and readiness for learning academic tasks, as supported by research on effects of deprivation, social isolation. Curriculum consists of providing enrichment such as sensory stimulation; early preacademic school skills experiences, field trips, music and art; emphasis on communication and play. May include parent training.	Informal assessment. Observation of child behavior in different situations. Developmental scales. Comparisons of perfomrance with average middle-class performances expected in the schools. Assess types and impact of deprivation; determine sources.	For infant and early education programs, "Head Start"; for students with profound and multiple disabilities.

Direct Instruction model	Educational skill deficit. Source of deficit not critical. Education should provide basic academic skills student needs to function in school environments and to benefit from schooling. Will also impact on psychological problems. Supported by most extensive comparative data base of all models.	Curriculum addresses basic academic skills: reading, writing, spelling, math computation, listening, language arts. in highly structured sequenced lessons set out in commercially published materials, including set methods of teacher presentation of material. Assessment instruments provided with curriculum materials.	For early education and primary-elementary ages, for children with mild mental retardation.
Criterion of Ultimate Functioning model	Skill deficit. Source of deficits not important. Education should provide skills student needs in the "ultimate environment"—skills needed to function independently as an adult in vocational, community, and domestic environments.	Direct observation of present skill levels in target criteria environments, discrepancy analyses to identify skills needed to be taught for competent adult independence, instruction, compensation, or prosthesis to achieve independent functioning in ultimate environments. "Top-down" approach.	For students with moderate and severe disabilities, and dual sensory impairments.

will involve assessing cognitive and metacognitive skills. The assessment of current functioning must be related to the curriculum, or else it will not be useful in establishing educational goals. For example, a developmental survey will not be of much use in either the caretaking model or a deficit model.

The curriculum approach that is adopted by a teacher or a program will be influenced by social expectations, by the training the teacher received, and by the availability of materials and resources required for implementation. The success of a particular curriculum model can also shape expectations. For example, after it has been demonstrated that students with severe disabilities can live and work in the community, changed expectations for others will affect curriculum development.

Practical Considerations

The fourth factor influencing the content of education is one of practicality in implementation, including the ease with which teachers can implement a curriculum and the availability and costs associated with it. Teachers who are initially trained in a particular curriculum model are likely to apply that model in the development of educational programs for their students. Retraining practicing teachers is often difficult, expensive, and lengthy; in addition, teachers, like most other people, are likely to be resistant to changing familiar procedures (Joyce & Showers, 1983).

Another element is the availability and quality of materials to support the curriculum. If assessment instruments are readily available, cheap, and easily interpreted, and if curricular materials also are easily available and attractive, implementation is facilitated. The availability of such instruments as the Denver Developmental Survey, and the ease of finding, relative appeal, and inexpensiveness of infants' and children's toys, have aided the adoption of developmentally based curricula. When assessment instruments and curriculum materials must be individually developed and designed by the classroom teacher, adoption and maintenance of the curriculum model is dependent on collegial, parental, and administrative support for the teacher's extra efforts.

Current Practices

Current practices in the United States are marked by the changing expectations for persons with disabilities, the characteristics of individual learners, the multidisciplinary approach to individualized educational goals, the variety of curriculum models, the nature of teacher preparation, and the availability of curriculum assessment instruments and materials. Students with sensory and physical disabilities with normal intellectual functioning are usually educated within the general education core curriculum with special instruction directed at remediating, minimiz-

3. Could students function as adults if they did not acquire the skill?
4. Is there a different activity that will allow students to approximate realization of the criterion of ultimate functioning more quickly and more efficiently?
5. Will this activity impede, restrict, or reduce the probability that students will ultimately function in community settings?
6. Are the skills, materials, tasks, and criteria of concern similar to those encountered in adult life? (p. 9)

The concept of the criterion of ultimate functioning consolidated the philosophy of educating students with severe disabilities in the 1970's, at the time of the Education for All Children Act. Most of its aims are still to be reached, in theory as well as in practice, but its influence on curriculum has been revolutionary.

One of the most remarkable changes in curriculum as a result of the implementation of the principle of the criterion of ultimate functioning is in the area of vocational preparation. During the 1970s, vocational curricula for students with disabilities consisted primarily of "career awareness programs" in which they visited, read, viewed films, and heard about various unskilled or semiskilled jobs. Or, alternatively, they participated in "vocational assessment programs", in which they were tested on various tasks associated with different unskilled or semiskilled jobs. Many students were excluded from even this level of vocational preparation. However, students who graduated from such vocational training programs were often not able to find or keep employment.

The criterion of ultimate functioning approach coupled with successful demonstrations that individuals with severe disabilities could be taught complex vocational tasks (Gold, 1972; Gold & Barclay, 1973) led to the development of vocational curriculum to teach a wide variety of job skills to students with severe disabilities. Curriculum designs for semiskilled and low-skilled jobs are available in *Vocational Habilitation of Severely Retarded Adults* (Bellamy, Horner, & Inman, 1979) and *Vocational Curriculum for Developmentally Disabled Persons* (Wehman & McLaughlin, 1980). The "ultimate environments" are now supported employment settings, enclave settings, and competitive work settings. In *Competitive Employment Issues and Strategies*, Frank Rusch (1986) has collaborated with other experts to describe strategies for identifying potential jobs, establishing work sites within the community to use during vocational education, assessing work behavior on-site, developing a curriculum for each job site, and analyzing work performance; Rusch also discusses issues related to instruction, generalization, and maintenance of work skills.

Normalization

The criterion of ultimate functioning, coupled with the principle of normalization, changed curriculum in other ways as well. During the

1970s, the principle of normalization affected curriculum by increasing the emphasis on skills to allow students to experience, and/or participate in, normal daily routines involved in waking, dressing, bathing, and eating, making choices and indicating desires (Bruininks & Warfield, 1978). These developments primarily affected school curriculum for students with the most severe disabilities, who began to enter public programs in 1974 and 1975. Specially prepared teachers were generally not available, so teachers who were trained to teach students with mild disabilities struggled to develop appropriate curricula or to adapt curricula from other groups of students. Teachers and professionals who produced some of the first curriculum materials for students with severe disabilities applied the principle of normalization in the design of curricula. *The Teaching Research Curriculum for Moderately and Severely Handicapped* (Fredericks et al., 1976); *The Programmed Environments Curriculum* (Tawney, Knapp, O'Reilly, & Pratt, 1979); *Student Progress Record Individualized Education Program* (State of Oregon, Mental Health Division, 1981); and the *Washington State Cooperative Curriculum* (Stewart, 1986) are examples of teacher-developed curricula that include substantial focus on teaching daily living skills. During the last decade, curricular materials to teach choice-making skills began to be developed and incorporated into some published materials (e.g., *Student Progress Record Individualized Education Program*, State of Oregon, Mental Health Division, 1981, pp. 219, 312, 327), although curriculum development for choice making skills lags far behind that for daily living skills.

During the 1980s, the principle of normalization as applied to curriculum was expanded and broadened to include a much wider spectrum of daily living skills, such as using the telephone, doing laundry, housekeeping, preparing meals, and so on. In addition, the variety and importance of the environments in which the student does and will function has been emphasized (e.g., Nietupski & Hamre-Nietupski, 1987). The *Community-Based Curriculum* (Falvey, 1986); *Individual Student Community Life Skill Profile System for Severely Handicapped Students* (Freagon, Wheeler, McDannel, Brankin, & Costello, 1983); and *An Individualized, Functional Curriculum Assessment Procedure* (Renzaglia & Aveno, 1986a, 1986b) are curricula that include such skills as using cosmetics, sorting clothing, choosing what to eat and when to eat it, maintaining a yard, and styling hair (Falvey, 1986, p. 93); using appropriate amounts of condiments, disposing of garbage, and initiating interactions for desired services (Freagon et al., 1983, p. 68); and shaving, cleaning and clipping nails, using deodorant, using and caring for glasses, and using and caring for hearing aids (Renzaglia & Aveno, 1986a, p. 3). *IMPACT: A Functional Curriculum Handbook for Students With Moderate to Severe Disabilities* (Neel & Billingsley, 1989) guides skill assessment, identification, and programming—incorporating instruction within normal routines of daily living and the functional intents of the learner's actions, skills, and behavior—to teach independence in school, family, and community settings. Rather than providing a set prescription of skills, *IMPACT* provides formats and guidelines for a team approach to individualized curriculum and individualized educational plan (IEP) development. These curricula also include skills to "normalize" leisure activities in preparation for community living. *Leisure and Recreation: Preparation for Independence, Integration, and Self-Fulfillment* (Voeltz, Wuerch, & Wilcox, 1982) and *The Activities Catalog: An Alternative Curriculum for Youth and Adults With Severe Disabilities*, which includes *A Comprehensive Guide to the Activities Catalog: An Alternative Curriculum for Youth and Adults With Severe Disabilities* (Wilcox & Bellamy, 1987a, 1987b), describe strategies for teaching a variety of leisure activities for each individual.

Integrated Therapy

The concept of integrating therapeutic goals and procedures within educational curricula is especially important for children with physical and communication disabilities. There is no evidence that providing physical, occupational, communication, or other forms of therapy on a pull-out model for a few minutes every day, or even for longer sessions during a week, has produced maintenance or improvement in the skill needed for integration. In many instances, prosthetic devices such as wheelchairs and computer-assisted speech, are routinely recommended when therapy goals have failed. In the United States, a truely integrated curriculum has not been developed. However, a Hungarian program has had remarkable success in teaching children with cerebral palsy to participate in normal educational programs without such prosthetics—to teach walking, sitting, standing, and talking in normal educational situations—using a completely integrated curriculum. The remarkable success of the program in Hungary, and the opening of Eastern Europe, have contributed to the rapid proliferation of Conductive Education programs around the world.

Conductive Education is a system of holistic education for children with motor disabilities developed in Hungary at the Petö Institute (Hari & Akos, 1988). The fundamental aim of Conductive Education is "'orthofunction' or, better, an orthofunctioning personality, i.e., an active, positive orientation to learning, an expectation that intention can, with persistence and a knowledge of one's own potential, lead on to achievement." (Sutton, in press, p. 1). This has been interpreted as education designed to produce the development of the skills by children with motor disabilities that are needed for them to "function as members of society, to participate in normal social settings appropriate to their age . . . without need for wheelchairs, ramps, special furniture or toileting arrangements" (Cottam & Sutton, 1986, p. 41). Because of evidence of the program's success in Hungary, programs utilizing Conductive Education principles, often led by Conductors trained in Hungary, are being established around the world (Bax, 1991; Bairstow, Cochrane, & Rusk, 1991; Sutton, in press).

A Conductive Education programme is directed by a specially trained person, a "conductor," who literally conducts the overt motor and verbal behaviours of the teachers working with the children in much the same way as the conductor of a symphony leads, controls, and directs the musicians as they play upon musical instruments. Under the guidance of the Conductor, each child is continuously guided physically and verbally by one or two persons to participate in exercises and practical activities of the normal school and living routines, throughout the program day. The content and procedures of communication, physical, orthopedic, and occupational therapy are continuously intertwined with functional skills training and academics. Although evaluative data are just beginning to be collected in several programs (Bax, 1991) evaluation at 6 months into one small program shows rapid acceleration in the acquisition of new skills related to sitting, standing, walking, communication and self-help by five of six preschool children with cerebral palsy and seizure disorders functioning at severely disabled levels (Liberty, Brodie, Young, & Berekely, 1991).

Mainstreaming

Educating students with disabilities in the same classroom as students without disabilities is normalization, because educating children with disabilities in the same way and place as children without disabilities "normalizes" their educational experiences. During the 1970s, the mainstreaming curriculum for children with severe disabilities emphasized creating opportunities for interactions with nonhandicapped peers (e.g., Voeltz, 1980, 1982, Voeltz, et al., 1982; Strain & Fox, 1981). During the last decade, curricula emphasized teaching all students the skills required for meaningful interactions. For example, *The Social Competence Curriculum Project: A Guide to Instructional Programming for Social and Communicative Interactions* (Peck, Schuler, Tomlinson, Theimer, & Haring, 1984) was developed to facilitate communication and socialization in the school and within the family, neighborhood, and community. A curriculum series for teaching primary and secondary students and adults without disabilities about disabling conditions, integration, and how to interact with individuals with disabilities, including suggested activities, was developed at the Severely Handicapped Integration Program at the University of Kansas (Campbell, Hinz, & Sasso, 1983; Clark & Cozad, 1983; Clark & Fiedler, 1983; Cozad, Fiedler, Novak, Simpson, & Werth, 1983; Cozad, Hintz, Novak & Campbell, 1983;

Novak, 1983), and also included a social skills curriculum for students with severe disabilities (Sasso & Simpson, 1983).

Prior to 1975, students with mild intellectual disabilities had generally been educated within regular programs until approximately age 12 or 13. Secondary schooling generally continued in separate classrooms, although integration in non-academic classes, such as art, music, and physical education was fairly common. Academic materials had been presented in a "watered down" version of the general curriculum in each subject matter area in both primary and secondary classrooms. Currently, many primary and secondary schools provide separate pull-out programs for specific skill remediation. Successful programs for the remediation of skill deficits did not, however, bring social acceptance in general education. In the 1980s, curricula designed to specifically teach skills needed for achievement and acceptance in general education classrooms were developed. For example, the goals of the *Walker Social Skills Curriculum: The ACCEPTS Program* (Walker et al., 1983) are to "facilitate the social development of handicapped children . . . to prepare them to meet the behavioral demands and expectations that exist in less restrictive settings . . . [and] to improve the social acceptance of handicapped children by their nonhandicapped peers" (p. 5). Teachers can instruct their students to use verbal mediation procedures and self-control skills to solve social, communication, and school problems, using the the *Think Aloud Programs* (Camp & Bash, 1988a,b,c,d), or to use strategy skills such as studying skills, test-taking skills, discussing in class skills, clarifying homework skills, and so forth using the *Social Skills for Daily Living* curriculum (Schumaker, Hazel, & Pederson, 1988). For example, in addition to providing a student with remedial drills on the content covered in science class, a strategy approach might involve teaching the student how to ask questions of the teacher, how to solicit feedback on assignments, and how to review the requirements of homework assignments.

Individuality

Until the mid-1970s, the concept of a curriculum was one of inclusiveness. Curricula were generally expected to include comprehensive coverage of the subject matter (e.g., vocational awareness) or developmental domain (e.g., gross motor skills), or be designed especially for a supposedly homogeneous group of students (e.g., for students with severe handicaps). However, the mandate and practice of individualizing education meant that not all children in the same class would or even should have similar, or even related, educational objectives. Therefore, it is unlikely that any single curriculum consisting of lists of objectives, would be comprehensive enough to meet the needs of a single classroom teacher

(Baldwin, 1976). Mainstreaming and integration have also reduced the probability that a single curriculum would be appropriate for all students in a classroom. Thus, curricula of the 1990's are much more likely to provide guidelines for the appropriate individualization of curriculum rather than a prescriptive list of skills.

One of the most significant changes over the last decade has to do with changes in the form rather than the content, of curricula. Curricula of the 1980s, unlike those of earlier decades, do not list specific objectives, instructional procedures, and materials for each skill within their scope. Instead, the materials for students with severe disabilities prescribe strategies for assessment, development of educational goals, and specification of objectives for each student (e.g., Freagon et al., 1983; Falvey, 1986). One of the most well-known systems is *Try Another Way* (Gold, 1980).

Commercial Curricula

Curricula for teaching basic academic skills for students with mild disabilities have become commercially available during the last decade. The *Peabody Rebus Reading Program* (Woodcock, Clark, & Davies, 1979) provides workbooks and readers for pre-primer instruction in which picture words (rebuses) replace spelled words. *Write Right—or Left* (Hagin, 1983); *D'Nealian Handwriting* (Thurber & Jordan, 1978); and *Learn to Write: Italic Style* (Duvall, 1981) were three new curricula designed to teach children with motor, neurophysiological, and learning problems to write, using letter forms adapted from manuscript style and cursive style writing. *Project Math* (Cawley, Goodstein, Fitzmaurice, Sedlack, & Althans, 1976) is a curriculum designed to teach basic mathematical skills to children with learning problems. The curriculum materials include all topics normally covered at the elementary level (c.f., geometry, sets, patterns, measurement, numbers, and fractions), beginning with manipulative exercises of concrete objects similar to those in a Montessori approach and progressing to abstract and symbolic levels.

One of the most systematically researched curricula in the basic skills of reading and math is based on "direct instruction," developed by Wes Becker, Doug Carnine, Siegfried Engelmann, and their colleagues at the University of Oregon. The *DISTAR Reading Program* (Engelmann & Bruner, 1984) is a very structured and systematic phonetically based beginning reading curriculum. The *Corrective Reading Program* (Engelmann, Becker, Hanner, & Johnson, 1978) provides material that is interesting for older students, grades 4–12, chronological ages 9 through 18, who are acquiring basic reading skills. *Direct Instruction Mathematics* (Silbert, Carnine, & Stein, 1981) covers basic math skills, including memorizing basic math facts; counting and place value skills; computations; story problems; fractions; decimals and percentages; measuring length, weight, and capacity; telling time; geometry; and study skills (maps, graphs, tables, statistics) for primary grades. Programs are also available in other languages, and have been adopted in more than 20 countries throughout the world.

The Direct Instruction curriculum has been extensively researched in the United States. A longitudinal study, Project Follow Through, across 139 school sites in the United States involved 9,255 children aged 6 to 7 (U.S. kindergarten and first grade) who were from "disadvantaged" backgrounds and predicted to be low achievers and were served in public educational programs for the disadvantaged. These students were compared with 6,485 disadvantaged students in other programs. Nine separate curricular approaches serving the 9,255 children were identified by program sponsors:

1. The Bank Street College model, which included a language-experience approach to reading.
2. The Florida parent education model, which involved having the parents of the disadvantaged children work with their children in the classroom and at home.
3. The language development (bilingual) model.
4. The University of Kansas behavior analysis model, which focused on systematic application of positive reinforment of achievement in small sequential steps of basic academic skills and careful monitoring of student progress.
5. The Open Education model derived from the British inschool school approach.
6. The cognitive-oriented curriculum, based on Piaget's model of cognitive process development.
7. The responsive education model, which incorporated some of the procedures of Montessori and Deutsch.
8 The Tucson early education model, designed to teach intellectual processes through child-directed choices.
9. Direct Instruction.

During the 10 year study, more than a dozen different measurement procedures were used to compare the children enrolled over a four year period in the nine programs, and an additional 6,485 children randomly sampled from other programs. Results indicated that Direct Instruction was the only model to show positive effects on the achievement of basic skills, and ranked first on positive impacts on cognitive measures in reading, comprehension, math concepts, and math problem solving—contrary to assumptions that the behavioral methodology would not result in improvements in conceptual skills (Abt Associates, 1976; 1977). Direct

Instruction also ranked first on affective measures. Additional measures of student achievement and intellectual development showed that children who began Direct Instruction at kindergarten age 6 showed educationally greater benefits than those who began at first grade, age 7; children in Direct Instruction showed significant gains in I.Q., which were evident through third grade, at age 9 and children with IQs below 80 showed significant improvement in academic skills (Becker & Carnine, 1980). Follow-up studies at fifth and sixth grade (ages approximately 10–12) showed significantly better performance by Direct Instruction children in comparison with students in other groups.

Despite methodological problems involved in the large study, the fact remains that no other curriculum model has withstood such research and scrunity and emerged with such strong support for its adoption. Direct Instruction remains the curricular model with the most direct and supportive empirical data base for its beneficial impact on the achievement of basic academic skills by young children. (In addition, see Becker, W. C., 1977; Gersten, Carnine, & Woodward, 1987.) For a critique and analysis of the Project Follow Through study, see House, Glass, McLean, & Walker, 1978.

Another program with a large evaluative base is Reading Recovery. Reading Recovery is a program of early detection and intervention for children with difficulties in reading and writing (Clay, 1985; 1987). Reading Recovery was developed in New Zealand between 1976 and 1983 to provide children with a "second chance" at learning to read and write if they have not made a successful start during the first year of standard instruction. During daily 30 minute lessons, individually designed and individually delivered, "Each child reads a new story book each day, and keeps about 20 of his recent books as his reading resource of easy reading" (Clay, 1987, p. 37). The children practice oral reading daily, which is observed and assessed by the teacher, who uses the performance data to determine the course of instruction and the content of special lessons. A great deal of positive feedback and success are provided to the children, who progress through the story books of gradually increasing difficulty until they are reading at the average level of their classmates. Achievement is graphed daily.

Evaluation of Reading Recovery is being conducted in Australia, the United States, and in New Zealand. Data collected by the Ministry of Education in New Zealand show that the percentage of children referred for Reading Recovery programmes increased from 6.5% in 1984 to 21% in 1988. However, despite the increasing enrollment, yearly about 96% of the children in Reading Recovery become independent readers at the average level of students in their classrooms within 12 to 20 weeks. About 32% of these will complete the Reading Recovery programme during the subsequent school year because of entering Reading Recovery late in the school year (Clay, 1990; Clay & Tuck, 1991). From 1984 to 1988, annually about 4% of the students in Reading Recovery failed to meet the criteria for independent average readers (Clay & Tuck, 1991). Nationally, less than 1% of the student population are referred to specialists for additional remediation of reading difficulties after Reading Recovery programmes (Clay, 1990). Two follow-up studies in New Zealand and the United States have shown that three years later gains are retained (Clay, 1990; Pinnell et al., 1988). According to Dr. Clay, "High success rates obtained in a short time are needed to make the programme cost-effective and a high quality programme based on sound training of the teachers is required to achieve these outcomes" (Clay, 1990, p. 64). Costs of the programme may be manipulated by controlling the number of children entering the program (i.e., providing Reading Recovery to the lowest 30% of readers will be more expensive in short-term costs than providing Reading Recovery to the lowest 5% of readers) (Clay, 1990). Reading Recovery programmes are also implemented in Australia, the United States with good effects despite problems in implementation (Clay, 1987; Clay 1990; Pinnell, et al., 1988), and are beginning in the United Kingdom.

Computers

The technology of computers began to significantly affect curriculum during the 1980s. Between 1981 and 1986, the percentage of U.S. schools with microcomputers for students rose from 18% to 96%; elementary schools from 11% to 95%, junior high schools from 26% to 99%, and senior high schools from 43% to 99% (Market Data Retrieval, 1987). The rapid growth has produced problems of hardware incompatibility as well as a proliferation of educational software rushed to meet a burgeoning market.

Computer software can increase the availability of individualized, repeated practice in basic skills. Students may work individually or in small groups with drills and practice, freeing the teacher to work with other children, and thus increasing the amount of instructional time. For students with mild disabilities, the extra drill and practice can be very beneficial (Lieber & Semmel, 1985). However, the extent to which computer software programs can replace teacher instruction in initial skill acquisition has not been determined, and, effectiveness will depend in large part on the particular nature of the computer-driven curriculum selected.

In order to sift through the available software, the Trace Resource and Development Center at the University of Wisconsin, and Closing the Gap, of Henderson, Minnesota have collaborated with DLM Teaching Resources to publish a guide, *Apple Computer Resources in Special*

Education and Rehabilitation (DLM Teaching Resources, 1988a). This book provides the following:

1. Information on how computers can affect the lives of disabled students.
2. Descriptions of more than 1,000 products, publications, and services that exist to support disabled individuals using Apple computers (including hardware and adaptive devices; software; and information resources such as organizations, publications, networks, and directories).
3. An alphabetical listing of the more than 400 manufacturers of these products, publications, and services.

Computer applications are divided into six areas of functional impairment: physical, hearing, vision, cognitive, behavior, deaf-blindness. (DLM Teaching Resources, 1988b, p. 109)

With little available research on the comparative effectiveness of computer-supported adaptations, guidelines for selecting educational software include (a) evaluating the program with particular students in mind and (b) considering the content and mode of instruction, the demands placed on the student (c.f., academic levels, physical demands for use of keyboard, speed demands, accuracy demands), the type of feed-back provided, documentation, and motivation. Lewis and Doorlag (1987) and the MicroSIFT project of the Computer Technology Program Northwest Regional Educational Laboratory (1986) provide detailed evaluation procedures for use with educational software.

One of the most promising uses of computer technology is the use of software applications, especially word-processing programs, to provide needed prostheses for students with disabilities that make writing, rewriting, and correction a physically burdensome task, and for students with dyslexia and other disabilities that inhibit the acquisition of academic skills. Applications such as spell checkers, grammar checkers, and built-in calculation formulas should permit students to direct attention to the development of concepts and content rather than worrying over mechanics of expression (Meng, 1990). Computer technologies are also providing prostheses for disabilities of speech and locomotion, as well as providing the microtechnological heart of other adaptations for physical and sensory disabilities.

Computer technology has also increased the ease with which teachers can analyze data on student performance and then identify and compose educational goals and instructional objectives for curriculum management. Some of the commercially available software programs include the *Functional Skills Screening Inventory* (Becker, H., Schur, Paoletti-Schelp, & Hammer, 1988); *Test for Auditory Comprehension of Language* (Carrow-Woolfolk, 1985); *Pre-Mod II: Diagnosis and Remediation of*

Behavior Problems (Kaplan & Kent, 1986); *IEP Generator* (EBSCO, 1989); and *UNISTAR II+* (Lillie & Edwards, 1984). Empirical data on the benefits ascribed to these programs (e.g., "saves time") versus traditional methods, or in comparison with each other, or in terms of impact on services to children, are not available.

Two computer-based curricula for students with disabilities have been shown to offer significant assistance to teachers. *Project R.I.D.E. (Responding to Individual Differences in Education* (Beck, 1990)) includes a computer bank and video library of tactics and curriculum for reducing behavior problems and for teaching school strategy skills to students in preparation for mainstreaming, or to solve mainstreaming problems, or as interventions prior to referral for special education services. School strategy skills include the following: stays on task; completes schoolwork on time; completes schoolwork satisfactorily; follows oral instructions; completes schoolwork; pays attention; improves attendance; follows written directions from text; develops better attitude toward school; organizes materials; completes homework; follows written directions, from the blackboard; follows delayed oral directions; decreases tardiness; gets help; completes homework, turns homework in; completes homework satisfactorily; and copies from blackboard or book (Beck, 1990). Tactics included in the computer bank were selected from research journals and rewritten in language easily understood by practicing teachers, using a menu format. Teachers identify the topic and are provided with several alternative strategies. After teachers choose a strategy, the description includes an introduction, steps to carry out and monitor the procedure, special considerations, and an original source reference for the tactic. The video library presents short scenarios of implementation of the tactic in actual classrooms on videotapes. *Project R.I.D.E.* was evaluated in elementary schools over a 3-year period and resulted in (a) a 56% reduction in referrals to special education, (b) an increase from 46% to 80% of referred children later identified as eligible for services (reduction in "false positives"), and (c) data on individual students that indicated improvement in performance on behavior problems and academic strategy skills (Beck & Weast, in press).

The *HOTS: Higher Order Thinking Skills Project*, designed by University of Arizona professor Stanley Pogrow, is a computer-based curriculum used in conjunction with a trained teacher and designed to improve four key thinking skills: metacognition, inference from context, decontextualization, and information synthesis (Pogrow, 1989; 1990). The curriculum is a 2-year, ungraded sequence for primary students in remedial math and reading instruction. Evaluation results from three schools published in the *Education Monitor* (Capitol Publications, July, 1989) indicate that "at Jamestown Elementary School in Pennsylvania 11 [remedial] students gained 5.6 years on the Stanford Diagnostic Reading Test from fall to spring, and 20% of the remedial fifth and sixth graders were beyond 12th-grade level on the posttests; at Mary Dill Elementary School in Altar Valley, Arizona, 36% of the [remedial] students made the school honor role; and at Katherine Current Elementary in Hopkins, Minnesota, 10% of the [remedial] students were rediagnosed as gifted at the end of the year" (p. 1). The HOTS and RIDE programs indicate that the combination of computer retrieval of curricular interventions with teacher decision-making for individual application may be a powerful and appropriate extension of resources available to practitioners.

Recent Research and Trends

In the previous sections, research into the effectiveness of particular curricula has been described, but curriculum research can also take other approaches. First, follow-up studies of how the graduates of programs do is increasingly being used to evaluate programs. This quantitative method of evaluating curriculum may provoke changes in curricula of the future. Second, studies evaluating the quality of individual curricula by the achievement of students in individualized curricula, may propel changes in curricula.

Follow-Up Studies

Follow-up studies look at the long-term effect of curriculum. Darlington, Royce, Snipper, Murray, and Lazar (1980) looked at children who had attended infant and preschool programs in the 1960s (N = 1,599). These programs were provided for children who were developmentally delayed but who showed no neurological basis for delay. At the time of the follow-up, the children were aged 9 through 19. When compared with control children who did not attend the preschool programs, graduates of the preschool programs were less likely to have been assigned to special education (14% vs. 29%) and less likely to have failed a grade (24% vs. 45%), indicating that the curricula did have a long-term benefit. The curricula were varied but were based primarily on "the Bank Street child development model, on Montessori's methods, on Piagetian theory, [and] on Bereiter-Engelmann method" (Darlington et al., p. 202). In studies that compared the effects of different curricular models, the Bereiter-Engelmann model, Direct Instruction (Engelmann et al., 1978; Engelmann & Bruner, 1984; Silbert et al., 1981), has shown consistency successful results in improving academic performance of different groups of children (Becker, W. C., 1977; Gersten et al., 1987).

Halpern, Close, and Nelson (1986) followed up 596 graduates of 64 different programs designed to prepare people with intellectual disabilities to live "semi-independently." All of the graduates were living on the west coast of the United States at the time of the follow-up. About 17% had

IQs below 55, about 52% had IQs between 56 and 70, and about 31% had IQs above 70. (In the latter group, clients were generally older, having qualified under pre-1970 definitions.) At the time of follow-up, 86% were living in an apartment, house, duplex, or mobile home—the same situations in which the majority of the non-disabled population live. Twenty-six percent lived alone, and 56% lived with either a roommate, spouse, boyfriend/girlfriend, or child. Thirty-four percent were employed in normalized situations, either in a competitive position (25%), a subsidized position (4%), or a temporary position (5%); 39% were employed at a sheltered workshop; and 29% were unemployed. More of those employed in competitive positions were satisfied with their work than those employed in sheltered work situations. At the time of the study, the average mean income from work for the disabled was $190.78 per month, as compared to the average income of $1,219.00 for a citizen in the same region of the country. However, when income from work was combined with income from government assistance ($289.95), family and friends ($193.30), and other sources ($143.85), the mean total was $428.81 per month (range $0–$1,328), still only about one third of average monthly income.

A national survey of 1,119 facilities providing job placement in competitive, supported, or sheltered employment produced information on 112,996 developmentally disabled adults (Kiernan, McGaughey, & Schalock, 1986). According to this survey, 57.6% worked in sheltered employment, 5.6% were enrolled in job-training, 3.7% worked in supported employment, and 10.6% were competitively employed. In a detailed survey of a sample of 28,617 adults, curricula aimed at a specific job or trade was found to reduce unemployment and increase competitive and supported employment placements for mild, moderate or severe persons with intellectual disabilities (Kiernan et al., 1986). Table 6.2 depicts the effect of vocational training on employment. Data from this study indicate higher mean earnings from employment than reported by Halpern et al. (1986); however, in both cases the earnings are below the United States poverty level, which was established at $464 per month.

Edgar (1987) surveyed 360 graduates, dropouts, and ageouts from public school special education programs and categorized their current status as either employed and/or in school, or as no activity. He found that only 28% of those who dropped out of school were employed versus 48% of those who completed school, providing a 20% gain in employment attributable to education, less than the Halpern et al. (1986) study.

The concentration on vocational outcomes apparent in these follow-up studies implies that the success of a particular special program or curriculum can be effectively judged by the level of employment it produces. The three studies report unemployment varying from 14.1% (Kiernan et al., 1986) to 29% (Halpern et al., 1986) to 36% (Edgar, 1987). Differences in outcome must be carefully considered. Differences may be

TABLE 6.2 Effects of Vocational Curricula

Disability level	Before education*	After education*	Change as a result of education
	A. Competitive employment		
Severe/profound	0%	35.8%	+35.8%
Moderate	7%	43.6%	+36.7%
Mild	39%	54.8%	+15.8%
	B. Supported employment		
Severe/profound	7.8%	29.9%	+22.1%
Moderate	1.7%	17.6%	+15.9%
Mild	2.1%	14.1%	+12.0%
	C. Unemployment		
Severe/profound	40.3%	11.9%	−28.4%
Moderate	18.9%	15.5%	−3.4%
Mild	24.2%	11.3%	−12.9%

* Percentage of persons within each disability level.
(adapted from Kiernan, McGaughey, & Schalock, 1986.)

attributed to many sources, including the sample size (i.e., the sample in the Edgar study is 10% of the sample size in the Kiernan et al. study), regional differences in employment patterns, racial differences in employment, and age differences in employment. In addition, it is most likely that there are in reality two groups of students lumped together to produce the various statistics: students who met vocational curricula criteria and those who did not. If students did not pass objectives, or if student programs did not include vocational preparation skills, or if students were educated in programs without properly qualified teachers, outcomes may inaccurately attributed to curricula, when in reality curriculum is but one factor in successful programs.

Several curriculum changes could come about if the impact of curricula are evaluated by the employment status of the graduates. First, programs would be likely to begin vocational preparation earlier, perhaps resulting in a more open conflict between functionalists, academicists, and developmentalists, which could strengthen curriculum development. Second, vocational education for an individual could become increasingly limited to preparation for one specific type of job. Unfortunately, even now, most programs offer preparation for very simple, repetitive, semiskilled positions—most frequently for jobs as kitchen workers, janitors, and benchwork or assembly line workers (Kiernan et al., 1986; Rusch, 1986). It has often been assumed that the disabled are "simple-minded" and therefore would be content with simple repetitive jobs. This isn't the case. At a meeting in Sweden in 1970, a conference of people with intellectual disabilities avowed as follows:

We demand more training in a wider range of vocational fields so that we can have larger freedom of choice in determining our vocations.
We want to choose our vocations ourselves and have influence over our education.
We demand more interesting jobs.
We do not want to be used on our jobs by doing the worst and the most boring tasks we do at present.
We demand that our capacity for work should not be underestimated. (Blatt, 1987, p. 101)

Limited curricula means limited opportunity to choose work. Even now, very few surveys of working adults ask if people like their jobs. When Halpern et al. (1986) asked this, 44% of those competitively employed and 63% of those in sheltered employment said they wished they could have a different job. Of those unemployed, 67% said they were bored without a job to go to.

Follow-up studies offer useful data on the lives of students after they leave school, but those data alone are not sufficient to evaluate curricula. Robert Edgerton, a pioneer in the field of independent living and author of *The Cloak of Competence*, recently concluded: "I feel safe in saying that there is still no consensus about how training or education programs might best be designed to improve community adaptation" (Edgerton, 1986, p. 227). Other data, perhaps including client satisfaction with their lives and schooling, would also be useful in evaluating the long term impact of programs. However, so many factors affect the quality of adult lives that follow-up data will only provide a rough estimate of the impact of curricula.

IEP Studies

Individualized education plan (IEP) studies evaluate the objectives included in IEPs.

Billingsley (1984) examined IEPs of 22 students with severe or profound intellectual disabilities over a 2-year period. There was an average of 22 objectives per student per IEP. Billingsley found that about two thirds of the objectives specified functional skills, but less than 6% specified that the skill would be performed outside of school setting. Skills which can not be performed outside of the school situation will have very limited usefulness in the individual's lifecycle. Newer curricula, however, tend to emphasize the necessity of cross-setting instruction and evaluation.

Hilton and Liberty (1986) studied the IEPs of 16 students in integrated secondary programs with severe or profound disabilities over a 9-year period. The number of objectives changed only slightly from year to year. However, as students aged, progressively fewer objectives involved the student in active responding (e.g., setting the table) and a progressively larger proportion required only passive participation (e.g., attending school assemblies). Also, no curriculum objectives were directed at interactions with non-disabled peers. All of the students were part of integrated programs in public high schools.

Hunt, Goetz, and Anderson (1986) compared 3 IEPs constructed by each of six teachers who taught in integrated settings with 3 IEPs by each of six teachers who taught in segregated settings. Teachers of students who went to school with nonhandicapped students were more likely to write objectives that were rated as high quality (i.e., age appropriate, generalized, and functional) than teachers of students in segregated settings.

Downing (1988) examined IEPs of 35 students with severe or profound intellectual disabilities from six states, aged 3 to 20 years. Downing compared the quality of IEP objectives for two categories of students in her sample. She found that students with voluntary control of one hand sufficient to grasp and manipulate an object had more instructional objectives (26 vs. 14), had more objectives with objectively observable performance criteria (68% vs. 34%), and were less likely to have vague or staff-oriented objectives than students who did not possess object manipulation skills.[1]

The IEP studies have suggested that deficiencies in IEP objectives are a result of the procedures used to develop them. Banbury (1987) points out parts of the curriculum development process that might be at fault for poor IEPs:

1. Parent participation may be procedural rather than substantive.
2. Almost one half of general education teachers do not participate in IEPs for students mainstreamed in their classrooms.
3. Many special education teachers consider IEPs to be excessively time-consuming and unrelated to classroom instruction.
4. Many teachers also oppose making a commitment to specified outcomes, which is required in preparing the criteria contained in IEP objectives.
5. Many teachers are not professionally trained in developing individual curricula.

Banbury recommends that parents and teachers improve their communication, and that school districts assist teachers in the development of IEPs through provision of curriculum resources and assistance, and through feedback and follow-through techniques for evaluating and revis-

---

1. Passive objectives were defined as "objectives that state what staff will do to student and/or provide general information on what activities will be provided (e.g., Steve will be positioned in a standing table for 30 minutes, or Steve will participate in leisure activities)" (Downing, 1988, p. 198).

ing instructional objectives and classroom practices. The newer curricula also emphasize changes in the process of IEP development.

Continued evaluation of curriculum through IEP analysis can result both in a strengthening of overall curriculum and in methods that will improve individualization of curricula. In the United States, the publication in popular newspapers and magazines of standardized academic achievement test scores of nonhandicapped students increased public awareness of serious problems in education (The National Commission on Excellence in Education, 1983). Although questions about the validity and sampling of published scores remain, the public has accepted test score measures, and these are even used to compare schools within a single school district. Special educators have argued against using achievement test scores to evaluate the progress of students with disabilities, but the evaluation of educational progress through the curriculum is a fair estimate of the "product" of educational programs.

The IEP *is* the curriculum for students with disabilities. Therefore, a measure of achievement for a student with an individualized curriculum (e.g., an IEP) would be the proportion of objectives passed each year. The intent of the enabling legislation is that the student make "satisfactory progress" (Education for All Handicapped Children Act of 1975). Recently, a judge defined "satisfactory progress" as passing "the majority" of objectives (*In re* Mandy C., 1985; *In re* Benjamin F., 1985; *In re* Keith S., 1985). It has been argued by school district officials that student progress from one year to the next, or across students, cannot be compared because the content of the objectives differ (Help for Retarded Children, 1986; Hill, 1986a, 1986b). IEP objectives, if properly written, describe the skills the student is expected to achieve in a school year, in a fashion similar to the objectives set in core curriculum for students in regular programs. Just as achievement test scores can record the level of reading or math achievement of a student in comparison with the curricular goals set for them, the proportion of IEP objectives passed can be a record of the achievement of a child with disabilities. Of course it is possible that the IEP is poorly written or not properly matched to the student's needs; achievement data will provide excellent feedback to the teacher and administrator about program and student needs so that such problems can be corrected. Comparisons made across children are relevant indicators of the degree of a programs' overall achievement, just as achievement test scores or university entrance scores or other measures are used to compare schools or programs of general education.

Hilton and Liberty (1986) reported on the proportion of objectives passed each year by students. The average dropped from 50% of IEP objectives passed by a student in the primary classes to 6% of objectives passed in the secondary school year. During the final year of the evaluation, when students were in the final years of the secondary program, none of the 16 students passed any objectives. A second group of students with less severe disabilities showed similar patterns of failure. In investigating factors related to the achievement of the students, Hilton and Liberty (1986) found that, because of a continuing shortage of teachers prepared to teach students with severe handicaps, the teachers preparing the current IEPs had not generally been professionally prepared to construct or implement curricula for students with severe handicaps, although all were certified under state guidelines and that most parents had not been involved in the construction of the IEPs from the beginning. The results of the Hilton and Liberty (1986) evaluation suggest that Banbury's (1987) conclusions affect not only the quality of the IEP objectives and the curriculum for the individual, but subsequent student achievement as well. Therefore, it is very important that IEPs be carefully constructed, or student achievement will certainly suffer.

Curriculum Strategies for Integrated Lifecycle Services

Curriculum development for individuals with disabilities has progressed from curricula that did little except list care to be provided to curricula that provide for skill development needed for semi-independent community living for adult graduates. Curriculum materials have progressed from sets of objectives supposedly suitable for all students in a segregated program to materials which carefully describe assessment and development procedures for individually tailored curriculum plans. Curriculum procedures have progressed from those specifying training in the classroom in a limited number of skills to training functional skills in a variety of environments, most notably environments in which individuals with disabilities can learn with individuals without disabilities. The development of curriculum for the lifecycle involves strategies which must be interwoven to produce a successful curriculum that prepares the student for community living. These strategies are described in the this section.

Professional Integration for Educational Planning

As Banbury (1987) has pointed out, parent participation in curriculum planning is unfortunately usually merely a matter of signing forms provided by the school. It is of the utmost necessity to involve parents from the very beginning in a substantial role. Beginning in the child's infancy, goals should be developed with parental involvement. As adolescence approaches, the child should become a full participant in the planning.

In addition to parents, professionals from many disciplines should participate in planning on a regular basis (Turnbull, Strickland, & Brantley, 1982). Professionals should be selected on the basis of the needs of the child. For example, if physical therapy is a vital component of the services needed by the child, then a physical therapist should participate in identifying educational goals. Likewise, if medical problems and/or medication need to be considered in planning education, a physician should participate in the educational planning. In this fashion, the needs of the child are used as a basis for creating a multidisciplinary team for educational planning. The team should jointly determine all objectives, with each professional contributing information and refinements. Currently, professionals often work independently, so that an IEP might contain objectives for physical therapy written by the physical therapist, communication objectives prepared by the speech and language therapist, and skill acquisition objectives prepared by the classroom teacher. An integrated IEP objective would be one in which information, suggestions, and techniques from each professional are combined. For example, the physical therapist should provide information, techniques, prosthetics, and so forth, for positioning the student throughout the day during instructional periods in skills and in communication. Physical therapy for 15 minutes a day, two or three times per week, is simply not as effective as proper positioning throughout every day. The physical therapist can also provide information on what types of physical responses are the easiest for the student to make—information that can be used by the communication specialist in designing a nonverbal communication program. The physical therapist can contribute information on relaxation and contractures during skill instruction for the objectives of the classroom teacher. The communication specialist can work with both the teacher and the therapist to ensure that communication objectives are implemented throughout the day. The classroom teacher can benefit from the information from both co-professionals, as well as assist the communication specialist in defining referent objects and events that are part of the student's daily routine.

Long-Term Goals With a Top-Down Approach

From the first day of education, curricula should be founded on a plan for fostering the development of skills and character for the individual's life cycle—a life to be lived with others in a community, which includes a normal school-based education. Adopting the top-down approach will provide a foundation for establishing the goals of education for each individual, for assessing the student to determine what to include in the curriculum, for selecting curriculum materials, and for the evaluation of student progress. Currently, the top-down approach is usually initiated in early adolescence and only for students with the most severe disabilities. Implementing this approach at the point of identification of the need for special education services, even as early as birth, would provide a focus of coordination for curriculum throughout the life cycle.

Long-term goals would be established for each step in the life cycle, including different levels of schooling as well as target environments for when the individual leaves school. Identifying long-term school goals might be as straightforward as identifying placement with nondisabled children in the next grade level in the community school, or entrance into a particular work-study vocational training program. In addition to goals regarding educational placement, goals regarding desirable outcomes of education for adult living would be identified. Of course, for young children, it will be impossible to detail exact environments for adult living and employment, but as the child grows up, goals such as "live independently" and "be employed" might evolve into "live in an apartment with a roommate" and "work at a photocopy center." Information on the student's likes and dislikes, skills and deficits, as well as on community resources, can be used to reformulate and define goals during scheduled evaluations, as discussed below.

The top-down approach can fit with any philosophical model of curriculum. For example, the top-down approach can easily incorporate developmental milestones. If one future educational goal is for the student to live in an apartment with a roommate, and one skill needed for that is loading a dishwasher, an analysis of the physical skills required will include most of the fine motor skills included in developmental curricula. In point of fact, almost all of the skills included in a developmental curriculum will be needed for integrated living. However, with a top-down approach, the rationale for selecting skills for instruction changes. The rationale for a developmental approach is usually to facilitate normal development in a non-normally developing child, but there is no direction or goal for what is to be accomplished if/when normal developmental milestones are achieved, or for what should be done if they are not. Adopting the top-down approach provides the foundation for the goal environments and situations targeted for achievement at the conclusion of formal education. It provides a criterion against which the selection of developmental milestones can be tested. Thus, the difference in educating infants and young children resulting from the top-down strategy might not be apparent in the content of specific objectives; it will, however, be apparent in the assessment, rationale, and progress evaluation of curriculum. (If the child were developing normally, specialized curricula would not even be considered.)

Ecological Assessments

The student's performance at the time at which curriculum is being planned must be compared with the performance needed in the "top" environments, whether those environments are a sheltered workshop, fifth grade, a resource room, or independent apartment living (Browder, 1987; Deno & Mirkin, 1977). An adequate assessment is one in which the student is given the opportunity to perform each skill sequence in the target setting, or in a simulation of the target setting, with the materials and natural distractions and features of that situation. Persons other than the teacher should be involved in the assessment, unless it is clear that the student will only perform for one or two people (this is a clear indication of the types of strategies needed in the educational setting). Prompts should be withheld until it is clear that the student is not going to perform without them (this is critical to sound educational planning).

Establishing Individual Educational Objectives

The next strategy in planning curriculum is to establish educational objectives for each individual. Long-range goals will be correlates of the goal environments identified in the top-down approach. Individual education objectives will define what the teacher and support staff will teach during the period between formal evaluations. Objectives specifying exactly what progress is aimed for during each school year support the educational goals.

Educators should take a proactive position in establishing procedures that support the individualization of objectives. Although goals may be similar across students, the heterogeneity of the disabled population usually means that the skill levels of individual students within a classroom group will vary considerably. Curriculum must be developed by comparing the skills the student needs to achieve the long-term goals with the skills he now has, and instructing or providing prosthetics or adaptives to fill the gap. This is a difficult task for many educators. As Banbury (1987) pointed out, many IEPs are deficient in individualization. In most classrooms, educational objectives are selected to fit into a schedule (e.g., playing a game is selected because the student is scheduled for physical education), or because of categorization of domains in a particular curriculum (e.g., one objective is written for communication, self-help, prevocational, gross motor) or for each academic skill area (e.g., reading, arithmetic, science, social studies) or because of resource allocations (e.g., the bus will take everyone bowling on Fridays, so bowling becomes an objective for each student). The establishment of long-term goals and the use of an ecological assessment procedure, in which the student's skills are compared with those required in the goal environments, would be the first step in ensuring individualization (cf. Brown et al., 1979; Deno, Mirkin, & Wesson, 1983; Fuchs, Fuchs, & Hamlett, 1989).

Balance Objectives for Instruction

A more careful and realistic approach is needed in establishing priority among objectives selected for the individual and between individuals. Instructional time is limited, and it is simply not realistic to expect that 15 objectives for 10 children can be instructed successfully on a daily basis.

A more thoughtful and pragmatic approach to selecting objectives and coordinating daily schedules will improve the achievement of children with disabilities.

Selecting Curricular Materials

Because the top-down approach does not require any particular curricular model, it is important to select curriculum materials that are directed at the specific skill that is to be instructed. All too often in practice, the reverse procedure is followed. A teacher sees an interesting set of materials or inherits from a previous teacher a set of materials, or a videotape, or some computer software, and if it is appealing, the teacher then writes objectives for teaching the material to the student. This is why one can now observe students with severe disabilities operating switches to make toy monkeys bang toy drums. Unfortunately, teachers are as susceptible to trends as anyone else, and curriculum fads continue to impede education. Develop the goals, and then find the materials.

IEP Progress Evaluations

During yearly progress evaluations, the goals will be refined, modified, or changed, based on a comparison between the student's current level of performance and that established for passing the objective. Then, each objective is evaluated as being passed or not. Following this evaluation-by-objective, decisions are made regarding the objectives to be instructed during the subsequent year.

In addition to establishing the yearly objectives, teachers, parents and administrators should discuss the student's achievement toward the long-term goals annually. If the student is passing objectives at a satisfactory rate each year, it would seem advisable to continue with the long-term goals previously established. If the student is passing goals at a faster rate, perhaps the expectations should be raised. If, in the worst case, the student's pass rate is low, then significant changes in instructional strategies are warranted. Rather than reduce goal expectations, more powerful instructional strategies can be implemented. If, however, several successive evaluations demonstrate continued problems, then the professional team may wish to consider revising the long-term goals. It may be helpful to keep a chart, similar to that shown in Figure 6.1, with the student's permanent record.

Overall Program Evaluation

A crucial strategy is to evaluate the overall success of the program. Program success can be evaluated by looking at the rate of passing IEP objectives over time and across students (as illustrated in Figure 6.2).

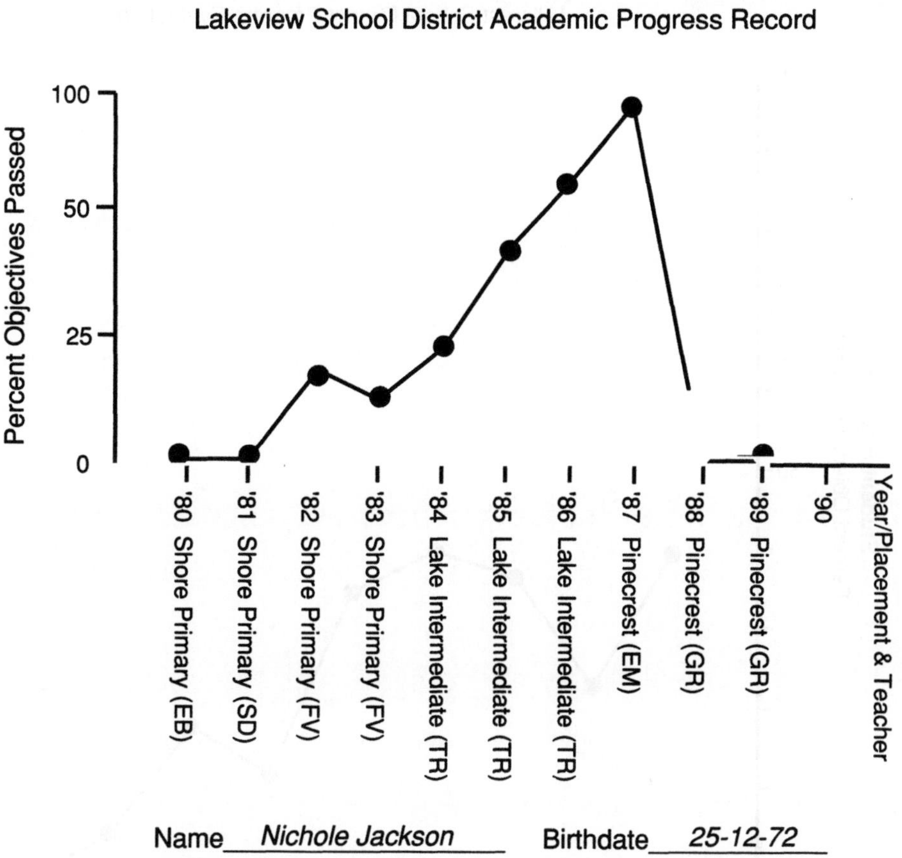

FIGURE 6.1. Illustration of longitudinal record of academic progress based on individualized education plan (IEP) of a student with profound intellectual disabilities and dual sensory impairments (adapted from Haring & Liberty, 1990).

There are some patterns that can be recognized and used to revise the program. First, if all students are passing almost all objectives, the program should be evaluated to determine whether students are being sufficiently challenged by the quality and quantity of the objectives set for or with them, and to determine whether expectations should be raised. One might also consider exporting the instructional and curricular strategies to weaker programs serving similar types of students. If on the other hand, almost all students are passing less than half of their objectives, the program should be evaluated to determine if objectives are individualized, if they are appropriate, and whether the most powerful teaching strategies are in use. Or if most students are passing less than 10% of

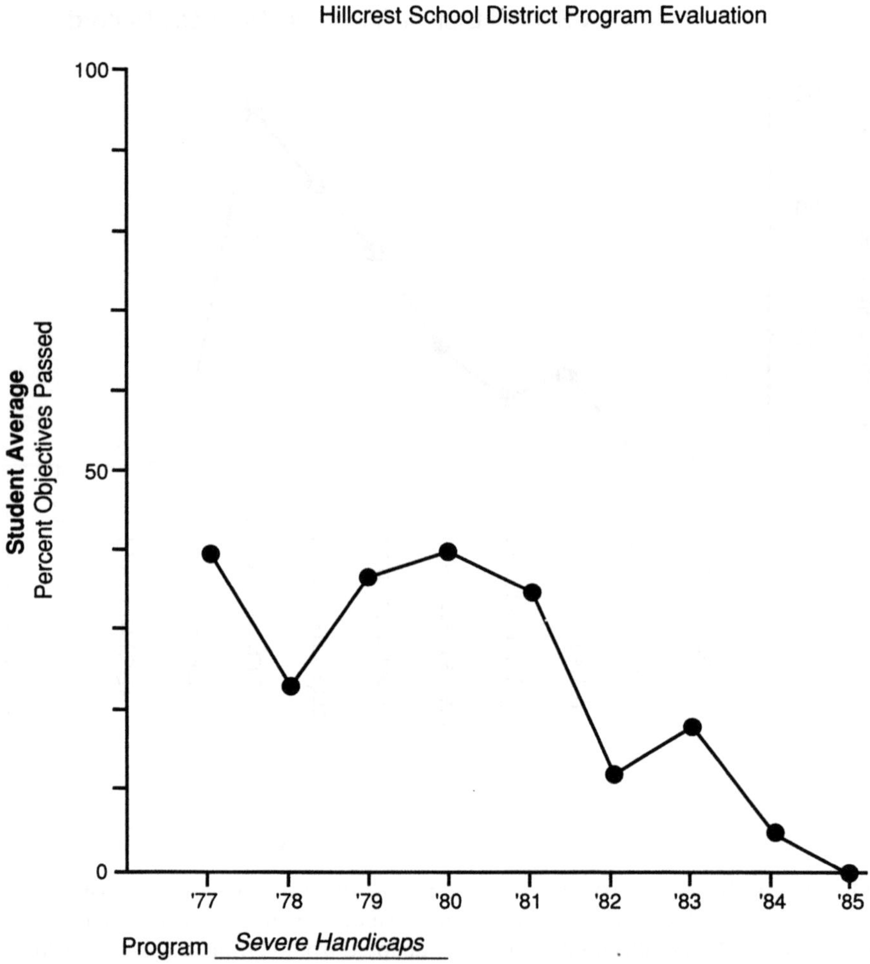

FIGURE 6.2. Example of actual longitudinal record of program success in instruction of learners with disabilities to meet individual goals and objectives (adapted from Hilton & Liberty, 1986).

their objectives, serious problems in the program should be identified and corrected as soon as possible.

Together, application of these strategies will improve the quality of each child's education by ensuring that curricula are truly individualized. In the short run, implementing such strategies may be time-consuming and difficult; in the long run, such techniques are the only conceivable route to graduating students with disabilities with the skills they need to be employed and accepted in their communities.

Future Trends and Issues

The drive toward integration and the development of powerful instructional strategies have propelled the significant changes in curriculum over the past two decades. They will continue to influence curriculum in the future, but with significant differences.

The impact of the powerful new instructional strategies for skill development has resulted in a proliferation of curricula for specific, observable, practical, skills—skills that can successfully be taught even to students with profound disabilities using the new teaching techniques. In the future, curricula will address skills that are more difficult to observe and quantify with current tools, and will include provisions for expanding skills across settings to increase their pragmatic value.

Pragmatic Integration

Curricula have been affected by the values that drive the push for integration—values reflected in the increasing availability of materials designed to educate people about individuals with disabilities, and their participation in the mainstream of education. In the future, curricula will increasingly reflect the pragmatics associated with integration—the problems encountered in communication, social skills, study skills, behavior problems, and the need for adaptations in the general curriculum.

Decision Making

Recently, curricula for teaching decision-making skills have been developed. Instruction in the use of self-instruction, self-monitoring, and self-reinforcement strategies is instruction in how to make decisions about managing one's own behavior (Lagomarcino, Hughes, & Rusch, 1989). These curricula will continue to be developed with increasing sophistication. In addition, for students with severe and profound disabilities, choice-making curricula are beginning of explore how one can teach decision-making skills to a more disabled group. Currently, such choice-making curricula provide only the opportunity to make minor decisions, such as which toy to play with or which music to listen to; but over time, systems to provide for the development of more powerful decision making should be developed (Liberty, 1989).

Adult Options

Curricula will also continue to be developed to reflect the increasing range of options available to adults with disabilities: not just curricula to prepare an individual for a variety of jobs, or types of workplaces, but curricula to increase independence and teach independent decision making in such areas as health care choices, clothing selection, deciding to work with a particular professional or accept a special service, financial decisions, and leisure time and employment choices.

Interactive Curricula

Integration of children with disabilities into settings and classrooms serving children without disabilities has served to highlight the areas where curricula must be developed: curricula to teach reciprocated communication skills to provide for interactive integration, not just one-way communication, or communication based on interpretation of behavior, and curricula to teach interactive reciprocal play, study, and learning skills. The development of such curricula will be preceded by research, because we have only begun to understand roles and relationships that occur in interactions. For example, in order to teach a student to engage and maintain a conversation with a peer, we must first understand the nature, structure, and sequence of conversation. The translation of current research into curricula will accelerate change.

Friendship Curricula

In the future, the integration and normalization emphasis, supported by the new instructional technologies, should result in expanding the social curriculum to include developing and maintaining reciprocal friendships with neighbors, classmates, and siblings, and in developing loving relationships as well. This is especially critical in early education programs, where a hug or a sign from a child with disabilities toward his parent would probably do more to maintain the quality of parent–child interactions than any intervention provided by an outside agency. We can also see, from studies of the elderly, the disabling effects of loneliness. What would be the purpose of teaching individuals with disabilities vocational skills and domestic skills, if the fundamental skills needed for interpersonal relationships were missing? This is a critical and complicated curricula area, but one that is now under development.

Holistic Curricula

In addition to reciprocal relationships, curricula will recycle to include the "whole child" once again. The appropriately increased attention to the perspective of the individual with disabilities, and the dimensions of study added by the adoption of the ethnographic research methodology, will focus attention on the emotional and moral development of the individual. Curricula designed to facilitate basic moral and ethical values of modern society will be developed—for teaching about lying, stealing, assault, due process protections, and so on. These are the shared values of society, and ones that must be included in an overall curriculum approach to lifecycle services.

As children disabled by abuse and neglect come to school in greater and greater numbers, and as the number of children classified as severely emotionally disturbed increases, it is becoming evident that education will not be successful until it is able to help these children develop emotionally. Even as debate continues on the best approach (e.g., behavioral vs. Freudian vs. Rogerian), and whether or not schools must pay for such services, teachers are trying to cope with children. Teachers find that they must deal with the emotional problems and the related impacts on self-concept before more conventional types of instruction are possible.

Most religions (e.g., Buddhism, Roman Catholicism, Episcopalianism) have not developed curricula for the religious or spiritual instruction for many people with disabilities, especially for people with intellectual disabilities. As moral education assumes greater importance in the education of children without disabilities, it is expected to affect children with disabilities as well, and religious and moral curricula will develop.

Conclusions

The changes in curricula mirror societal changes in the roles and perceptions of individuals with disabilities. Curriculum is in the process of evolving from concern with controlling behavior of individuals with disabilities and reinforcing caretakers by obedience, cleanliness, and passivity, to a curriculum designed to provide power to people with disabilities. Instead of asking the disabled child to choose between two toys, the child will be able to decide where, when, how, and with whom he wants to play. Instead of assigning students to a sheltered workshop, work-related curricula will be geared to the choices and preferences of the individual, not just to his skills and needs. Instead of ignoring emotional and sexual development, curricula will help the individual develop as fully as possible in all areas. In the past, curriculum and instruction have worked to counter independence by fostering learned helplessness and prompt dependence (Dweck, 1975). Now, however, curriculum and instruction are changing to focus on independence from the perspective of the person with disabilities. Increasingly, people with disabilities will work with people without disabilities in establishing areas for research and in public policy development.

Power to the people is more than just a slogan. It is a reality that is accelerating in the United States, as people with disabilities enter the mainstream of politics and public life. This is one triumphant sign that the struggle to match individual curricula to individual needs within the context of a changing society struggling toward equality is beginning to succeed.

Summary

Curriculum development is influenced by the societal expectations for the development and eventual role of disabled individuals, by the educational goals for the individual student, by the approach to curriculum, and by practical considerations. Current curricular practices in the United States reflect the multiplicity imposed by individualization and changing expectations. Recent research has emphasized outcome measures to gauge the effectiveness of curriculum and instruction, while using critical examination of individual education plans to provide overall pictures of the quality of current curriculum decisions. Developing a curriculum for integrated lifecycle services will include fostering spirited family and multidisciplinary team participation, as well as the participation of the individual with disabilities in a more active role; developing longitudinal and comprehensive planning; and adopting evaluation standards to provide for timely adjustments and changes. As individuals with disabilities play, learn, and work in our community neighborhoods, day-care centers, schools, and businesses, our curriculum will become more individualized and diverse, at once focusing pragmatically on the skills and competencies needed by the individual, and on the growth and development of the "whole person." The lifecycle approach will include not only the dimension of time but also the dimensions of self.

References

Abt Associates. (1976). *Education as experimentation: A planned variation model* (Vol. 3). Cambridge, MA: Author.

Abt Associates. (1977). *Education as experimentation: A planned variation model* (Vol. 4). Cambridge, MA: Author.

Aeschleman, S.R., & Schladenhauffen, J. (1984). Acquisition, generalization and maintenance of grocery shopping skills by severely mentally retarded adolescents. *Applied Research in Mental Retardation*, *5*, 245–258.

Bairstow, P., Cohrane, R., & Rusk, I. (1991). Selection of children with cerebral palsy for Conductive Education and the characteristics of children judged suitable and unsuitable. *Development Medicine and Child Neurology*, *33*, 984–992.

Baldwin, V.I. (1976). Curriculum concerns. In M.A. Thomas (Ed.), *HEY, don't forget about me! Education's investment in the severely, profoundly, and multiply handicapped* (pp. 64–73). Reston, VA: Council for Exceptional Children.

Banbury, M. (1987). The IEP revisited: A look at the concept and the reality. In A. Rotatori, M. Banbury, & R.A. Fox (Eds.), *Issues in special education* (pp. 42–50). Mountain View, CA: Mayfield.

Baumgart, D., Brown, L., Pumpian, I., Nisbet, J., Ford, A., Sweet, M., Messina, R., & Schroeder, J. (1982). Principle of partial participation and individualized adaptations in educational programs for severely handicapped students. *The Journal of the Association for the Severely Handicapped*, 7(2), 17–27.

Bax, M. (1991). Conductive Education. *Developmental Medicine and Child Neurology*, *33*, 941–942.

Beck, R. (1990). *Responding to Individual Differences in Education*. Longmont, CO: Sopris West Publishing Co.

Beck R. (1991). Project RIDE. *Teaching Exceptional Children*, *23*(2), 60–61.

Beck, R., & Weast, J.D. (in press). Project R.I.D.E.: A staff development model for accommodating "at risk" students. *Phi Delta Kappan*.

Becker, H., Schur, S., Paoletti-Schelp, M., & Hammer, E. (1988). *Functional skills screening inventory: Criterion referenced behavioral checklist* [Computer program]. Portland, OR: ASIEP Education Company.

Becker, W.C. (1977). Teaching reading and language to the disadvantaged: What we have learned from field research? *Harvard Educational Review*, *47*(4), 518–543.

Becker, W.C., & Carnine, D.W. (1980). Direct instruction: An effective approach to educational intervention with the disadvantaged and low performers. In B.B. Lahey & A.E. Kazdin (Eds.), *Advances in clinical child psychology* (Vol. 3, pp. 429–473). New York: Plenum.

Bellamy, G.T., Horner, R.H., & Inman, D.P. (1979). *Vocational habilitation of severely retarded adults: A direct service technology*. Baltimore: University Park Press.

Billingsley, F.F. (1984). Where are the generalized outcomes? An examination of instructional objectives. *Journal of the Association for Persons With Severe Handicaps*, *9*(3), 186–192.

Blatt, B. (1987). *The conquest of mental retardation*. Austin, TX: Pro-Ed.

Browder, D.M. (1987). *Assessment of individuals with severe handicaps*. Baltimore: Paul H. Brookes.

Brown, L., Branston, M.B., Hamre-Nietupski, S., Pumpian, I., Certo, N., & Gruenewald, L.A. (1979). A strategy for developing chronological age appropriate and functional curricular content for severely handicapped adolescents and young adults. *Journal of Special Education*, *13*, 81–90.

Brown, L., Nietupski, J., & Hamre-Nietupski, S. (1976a). Criterion of ultimate functioning. In M.A. Thomas (Ed.), *HEY, don't forget about me! Education's investment in the severely, profoundly, and multiply handicapped* (pp. 2–15). Reston, VA: Council for Exceptional Children.

Brown, L., Nietupski, J., & Hamre-Nietupski, S. (1976b). The criterion of ultimate functioning and public school services for severely handicapped students. In N. Certo, K. Belmore, T. Crowner, & L. Brown (Eds.), *Madison Avenue alternative for zero exclusion: Papers and programs related to public school serivce for secondary age severely handicapped students* (Vol. 6, Part 1). Madison, WI: Department of Specialized Educational Services, Madison Public Schools.

Bruininks, R.H., & Warfield, G. (1978). The mentally retarded. In E. L. Meyen (Ed.), *Exceptional children and youth: An introduction*. Denver, CO: Love.
Bulletin of Conductive Education, Queensland, Australia: Special Education Resource and Development Centre, 72 Cornwall Street, Annerley, Queenstown.
Camp, B.W., & Bash, M.A.S. (1988a). *Think aloud: Classroom program (Grades 1–2)*. Champaign, IL: Research Press.
Camp, B.W., & Bash, M.A.S. (1988b). *Think aloud: Classroom program (Grades 3–4)*. Champaign, IL: Research Press.
Camp, B.W., & Bash, M.A.S. (1988c). *Think aloud: Classroom program (Grades 5–6)*. Champaign, IL: Research Press.
Camp, B.W., & Bash, M.A.S. (1988d). *Think aloud: Small group program*. Champaign, IL: Research Press.
Campbell, M.M., Hintz, P.E., & Sasso, G.M. (1983). *Severely Handicapped Integration Program: Attitude change curricula* (Vol. 4, junior high level). Kansas City, KS: University of Kansas, Department of Special Education, Severely Handicapped Integration Project.
Capitol Publications. (1989, July). *Education Monitor: The National Digest of Education Information*.
Carrow-Woolfolk, E. (1985). *Test for auditory comprehension of language (TACL–R)* (rev. ed.). Allen, TX: DLM Teaching Resources.
Cawley, J., Goodstein, H., Fitzmaurice, A., Sedlak, R., & Althans, V. (1976). *Project math: A program of the mainstream series*. Wallingford, CT: Educational Services.
Clark, P.A., & Cozad, S.K. (1983). *Severely Handicapped Integration Program: Adult curriculum and mini-modules* (Vol. 2). Kansas City, KS: University of Kansas, Department of Special Education, Severely Handicapped Integration Project.
Clark, P.A., & Fiedler, C.R. (1983). *Severely Handicapped Integration Program: Attitude change curricula* (Vol. 5, senior high level). Kansas City, KS: University of Kansas, Department of Special Education Severely Handicapped Integration Project.
Clay, M. (1985). *The early detection of reading difficulties*. Auckland: Heinemann Publishers.
Clay, M. (1987). Implementing Reading Recovery: Systemic adaptations to an educational innovation. *New Zealand Journal of Educational Studies*, *22*(1), 55–58.
Clay, M. (1990). The Reading Recovery Programme, 1984–1988: Coverage, outcomes and Education Board district figures. *New Zealand Journal of Educational Studies*, *25*(1), 61–70.
Clay, M., & Tuck, B. (1991). *A study of Reading Recovery subgroups*. Unpublished research report. Wellington: Ministry of Education.
Cottam, P.J., & Sutton, A. (1986). *Conductive Education: A system for overcoming motor disorders*. London: Croom Helm. p. 41
Cozad, S., Fiedler, C.R., Novak, C.G., Simpson, R.L., & Werth, K.B. (1983). *Severely Handicapped Integration Program: Introduction and resources* (Vol. 1). Kansas City, KS: University of Kansas, Department of Special Education, Severely Handicapped Integration Project.

Cozad, S., Hintz, P.E., Novak, C.G., & Campbell, M.M. (1983). *Severely Handicapped Integration Program: Interaction activities* (Vol. 6). University of Kansas, Department of Special Education, Severely Handicapped Integration Project.

Darlington, R.B., Royce, J.M., Snipper, A.S., Murray, H.W., & Lazar, I. (1980). Preschool programs and later school competence of children from low-income families. *Science*, *208*(11), 202–204.

Deno, S.L., & Mirkin, P.K. (1977). *Data-based program modification: A manual.* Reston, VA: Council for Exceptional Children.

Deno, S.L., Mirkin, P.K., & Wesson, C. (1983). How to write effective data-based IEPs. *Teaching Exceptional Children*, *16*, 99–104.

DLM Teaching Resources. (Eds.). (1988a). *Apple computer resources in special education and rehabilitation.* Allen, TX: Author.

DLM Teaching Resources. (1988b). *1988 Comprehensive Catalog.* Allen, TX: Author.

Downing, J. (1988). Active versus passive programming: A critique of IEP objectives for students with the most severe disabilities. *Journal of the Association for Persons with Severe Handicaps*, *13*(3), 197–201.

Duvall, B. (1981). *Learn to write: Italic style.* Great Falls, MT: Can Do.

Dweck, C.S. (1975). The role of expectations and attributions in the alleviation of learned helplessness. *Journal of Personality and Social Psychology*, *31*(4), 674–685.

EBSCO. (1989). *IEP generator* [Computer program]. *EBSCO curriculum materials: Instructional programs and materials* [Computer Program]. Birmingham, AL: Author.

Edgar, E. (1987). Secondary programs in special education: Are many of them justifiable? *Exceptional Children*, *53*(6), 555–561.

Edgerton, R. (1986). [Review of *On my own: The impact of semi-independent living programs for adults with mental retardation*]. *Journal of the Association for Persons with Severe Handicaps*, *11*(3), 225–227.

Education for All Handicapped Children Act of 1975, §602, 20 U.S.C. §1402.

Engelmann, S., Becker, W., Hanner, S., & Johnson, G. (1978). *Corrective reading program.* Chicago: Science Research Associates.

Engelmann, S., & Bruner, E. (1984). *DISTAR reading program.* Chicago: Science Research Associates.

Falvey, M.A. (1986) *Community-based curriculum: Instructional strategies for students with severe handicaps.* Baltimore: Paul H. Brookes.

Freagon, S., Wheeler, J., McDannel, K., Brankin, G., & Costello, D. (1983). *Individual student community life skill profile system for severely handicapped students.* DeKalb, IL: Northern Illinois University and DeKalb County Special Education Association.

Fredericks, H.D., Riggs, C., Furey, T., Grove, D., Moore, W., McDonnell, J., Jordan, E., Hanson, W., Baldwin, V., & Wadlow, M. (1978). *The Teaching Research curriculum for moderately and severely handicapped* (3rd ed.). Springfield, IL: Charles C. Thomas.

Fuchs, L.S., Fuchs, D., & Hamlett, C.L. (1989). Effects of instrumental use of curriculum-based measurement to enhance instructional programs. *Remedial and Special Education*, *10*(2), 43–52.

Gersten, R., Carnine, D., & Woodward, J. (1987). Direct instruction research: The third decade. *Remedial and Special Education*, *8*(6), 48–56.

Gold, M.W. (1972). Stimulus factors in skill training of the retarded on a complex assembly task: Acquisition, transfer, and retention. *American Journal of Mental Deficiency*, *76*, 517–526.

Gold, M.W. (1980). *Try another way: Training manual*. Champaign, IL: Research Press.

Gold, M.W., & Barclay, C.R. (1973). The learning of difficult visual discriminations by the moderately and severely retarded. *Mental Retardation*, *11*(2), 9–11.

Hagin, R.A. (1983). Write right—or left: A practical approach to handwriting. *Journal of Learning Disabilities*, *18*, 266–271.

Halpern, A.S., Close, D.W., & Nelson, D.J. (1986). *On my own: The impact of semi-independent living programs for adults with mental retardations*. Baltimore: Paul H. Brookes.

Hari, M., & Akos, K. (1988). *Conductive Education*. London: Routledge.

Help for retarded children. (1986, November 19). *The Oregonian*, p. B6.

Hill, A. (1986a, Novermber 21). Study faulting handicapped instruction under fire. *The Oregonian*, p. 1.

Hill, A. (1986b, December 17). Report on handicapped adopted. *The Oregonian*, p. E10.

Hilton, A., & Liberty, K.A. (1986, Novermber). *Analysis of progress of integrated secondary students with profound mental retardation*. Paper presented at the Association for Persons with Severe Handicaps Annual Convention, San Francisco, CA.

Hirsch, E.D. Jr. (1989). The primal scene of education. *The New York Review of Books*, *36*(3), 29–35.

House, E.R., Glass, G.V. McLean, L.D., & Walker, D.C. (1978). No simple answer: Critique of the "Follow Through" evaluation. *Harvard Education Review*, *48*, 128–160.

Hunt, P., Goetz, L., & Anderson, J. (1986). The quality of IEP objectives associated with placement on integrated versus segregated school sites. *Journal of the Association for Persons with Severe Handicaps*, *11*(2), 125–130.

In re Mandy C., Administrative law judge post-hearing brief (Special Education Cause No. 85–16, 1985).

In re Benjamin F., Administrative law judge post-hearing brief (Special Education Cause No. 85–22, 1985).

In re Keith S., Administrative law judge post-hearing brief (Special Education Cause No. 85–17, 1985).

Joyce, B., & Showers, B. (1983). *Power in staff development through research on training*. Alexandria, VA: Association for Supervision and Curriculum Development.

Kaplan, J., & Kent, S. (1986). *Pre-mod II: Diagnosis and remediation of behavior problems* [Computer program]. Portland, OR: ASIEP Education Company.

Kiernan, W.E., McGaughey, M.J., & Schalock, R.L. (1986). *Employment survey for adults with development disabilities: A national survey*. Boston: Developmental Evaluation Clinic, Children's Hospital.

Kugel, R.B., & Wolfensberger, W.E. (1969). *Changing patterns in residential services for the mentally retarded.* Washington, DC: U.S. Government Printing Office.

Lagomarcino, T.R., Hughes, C., & Rusch, F.R. (1989). Utilizing self-management to teach independence on the job. *Education and Training in Mental Retardation, 24*(2), 139–148.

Lewis, R.B., & Doorlag, D.H. (1987). *Teaching special students in the mainstream* (2nd ed.) Columbus, OH: Charles E. Merrill.

Liberty, K. (1989). *Answering questions with yes or no.* Unpublished manuscript, University of Washington, College of Education, Seattle, WA.

Liberty, K.A., Brodie, J., Young, D., & Berkeley, M. (1991, November). *Evaluation of Conductive Education for Children with Motor Disabilities: First Results from the Dunedin Programme.* Paper presented at: the annual conference of the New Zealand Association for Research in Education, Dunedin.

Lieber, J., & Semmel, M. (1985). Effectiveness of computer application to instruction with mildly handicapped learners: A review. *Remedial and Special Education, 6*(5), 5–12.

Lillie, D.L., & Edwards, J.D. (1984). *UNISTAR II+* [Computer program]. Portland, OR: ASIEP Education Company.

Market Data Retrieval. (1987). *Microcomputers for student instruction in elementary and secondary school: 1981 to 1986* [Published and unpublished data]. Shelton, CT: Market Data Retrieval.

Meng, B. (1990, September). With a little help from my Mac. *Macworld*, pp. 181–188.

MicroSIFT Project, Computer Technology Program, Northwest Regional Educational Laboratory (1986). *Evaluator's guide for microcomputer-based instructional packages (sixth revision).* Eugene, OR: International Council for Computers in Education.

National Commission on Excellence in Education. (1983). *A nation at risk: The imperative for education reform.* Washington, DC: U.S. Government Printing Office.

Neel, R.S., & Billingsley, F.F. (1989). *IMPACT: A functional curriculum handbook for students with moderate to severe disabilities.* Baltimore: Paul H. Brookes.

Nietupski, J.A., & Hamre-Nietupski, S.M. (1987). An ecological approach to curriculum development. In L. Goetz, D. Guess, & K. Stremel-Campbell (Eds.), *Innovative program design for individuals with dual sensory impairments.* (pp. 225–253). Baltimore: Paul H. Brookes.

Nietupski, J., Welch, J., & Wacker, D. (1983). Acquisition, maintenance and transfer of grocery item purchasing by moderately and severely handicapped students. *Education and Training of the Mentally Retarded, 18*, 279–286.

Nirje, B. (1969). The normalization principle and its human management implication. In R.B. Kugel, & W. Wolfensberger (Eds.), *Changing patterns in residential services for the mentally retarded.* Washington, DC: U.S. Government Printing Office.

Novak, C.G. (1983). *Severely Handicapped Integration Program: Attitude change curricula* (Vol. 3, elementary level). Kansas City, KS: University of Kansas, Department of Special Education, Severely Handicapped Integration Project.

Peck, C.A., Schuler, A.L., Tomlinson, C., Theimer, R.K., & Haring, T. (1984). *The Social Competence Curriculum Project: A guide to instructional programming for social and communicative interactions*. Santa Barbara, CA: University of California, Graduate School of Education, Special Education Research Institute.

Pinnell, G., Deford, D., & Lyons, C. (1988). *Reading Recovery: Early intervention for at risk first graders*. Arlington, VA: Educational Research Service.

Pogrow, S. (1989). HOTS: Higher order thinking skills project. In U.S. *Educational Programs That Work* (15th ed., Education Department, National Diffusion Network). Longmont, CO: Sopris West, Inc.

Pogrow, S. (1990). Challenging at-risk students: Findings from the HOTS program. *Phi Delta Kappan*, *72*, 389–397.

Renzaglia, A., & Aveno, A. (1986a). *Curriculum assessment forms for an individualized, functional curriculum assessment procedure for students with moderate to severe handicaps: Domestic, leisure, and community domains*. Charlottesville, VA: University of Virginia, Curry School of Education.

Renzaglia, A., & Aveno, A. (1986b). *Manuals for the administration of an individualized, functional curriculum assessment procedure for students with moderate to severe handicaps: Domestic, leisure, and community domains*. Charlottesville, VA: University of Virginia, Curry School of Education.

Rusch, F.R. (1986). *Competitive employment issues and strategies*. Baltimore: Paul H. Brookes.

Sasso, G.M., & Simpson, R.L. (1983). *Severely Handicapped Integration Program: Socialization programs for handicapped students* (Vol. 7). Kansas City, KS: University of Kansas, Department of Special Education, Severely Handicapped Integration Project.

Schumaker, J.B., Hazel, J.S., & Pederson, C.S. (1988). *Social skills for daily living*. Circle Pines, MN: American Guidance Services.

Silbert, J., Carnine D., & Stein, M. (1981). *Direct instruction mathematics*. Columbus, OH: Charles E. Merrill.

State of Oregon, Mental Health Division (1981). *Student progress record: Placement action form & individualized education program*. Salem, OR: State of Oregon Mental Health Division, Programs for Mental Retardation and Developmental Disabilities.

Stewart, J.E. (Ed.). (1986). *Washington State Cooperative Curriculum* (4th ed.). Seattle, WA: Shoreline School District.

Strain, P.S., & Fox, J.J. (1981). Peer social initiations and the modification of social withdrawal: A review and future perspective. *Journal of Pediatric Psychology*, *6*, 417–433.

Sutton, A. (in press). Conductive Education: A complex question for psychology. In P. Jones, (Ed.) *Psychology and Physical Disability*. p. 1.

Tawney, J.W., Knapp, D.S., O'Reilly, C.D., & Pratt, S.S. (1979). *Programmed environments curriculum*. Columbus, OH: Charles E. Merrill.

Thurber, D.N., & Jordan, D.R. (1978). *D'Nealian handwriting*. Palo Alto, CA: Scott, Foresman.

Turnbull, A.P., Strickland, B.B., & Brantley, J.C. (1982). *Developing and implementing individualized education programs* (2nd ed.) Columbus, OH: Charles E. Merrill.

Voeltz, L.M. (1980). Children's attitudes toward handicapped peers. *American Journal of Mental Deficiency*, *84*, 455–464.

Voeltz, L.M. (1982). Program and curriculum innovations to prepare children for integration. In N. Certo, N. Haring, & R. York (Eds.), *Public school integration of the severely handicapped: Rational issues and progressive alternatives*. (pp. 155–184). Baltimore: Paul H. Brookes.

Voeltz, L.M. Wuerch, B.B., & Wilcox, B. (1982). Leisure and recreation: Preparation for independence, integration, and self-fulfillment. In B. Wilcox, & G. T. Bellamy (Eds.), *Design of high school programs for severely handicapped students*. (pp. 175–209). Baltimore: Paul H. Brookes.

Walker, H.M., McConnell, S., Holmes, D., Todis, B., Walker, J., & Golden, N. (1983). *The Walker social skills curriculum: The ACCEPTS program*. Austin, TX: Pro-Ed.

Wehman, P., & McLaughlin, P.J. (1980). *Vocational curriculum for developmentally disabled persons*. Baltimore: University Park Press.

Wilcox, B., & Bellamy, G.T. (1987a). *The activities catalog: An alternative curriculum for youth and adults with severe disabilities*. Baltimore: Paul H. Brookes.

Wilcox, B., & Bellamy, G.T. (1987b). *A comprehensive guide to the activities catalog: An alternative curriculum for youth and adults with severe disabilities*. Baltimore: Paul H. Brookes.

Woodcock, R.W., Clark, C.R., & Davies, C.O. (1979). *Peabody rebus reading program*. Circle Pines, MN: American Guidance Service.

7
Promoting Development and Integration of Infants Experiencing Neonatal Intensive Care

FORREST C. BENNETT AND MICHAEL J. GURALNICK

With the advent in the early 1960s of neonatal intensive care technology for low birthweight, premature, and other biologically vulnerable and medically fragile infants, there has been an associated professional, parental, and general public interest in the health and developmental outcomes of the survivors of this highly specialized care. Concerns about the short- and long-term neurodevelopmental prognoses for graduates of neonatal intensive care have increased as the accepted medical intervention strategies—such as mechanical ventilation, continuous positive airway pressure (CPAP), parenteral nutrition, central nervous system shunting, and drainage procedures—have become continually more complex and more aggressively utilized.

This growing concern has been accompanied by an increase in both the number of clinicians involved and the number of programs that are implementing specific interventions aimed at optimizing the developmental recovery during the following neonatal hospitalization. Increasingly, these efforts have affected the home environment, where family and community are taking over the support for these survivors of "high-tech" care. This chapter delineates the scope and magnitude of these issues, addresses the most prominent clinical challenges that confront professionals in neonatal developmental care, and critically examines the results of intervention research.

Nature of the Population and Associated Problems

There are approximately 240,000 low birthweight ($\leq$2,500 g) infants born each year in the United States, constituting 6% to 7% of all births. As a subdivision within this group, approximately 1% to 2% of all births are classified as very low birthweight ($\leq$1,500 g). The incidence of both low birthweight and very low birthweight in nonwhite populations is more than twice that encountered in the white population. Because the estimated low birthweight incidence has remained discouragingly stable over the past 20 to 25 years, contemporary reductions in neonatal mortality are steadily increasing the prevalence of biologically vulnerable infants and toddlers in the overall population. Much medical, legal, ethical, and economic debate continues to occur over the effects of neonatal intensive care on the long-term health and neurodevelopmental status of low birthweight survivors. Most investigators are in current agreement that the single clearest outcome of this technically enhanced care has been a dramatic and continuing reduction in neonatal mortality since the early 1960s, particularly for very low birthweight infants since the mid-1970s (Hack, Fanaroff, & Merkatz, 1979; Lee, Paneth, Gartner, Pearlman, & Gruss, 1980; McCormick, 1985). Simply stated, with present standards of practice in the neonatal intensive care unit (NICU), many more very premature, very low birthweight infants are surviving than was the case even 5 to 10 years ago. A 40% survival rate for infants with a birthweight between 500 and 750 g recently has been reported (Hack & Fanaroff, 1986). Figure 7.1 (Bennett, 1987) illustrates this dynamic phenomenon and emphasizes that although survival continues to increase in all low birthweight categories, the greatest impact of neonatal intensive care technology in recent years has clearly been on the smallest, sickest, and most medically fragile infants.

With continued reductions in the neonatal mortality of low birthweight, premature infants, serious concerns persist that this improved survival may be accompanied by an increase in the number of children with permanent health and/or neurodevelopmental impairments. Health complications that frequently result in prolonged and repeated medical care and hospital usage include bronchopulmonary dysplasia (i.e., chronic lung disease, which has an approximately 20% prevalence following severe respiratory distress syndrome); progressive hydrocephalus; necrotizing enterocolitis (i.e., acute bowel disease, which may necessitate intestinal resection); recurrent apnea requiring cardiorespiratory monitoring; and failure to thrive.

The major neurosensory handicapping conditions associated with prematurity are cerebral palsy (particularly the spastic diplegia type); mental or developmental retardation; sensorineural hearing loss; and visual impairment (primarily the consequence of retinal scarring, i.e., retinopathy of prematurity). These handicaps frequently occur together in the same child and are occasionally complicated by a chronic seizure disorder. They are usually clinically apparent by 2 years of age and vary in severity from mild to profound. As a group, their prevalence increases with decreasing birthweight and gestational age; the handicap rate in males consistently exceeds that in females. Table 7.1 (Bennett, 1988) provides current combined prevalence estimates and ranges by birthweight group for these chronic neurosensory impairments. Epidemiological investigations appear to document that reductions in neurodevelopmental morbidity have *not* paralleled or kept pace with reductions

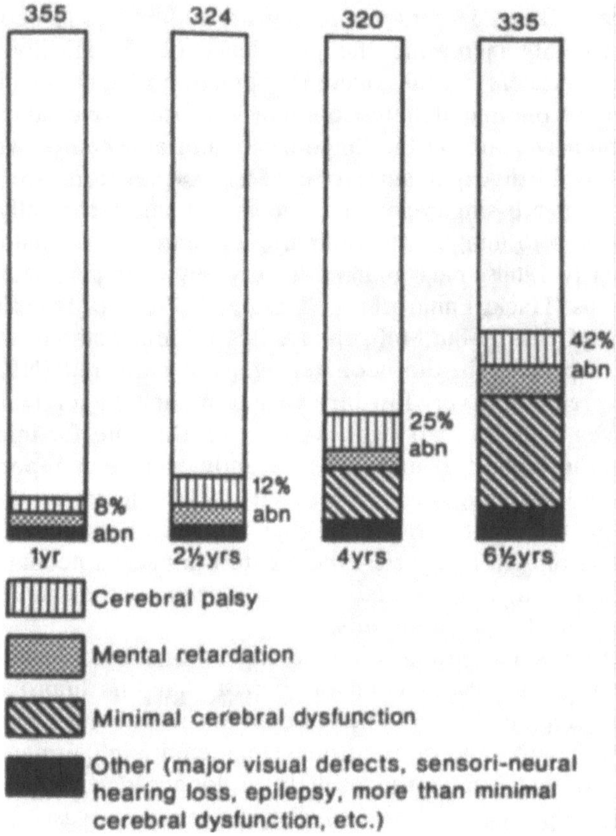

FIGURE 7.1 Comparison of NICU survival for mid-1970s and mid-1980s.

Reprinted, by permission, from Guthrie: Neonatal Intensive Care, Churchill Livingstone, New York, 1988.

in neonatal mortality. In fact, actual increases in both the incidence and prevalence of major handicaps have recently been reported among the smallest and sickest survivors (Hagberg, Hagberg, & Olow, 1984; Paneth, Kiely, Stein, & Susser, 1981).

Although major handicapping sequelae are the easiest for NICUs to quantify and report, numerous long-term follow-up studies clearly indicate that so-called minor neurodevelopmental and neurobehavioral sequelae are at least as prevalent, if not more so, in surviving low birthweight, premature infants. These relatively minor developmental sequelae become increasingly apparent in a variety of clinical manifestations with advancing age during the first 6 years of life (Bennett, 1984). These early, often subtle, developmental and behavioral delays and differences are not necessarily outgrown but frequently portend future

TABLE 7.1 Surviving low birthweight infants with one or more major handicaps. Reprinted, by permission, from Guthrie: Neonatal Intensive Care, Churchill Livingstone, New York, 1988.

Birthweight (g)	Major Handicapping Conditions
1,501–2,500	8 (5%–20%)
1,001–1,500	15 (5%–30%)
≤1,000	25 (8%–40%)

school dysfunction and may therefore become major impediments to normal academic and social progress (Blackman, Lindgren, Hein, & Harper, 1987). Collectively, these problems, which typically manifest themselves during the preschool and early school years, have been termed the "new morbidity" of NICU graduates.

Specific types of "minor" developmental sequelae include borderline intelligence (Rubin, Rosenblatt, & Balow, 1973); speech and language disorders (Largo, Molinari, Comenale-Pinto, Weber, & Duc, 1986); persistent neuromotor abnormalities including difficulties with balance and coordination (Nickel, Bennett, & Lamson, 1982); and perceptual problems (Klein, Hack, Gallagher, & Fanaroff, 1985). Specific areas of suboptimal behavioral style and performance include neonatal behavior (Kurtzberg et al., 1979); infant and toddler temperament (Field, 1983); emotional maturity (Malatesta, Grigoryev, Lamb, Albin, & Culver, 1986); social competence (Crnic, Ragozin, Greenberg, Robinson, & Basham, 1983); and selective attention (Dunn, 1986). As with major handicaps, the overall prevalence of these "minor" handicapping conditions increases with decreasing birthweight and gestational age, and is also greater in male survivors. Current prevalence estimates in very low birthweight infants vary between 15% and 25%. Accordingly, when the 15% to 20% prevalance of major handicaping conditions is also considered, between 35% and 45% of very low birthweight survivors demonstrate a residual neurodevelopmental problem that compromises their age-expected function. Dunn et al. (1980), in one of the most extensive longitudinal follow-up studies in this area, reported minimal cerebral dysfunction (i.e., "minor" developmental and behavioral abnormalities) to be the single most prevalent (20%) handicapping syndrome at school age in a population of over 300 low birthweight premature children. Furthermore, the authors stressed the difficulty in adequately predicting or identifying such dysfunctions prior to school entry at age 5. This important group of sequelae is consequently liable to be missed when the outcome of NICU graduates is assessed before that age. Figure 7.2 illustrates this diagnostic evolution and increase in developmental/behavioral problems over time.

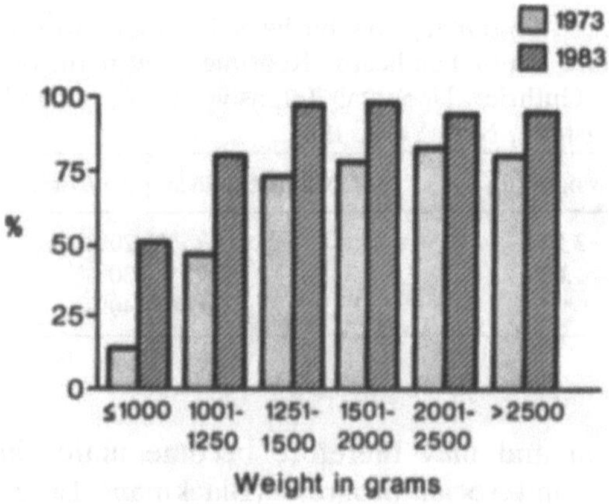

FIGURE 7.2 Evolution of developmental dysfunction in preterm/low birthweight children.

Modified from H.G. Dunn et al., (1980), Neurological, psychological, and educational sequelae of low birthweight. *Brain and Development*, *2*, p. 62.

Most of the major and minor neurodevelopmental sequelae associated with prematurity and low birthweight are also related to the severity of perinatal/neonatal illness; that is, low birthweight infants experiencing a prolonged hospital course with many medical complications have an increased likelihood of developing some type of developmental dysfunction. Specific events or observations highly associated with suboptimal outcomes include intrauterine growth retardation, intrauterine or intrapartum infection, severe asphyxia, neonatal meningitis/encephalitis, intracranial hemorrhage, neonatal seizures, and severe chronic lung disease with prolonged mechanical ventilation and oxygen requirements. However, it must be emphasized that despite the large number of positive group associations in follow-up studies, individual neurodevelopmental outcome remains very difficult to predict with accuracy in the NICU. Infants with apparently similar neonatal courses may develop remarkably differently. This repeated observation should be a source of both caution and hope to those making critical neonatal care decisions, to those providing hospital-based developmental and family interventions, and to those conducting follow-up evaluations. Counseling and interventions directed at those infants and toddlers who are also at increased risk environmentally (e.g., due to poverty, low socioeconomic status, a single parent, a teenage mother), that is, so-called doubly vulnerable, and specifically focused toward parent training would seem to demand high priority because of the documented importance of family and psychosocial variables in the ultimate prognosis for low birthweight and other medically fragile infants (Escalona, 1982).

The NICU Environment

The contemporary tertiary-care (Level III) NICU is a unique, lifesaving, intensive-medical-care world experienced by the low birthweight, premature newborn for an average duration of 1 to 3 months, and occasionally longer, depending on the degree of prematurity and the extent of complications. Proper care of the many medical complications of prematurity and other medically fragile conditions requires marked invasiveness and disruption of diurnal sleep/wake patterns through the use of isolettes. The infant may experience continuous bright lights; loud noises; mechanical respirators; indwelling catheters for the administration of fluid and calories and for blood sampling; gastric and intestinal tubes for feeding; prolonged phototherapy with eye patching; multiple needle punctures for blood, urine, and cerebrospinal fluid collections; multiple radiologic and ultrasound procedures; countless different examiners and nurses with repetitive, disruptive handling; and, at best, significantly restricted opportunities for normal parent–infant interaction (Gottfried, Hodgman, & Brown, 1984). Dr. Jerold Lucey (1977), a prominent neonatologist, has painted a stark but quite realistic picture of the NICU resident:

> Picture yourself in a brightly lit room, nude, defenseless, and your eyes hurting from silver nitrate. You are blindfolded, chilly, and surrounded by a tepid fog. You are gasping for air, fighting to breathe, and choking and gagging every so often on mucus. You are unable to clear your throat or cough. A mask is placed over your face, and blasts of air are forced into your lungs. Somebody sticks a catheter into your mouth, occasionally too far, causing you to retch or vomit. You are startled and frightened by loud, strange noises (beepers, voices, roaring respirators, telephones, radios, incubator noise). Some giant is pouring food into a tube which has been forced through your nose or throat into your stomach. It is uncomfortable and obstructs your nasal airway. You are probably nauseated; you are certainly not hungry, but you are expected to eat—and soon.
>
> You have a headache, probably the worst one of your life. You are sleep deprived. Every time you doze off, somebody gets worried about you. They think you are in a coma. You have to be very careful to breathe very regularly. You are not allowed the multiple long pauses (15 seconds or more) of a sleeping, dreaming adult. If you do pause, a bell goes off, waking you up, and somebody slaps your feet or pulls your hair to see if you will or can cry. If you are exhausted or unresponsive, you are in trouble. If you have any jerky movements, you are suspected of having a convulsion.
>
> Every few hours somebody cuts your foot or sticks a needle into your scalp or one of your arteries. Your arms and legs are taped down to boards. Electrodes are attached to your chest. You are immobilized. You may even have an itch, but you can't scratch. Cool, rude hands probe your abdomen ever so often, feeling for your liver, kidneys, or bladder. After a few days of this "intensive" care you are exhausted and you may need assistance to continue breathing just because you are too tired to do it on your own. (pp. 1064–1065)

This markedly atypical "life-style" is commonplace for those infants who, because of complex medical and/or surgical needs, require extended or repeated intensive care hospitalizations and, in the severest of cases, may spend the bulk of their first years of life in and out of such settings. Considering these factors, the suggestion that the contemporary treatment of newborns receiving intensive care may be responsible for newly recognized complications, and may contribute to the developmental deficits associated with prematurity and other medically fragile conditions, is certainly not surprising.

A major philosophical debate of the past 15 to 20 years concerning the appropriate developmental interpretation of the NICU environment has markedly influenced the rationale and direction of neonatal and other hospital-based developmental intervention approaches (Meisels, Jones, & Stiefel, 1983). Does this unusual medical setting constitute a source of (a) sensory deprivation, requiring a variety of added stimulations; (b) constant overstimulation, requiring less handling and less intervention of all types, and more time for protected, uninterrupted sleep; or (c) an inappropriate pattern of interactions rather than simply too much or too little stimulation, and including aspects of both deprivation and overstimulation?

Most recent ecologic investigations of the NICU support the third viewpoint (Gottfried & Gaiter, 1984; Gottfried, Wallace-Lande, & Sherman-Brown, 1981). Pertaining strictly to physical stimulations, these careful observational studies indicate that NICU residents are not sensorially deprived, but in fact receive large amounts of ongoing stimulation. Infants monitored in these studies were continuously exposed to cool-white fluorescent lighting with illumination not varying across day and night. Likewise, recording of the acoustic environment revealed continuously high sound levels, higher than in a home or even a busy office. Isolettes provided little to no sheltering from this collection of visual and auditory insults, since recordings of light and sound were virtually identical both outside and inside the incubator. Recent reports suggest possible links between these light and noise excesses and subsequent visual and hearing deficits in NICU graduates (Glass, Avery, & Siva Subramanian, 1985; Long, Lucey, & Philip, 1980). NICU observational studies also indicated that infants have extensive contacts with caregivers. However, almost all contacts were with staff members. In spite of open visiting policies, a minimal percentage of contacts involved family members. The contacts were brief (2 to 5 minutes in duration) and occurred on the average of every 18 to 30 minutes. Virtually all of the contacts involved medical or nursing care with some form of handling.

In contrast to the high magnitude of visual, auditory, and tactile stimulation, these time–motion studies found that NICU residents had infrequent social experiences. Despite the fact that medically fragile infants were in contact with other persons, they seldom received social types of stimulation. The preponderance of contacts between caregivers and sick infants was nonsocial; if social stimulation occurred, it was embedded within routine nursing care and not initiated independently. In more than half the instances in which infants cried during contacts, caregivers did not attempt to soothe them. Additionally, the integration of social and sensory experiences was not impressively high. Often infants were handled but not talked to, and were positioned in such a way that they could not see caregivers. Quite often, social stimulation was given without regard for the infant's behavioral state. For example, in no more than approximately one half of the situations in which social events occurred did the infants have their eyes open. Surprisingly, even in the intermediate care (i.e., for infants growing and gaining weight, with less acute needs) nurseries assessed, the large majority of contacts were devoid of social events. Social touching of, rocking of, or talking to infants, all of which are felt to be developmentally advantageous, occurred during less than one third of all contacts.

In summary, with respect to social stimulation, it appears that many medically fragile infants may indeed be deprived throughout their course of hospitalization. Despite the constant bombardment by visual, auditory, and tactile physical stimuli that it provides, the NICU is often a startlingly nonsocial environment, especially for the smallest and sickest residents. Unfortunately, there is also frequently little or no organization, rhythmicity, or developmentally appropriate pattern of physical and social stimulation incorporated into the plan of intensive care.

Published Practices of Hospital-Based Neonatal and Postneonatal Developmental Interventions

Early Approaches

The theoretical rationale and models guiding early, hospital-based, developmental intervention programs continue to evolve over time. This ongoing evolution of purpose has dramatically altered the focus and form of current intervention strategies, specific procedures, and supporting organizational structures. Throughout the 1970s, three principal objectives variously influenced the types and emphases of developmental intervention efforts: (a) to attempt to normalize and humanize the disruptive effects of the NICU environment so that it more closely resembled the environment of healthy, full-term infants; (b) to correct for presumed sensory deprivation associated with prolonged NICU care by means of specific stimulations; and (c) to compensate for intrauterine experiences lost as a result of premature birth. The determination of which of these three philosophies was functionally dominant in terms of both clinical practice and research activities at a given NICU was predicated on personal, local interpretations of the developmental needs of hospitalized, medically fragile infants.

Although a review of published efficacy investigations reveals great interstudy variability in terms of the specific developmental interventions (independent variables) utilized, practically all reporting centers in the 1970s employed early supplemental stimulation, environmental modification, or both in one or more of four major sensory areas (Field, 1980). In fact, the majority of investigations are of multimodal (i.e., combined) sensory manipulations in more than one circumscribed area. They are almost exclusively infant-focused, that is, based on "doing something" of a presumed stimulating nature to sick or recovering NICU residents. Nurses in the NICU have been the principal intervention agents in most reports. Other providers include physical therapists, occupational therapists, early childhood special educators, and infant developmental specialists from a variety of training backgrounds who focus on the specific needs of the recovering neonate.

The four major sensory modalities variously incorporated into NICU developmental intervention programs include (a) visual stimulation (e.g., decoration of the surroundings, mobiles with brightly colored objects); (b) auditory stimulation (e.g., singing, music boxes, recordings of the mother's voice and/or heartbeat), (c) tactile stimulation (e.g., non-nutritive sucking, flexing, massaging, handling, positioning); and (d) vestibular-kinesthetic stimulation (e.g., rocking and the use of oscillating beds, including waterbeds). Countless different combinations of these infant-focused interventions have been described and analyzed (e.g., massaging, handling, and rocking; use of a rocking bed and heartbeat recording; visual decoration and body rubbing; and bright mobiles, massaging, rocking, singing, and music boxes—thus representing all four sensory modalities in this case). As can be appreciated, the number of individual protocols is almost limitless, and intervention programs further vary in terms of their specificity (or lack thereof) within a given sensory area. For example, one program may utilize a variety of vestibular stimulations in differing degrees and sequences, whereas another may have chosen to assess the effects of vestibular stimulation as specifically provided by a motorized hammock or, alternatively, by an oscillating waterbed. Such marked variability between individual intervention programs seriously impairs both the interpretation and generalizability of their outcomes.

As with the specific combinations of sensory stimulations, great variability also exists in the reported onset, frequency, and duration of interventions. The timing of initial developmental intervention varies from immediately after birth, to some relatively arbitrary starting point such as 14 days of age, to the time when the infant is deemed physiologically stable. Likewise, even though most studies have provided an intervention program taking place at least several times daily, some stimulations were given only during feedings, some were prescribed every 15 minutes regardless of the infant's readiness or state of alertness, and others were contingent on the infant's own activity and responsiveness. In terms of duration, typical intervention endpoints have included term gestational age, attainment of normal birthweight, or nursery discharge. Furthermore, although most developmental interventions with NICU residents have focused exclusively on manipulating the environment during the infant's initial hospitalization, in recent years an increasing number of programs also provide intervention protocols for parents that continue after hospital discharge into the home.

The comparison of efficacy studies involving NICU developmental interventions is further hampered by limited information about subject selection and sample characteristics. Many studies have exclusively involved families of low socioeconomic status with predominantly young, unmarried mothers. Unfortunately, most have also involved relatively healthy NICU residents; infants who may theoretically benefit the most from intervention—such as those of extremely low birthweight (≤1,000 g) and those experiencing numerous medical complications—are quite underrepresented in most published investigations. Thus, the bulk of experimental evidence in this area has been accumulated from infants who, biologically and medically, are at relatively lower risk (i.e., larger and healthier) but environmentally are at higher risk (i.e., more socioeconomically disadvantaged). Additionally, study differences abound in such basic infant characteristics as birthweight and gestational age means and ranges, types and severity of medical complications, and duration of hospitalization and in such family demographic characteristics as race and socioeconomic status.

NICU intervention investigations have employed a wide variety of dependent outcome measures. These can be grouped into three broad categories: developmental, medical, and parental. The various developmental outcome measures utilized include (a) performance on standardized neurodevelopmental and neurobehavioral evaluations; (b) performance on specific cognitive-sensory tasks (e.g., visual orienting, auditory responsivity, recognition memory); (c) sleep/wake state organization; (d) temperament characteristics such as activity level and irritability; (e) and neuromotor criteria such as muscle tone and volitional movement. The dependent medical variables that are typically assessed are weight gain, head growth, oxygen requirements, frequency of apnea, frequency of vomiting, and length of hospitalization. Parental outcome measures have included the frequency of parental visitation and evaluation of the quality of the parent–infant interaction. In sum, critical appraisal of the NICU developmental intervention studies of the 1970s involves a search for effects within a complex mixture of structural, methodologic, sampling, and outcome variables (Bennett, 1987).

As might be anticipated, the reported results of these early studies are as various as the methodologies employed, and the outcomes reveal great variability in terms of their exact nature, extent, significance, and duration. One or more positive developmental, medical, and/or parental outcome is reported in almost every scientifically credible infant-focused study published during the 1970s. However, the benefits of one particular intervention protocol are often not replicated in other investigations, and because of frequently contradictory results, only limited generalizations can be made from most of the individual, isolated outcomes. In most of these early stimulation studies, the actual interventions occurred exclusively while the infant was hospitalized in the intensive care or intermediate care nursery and were administered by hospital staff alone without direct parental involvement.

Two major studies, utilizing very similar multimodal stimulations in all four sensory areas, reported conflicting results. Scarr-Salapatek and Williams (1973) found significantly greater weight gain and superior performance in measures of neonatal behavior for experimental group infants who received visual (mobiles, human faces); tactile (handling, patting); vestibular-kinesthetic (rocking); and auditory (talking) interventions. In contrast, Leib, Benfield, and Guidubaldi (1980) reported no significant improvements in the identical outcome measures following the same types of approaches. The two studies did both report significantly higher scores on assessments of mental and motor development during the first year of life for experimental infants. But even this general agreement in findings must be cautiously interpreted because of its short-term nature, and also because of other studies (Brown et al., 1980) showing essentially no infant performance benefits following similar sensory stimulations.

Current Approaches

Because of the continued lack of consensus about the effectiveness of NICU developmental interventions based solely on an infant stimulation model, there was a clear shift in focus and orientation during the 1980s toward more family-centered interventions emphasizing and facilitating interactions between parents and medically fragile infants (Ramey, Bryant, Sparling, & Wasik, 1984). This more recent, parent-focused model attempts both to facilitate the fragile infant's optimal social functioning and to directly train parents to recognize the important stress and stability signals of their sick infant. NICU interventions aimed at improving the parent–infant relationship have taken various forms, usually including a component of infant preparation and readiness for such intimate contact and a component of parent instruction in initiating dialogue and responding appropriately to the fragile infant's communicative overtures. With this contemporary evolution to more parent-focused strategies, parents and other family members are, naturally, increasingly involved in all NICU developmental interventions.

As an additional impetus to avoid a purely stimulation approach, Gorski, Hole, Leonard, and Martin (1983) and others (Long, Philip, & Lucey, 1980) have carefully documented potentially adverse side effects of indiscriminate intervention. The link between repeated, intrusive handling of the physiologically fragile infant and such deleterious complications as hypoxia (i.e., diminished oxygen supply); apnea (i.e., intermittent cessation of breathing); bradycardia (i.e., slow heart rate); and vomiting has been demonstrated. Increasing numbers of detailed investigations into the typical "life" and ecology of the NICU emphasize both the instability of the sick infant's autonomic nervous system and the surprising ease of exacerbating this instability by continual and unpredictable disruptions of quiet sleep. For example, when the fragile infant becomes overloaded with stimuli, he or she may withdraw, become rigid, or demonstrate signs of autonomic nervous system dysfunction. As a result, the infant becomes unavailable to its environment in terms of obtaining information or giving positive feedback, which in turn may cause the parents and other caregivers to feel less competent and effective. Thus, it becomes critical for fragile infants to engage in interactions without experiencing great physiologic, motor, and state regulatory costs.

Armed with this important information, contemporary NICU developmental intervention programs increasingly promote an "infant protection" approach, which minimizes unnecessary handling and times contacts to coincide with infant readiness. Als et al. (1986) have reported very encouraging results based on this type of highly individualized approach in a small group of very low birthweight infants with bronchopulmonary dysplasia (i.e., chronic lung disease). Experimental group infants receiving individualized care had significantly briefer stays on the respirator, improved feeding behavior, better behavioral regulation, and higher mental and motor developmental scores in comparison to control infants receiving standard NICU care. Als et al. taught and trained the incorporation of individualized nursing care plans into the daily routines of the intensive and intermediate care nurseries. The specific components of this "environmental neonatology" model include (a) reduction of excessive environmental stimulations (e.g., light, noise, traffic); (b) a minimal handling protocol; (c) use of facilitative positioning; (d) promotion of self-regulation and state control; (e) timing of daily routines to match autonomic readiness; and (f) parent support and behavioral observation training. As a result of Als et al.'s and others' ongoing efforts in this area, an increasing number of NICUs across the United States are modifying their current practices in light of these new concepts and directions.

The most consistent finding of 1980s studies that were partially or completely parent-focused involved the positive facilitation of parent–infant interactions. Almost all of these studies (Bromwich & Parmelee, 1979; Field, Widmayer, Stringer, & Ignatoff, 1980) reported at least some significant, objective enhancement of the mother–infant relationship, with only Brown et al. (1980) failing to detect any group differences in interactional quantity or quality. Several of these studies also involved home-based interventions following hospital discharge. Some of the most sustained intervention effects were best demonstrated in those relatively few programs that continued their efforts through the transition process and into the infant's home, with close and considerable parental involvement. Bromwich and Parmelee (1979) provided both free medical and nursing care, including home visitation by nurses and educational intervention by developmental home visitors; Field et al. (1980) provided home visitation by trained interventionists to both educate and support mothers. Brown et al. (1980), discussing their failure with a combined infant- and parent-focused approach to involve socially disadvantaged mothers with their hospitalized infants, enumerated such intervention impediments as mothers' lack of transportation to and from the hospital, need to care for older children at home, inability to leave home because of cultural concerns of their own mothers, and crises of daily living (e.g., inadequate or no housing, lack of financial support). These very realistic observations should serve both to keep individual, limited NICU interventions in perspective and to challenge investigators to develop innovative, comprehensive, coordinated approaches to the complex but essential task of optimizing the developmental and behavioral outcome of low birthweight, premature infants.

Transitions to Posthospital Environments: Family-Focused Intervention

The transition from the highly technological environment of the NICU to home and to the community provokes one of the most stressful moments for families. In addition to the added burden of having a new baby to care for, this stress is increased by those characteristics of children at biologic risk described earlier in this chapter such as sleeping and feeding difficulties, less organization, and general irritability, as well as a continuing need for health care for many infants (see McCormick, Stemmler, Bernbaum, & Farran, 1986; TeKolste & Bennett, 1987). When these factors are combined with the uncertainty that parents feel about the developmental outcome of their child, it is easy to see why the transition to home is so hazardous.

The critical analysis and theoretical framework provided by Sameroff and Chandler (1975), suggesting that the impact of biologic risk factors could be mitigated by sensitive transactions with caregiving environments, have served as important factors for family-focused interventions. Although various refinements of this fundamental principle continue to emerge, research findings support the connection between risk factors and caregiving environments. For example, a long-term follow-up of very low birthweight children revealed that the degree of neonatal illness was associated with whether or not a normal outcome occurred. However, the severity of an infant's disability itself was associated with parent education and all that that implies about the nature of the caregiving environment (Hunt, Cooper, & Tooley, 1988). In fact, for indigent high-risk newborns cared for in far less than optimal circumstances, the incidence of significant developmental delays is extremely high, affecting as many as one third of the children (Lasky et al., 1987). The results of the latter study do not appear to be linked to the quality of prenatal care, to atypical referral populations, or to race; they continue to suggest that it is the combination of biologic risk and an unfavorable home environment that produces these unusually poor outcomes.

In a very real sense, the problems posed by a child at biologic risk challenge parents' confidence in their ability to care for their child at home and to establish a warm and developmentally supportive relationship, even in environments that appear favorable. As a consequence, the potential exists for mitigating some of the effects of risk factors on developmental outcome through facilitating and supporting certain aspects of the caregiving environment for most families. Moreover, this transition point constitutes the initial experiences that families have with the nonhospital community and its service system. The manner in which professionals interact with families, the quality of their technical skills, their attitudes with regard to the parent–professional relationship, and their encouragement of families to maintain community involvement establishes an important frame of reference for families.

Recent efforts in family-focused preventive interventions for children at biologic risk are characterized by a number of important features (see Guralnick, 1989). These include an effort to provide a supportive parent–professional relationship to enhance the confidence and competence of families in caring for their children and to ensure that families take a productive, active role in all aspects of decision making. How this can be accomplished, what strategies are used, what constitutes the content and framework for preventive intervention efforts, and what the impact is of these programs on parents and children are all issues that will be examined in this section.

Parent-Focused Interventions

It is only relatively recently that developmental models (e.g., Goldberg, 1977) emphasizing ways of improving parental confidence, support, and responsiveness to biologically at-risk infants have been translated into specific intervention programs. The pioneering work by Bromwich (Bromwich & Parmelee, 1979) and Kathryn Barnard and her colleagues (1987) at the University of Washington's Child Development and Mental Retardation Center has provided important models for preventive intervention programs for preterm infants. Barnard's group, in particular, has continued to carefully evaluate a program designed primarily for healthy preterm infants. Much of that work has been incorporated into the current version of Nursing Systems Toward Effective Parenting–Preterm (NSTEP–P) concept and protocol manuals (Johnson-Crowley & Sumner, 1987a, 1987b) and has been extensively field-tested (Barnard et al., 1987). This program is designed explicitly to be sensitive to the unique needs of parents yet to impart the necessary information and skills to assist parents to effectively care for their premature child. The intervention protocol generally calls for one hospital visit plus eight additional home visits over the course of a 6-month period. During these visits, four major content areas—health and related concerns, state modulation, behavioral responsiveness, and parent support and community resources—are covered.

The Mother–Infant Transaction Program (MITP) developed by Rauh (1979), was designed to improve the adaptations of mothers to their at-risk infant by:

> (a) Enabling the mother to appreciate her infant's unique behavioral characteristics; (b) sensitizing her to the infant's cues, particularly those that signal stimulus overload, distress, or readiness for interaction; and (c) teaching her to respond appropriately to those cues so as to facilitate mutually satisfying interactions. (Rauh, Achenbach, Nurcombe, Howell, & Teti, 1988, p. 546)

Implemented by a neonatal intensive care nurse, the program encompasses a total of 11 one-hour sessions—7 prior to hospital discharge and 4 in the home. All sessions are to be completed before 90 days post discharge (Rauh et al., 1988). The MITP begins with a demonstration of the Brazelton Neonatal Assessment Scale (1973), a strategy that encourages an exploration of parents' perceptions of their infant, their fears, anxieties, and the levels of support provided by family members. The following session is designed to improve parents' knowledge and sensitivity to their infant's innate reflex systems, including respiration, skin circulation, extremity movement, facial movement, and visceral activity. Indications of well-organized and excited states for these five areas as well as techniques that will minimize overly excited states and promote organization are presented. The mother's role in fostering organization is emphasized in a subsequent session focusing on the motor system (posture, tone, and movement). Again, efforts are made to alert mothers to indications of the infant's level of organization, to reduce stress, and to foster organized behavior. Sessions 4 and 5 are devoted to indicators of the infant's state and the varying degrees of the infant's responsiveness in each state. In addition, how infants self-regulate and how mothers can match their interactions to promote well-organized levels and alertness are also part of this session. In Session 6, mothers are shown how they can integrate knowledge of their children's abilities into caretaking activities of changing, feeding, bathing, and waking. Suggestions to minimize problems for easily stressed infants are provided to mothers for each caretaking area. The final in-hospital session reviews the prior activities and is designed to further prepare the mother to appropriately initiate interactions following discharge. Synchronizing mothers' interactions to support their infant's organization is the central focus.

The four sessions in the home are designed to continue to foster competent parenting in the new environment, "being careful to support [the mother's] sense of control and self-confidence" (Rauh, 1979, p. 14). Additional strategies to enhance mutual play through visual, auditory, and tactile modalities are discussed, including imitation, the use of bright objects for focusing and following, and soothing through rhythmic touching.

In the final two sessions, the concept of infant temperament is introduced. Mothers are assisted in identifying the behavioral patterns of their child and in improving the fit between their interactions and their child's style. Continued emphasis is placed on the mother's initiative in solving problems related to this fit and understanding that difficult temperaments are not caused by parents themselves. The final session consists of a review and provides an opportunity for feedback.

A similar approach, focusing primarily on severely handicapped medically fragile children, is being carried out at the University of Washington's Child Development and Mental Retardation Center. Referred to as the Transactional Family Systems Model (TFSM), a team consisting of a pediatric/perinatal nurse clinician, a pediatric physical or occupational therapist, and an infant educator provides services on a weekly basis to families upon discharge from the neonatal intensive care unit until the child receives regular services from a developmental center. As was the case for the MITP, the emphasis of the TFSM is on improving parental competence and confidence and on promoting satisfying and enjoyable parent–child interactions. This is accomplished in the following five ways:

1. Educating parents in the significance of four types of communication available to the infant (i.e., autonomic or automatic, motoric, state organizational, and attentive/interactional or social).
2. Assisting parents to define and read behavioral cues (i.e., approach, stress, and self-regulatory behaviors) through observation and guided interpretation of their infant's behavior.
3. Training parents to assess, predict, elicit, and respond in an appropriate contingent manner.
4. Assisting parents through guided practice and encouragement to independently change their interactional style to more naturally mesh with that of their developing baby.
5. Encouraging parents to highlight each small developmental step and to see how each incremental step fits into the larger developmental picture. (modified from Hedlund, 1987)

Outcomes of Intervention

Accordingly, the programs described above, as well as others such as the Social Interaction Assessment and Intervention (McCollum, 1984) and the Transactional Model of Early Home Intervention (Barrera, Rosenbaum, & Cunningham, 1986), have a number of common elements. These include (a) their parent-focused nature; (b) interventions designed to build parents' confidence and competence; (c) an emphasis on the infant's self-regulation; and (d) efforts to improve parents' sensitivity to their child's cues to communicate, to promote satisfying "dialogues," and to encourage a match between parent and child interactional styles. In recent years a number of well-designed studies have evaluated the effects of many of these parent-focused interventions and have sought to determine some of the factors that may mediate any changes that might have occurred. A comprehensive review is beyond the scope of this chapter. However, a summary of findings from a few recent studies, particularly those that attempted to assess how parents may have mediated any changes, should provide a fair representation of outcome patterns.

The MITP curriculum has actually been carefully evaluated (Rauh et al., 1988) and did include a number of parent-related measures. In this study, a well-defined cohort of low birthweight infants (less than 2,250 g and a gestational age of under 37 weeks) was randomly assigned to a group receiving the MITP curriculum or to a group receiving conventional care. A full-term control group was also available for comparison.

An additional important feature of this study was the fact that the evaluation of impact of this 11-hour preventive intervention program, ending 3 months after the child went home, was evaluated over a 4-year period. Remarkably, the low birthweight group receiving the MITP curriculum scored nearly 13 points higher on the McCarthy Scales of Children's Abilities at 4 years of age than the low birthweight control group. In fact, whereas the treatment and full-term children were not distinguishable from one another in terms of cognitive development by age 4, the low birthweight control group followed the more typical developmental pattern of declining performance over time.

In order to examine possible mediating factors, measures of parent self-confidence in relationship to competent parenting and satisfaction with the mothering role were assessed at 6 months. The outcomes of these scales revealed that, in fact, treatment group mothers considered themselves more self-confident and were more satisfied with their role as parents than control group mothers. These findings are consistent with the contention that it is this confidence in their ability to parent their developmentally at-risk children fostered by the MITP that may have been responsible for the long-term effects.

Similar, although more short-term, results by Resnick, Armstrong, and Carter (1988) also supported the finding that substantial differences in cognitive development occur as a result of preventive intervention efforts.

The intervention activities were both parent-centered and infant-centered (e.g., stimulation and exercise). However, perhaps most important for this discussion is the fact that a variety of measures of parent–child interaction revealed that a close association existed between growth in cognitive development and positive parent–child interactions. Moreover, although it is not possible to separate out the child-focused from the parent-focused components of this study, research by Barrera et al. (1986) suggested the greater value of parent–infant intervention programs.

Individualizing

This pattern of outcomes is centainly consistent with the developmental framework described earlier; that is, the centrality of fostering parent–child relationships and ensuring that parents become confident in their abilities to solve the numerous developmental and relationship problems that are likely to arise. Despite the overall encouraging patterns, considerable variability in outcome has been found. There are many factors, such as initial level of stress or disorganization of the home, available resources, and perhaps severity of child's actual or potential disability, that can moderate the efforts of these general intervention programs. In fact, more recently, Affleck, Tennen, Rowe, Roscher, and Walker (1989) demonstrated how the effects of a hospital-to-home transition program varied in relation to parents' perceived need for support. For parents with a need for high levels of support, the program had positive effects on perceptions of personal control, sense of competence, and responsiveness to their infant. However, for those parents with a perceived need for support below the average level, the program had a negative impact on some of the variables.

Possible explanations for the negative findings include the alternative that in some cases, intervention may be overly intrusive to parents and may actually form a threat to their self-confidence (Affleck et al., 1989). Other parents could question the implication that an optimistic child outcome is unlikely without intervention and implementation of those preventive intervention programs. The major principles, framework, and methods appear sound and results are highly encouraging. However, the identification of those nonprogram factors that must be considered, how they are assessed, and how they modify our interventions are essential problems for future research.

Summary

The dramatic growth and success of neonatal intensive care technologies during the past 25 years have resulted in the survival of ever smaller and sicker infants. These "new survivors" frequently share a wide variety of health and developmental vulnerabilities. In an attempt to prevent or ameliorate these documented morbidities, a heterogeneous array of developmental interventions has been suggested, implemented, and evaluated. These approaches range from early, infant-focused nursery stimulations to long-term family education and support services. They increasingly utilize an interdisciplinary mix of child-care professionals with diverse training and experience. They increasingly involve parents as the necessary principal agents of eventual outcome and successful community integration. The accumulated clinical research in this rapidly expanding area has already taught us much about the nature and intensity of those interventions most likely to be effective for this unique population.

However, there remains much yet to be learned. We need more precise means of assessing biologic/neurologic risk. Physicians, nurses, therapists, and educators need to unite their focus in the next decade on identifying appropriate "brain care" guidelines for infants experiencing neonatal intensive care or other prolonged hospitalizations. All developmental intervention plans for biologically fragile infants must now take into consideration the frequently coexisting environmental problems of poverty, substance abuse, single parenthood, unemployment, and/or homelessness. These contemporary multiple vulnerabilities must be recognized and addressed as part of the coordinated service provisions described in Public Law 99–457. Without this type of comprehensive, realistic approach, more narrow interventions are unlikely to effectively improve the long-term developmental and behavioral prognosis of low birthweight, premature, and other medically fragile infants.

References

Affleck, G., Tennen, H., Rowe, J., Roscher, B., & Walker, L. (1989). Effects of formal support on mothers' adaptation to the hospital-to-home transition of high-risk infants: The benefits and costs of helping. *Child Development*, *60*, 488–501.

Als, H., Lawhon, G., Brown, E., Gibes, R., Duffy, F., McAnulty, G., & Blickman, J. (1986). Individualized behavioral and environmental care for the very low birthweight preterm infant at high risk for bronchopulmonary dysplasia: Neonatal intensive care unit and developmental outcome. *Pediatrics*, *78*, 1123–1132.

Barnard, K.E., Hammond, M.A., Sumner, G.A., Kang, R., Johnson-Crowley, N., Snyder, C., Spietz, A., Blackburn, S., Brandt, P., & Magyary, D. (1987). Helping parents with preterm infants: Field test of a protocol. *Early Child Development and Care*, *27*(2), 255–290.

Barrera, M.E., Rosenbaum, P.L., & Cunningham, C.E. (1986). Early home intervention with low-birth-weight infants and their parents. *Child Development*, *57*, 20–33.

Bennett, F.C. (1984). Neurodevelopmental outcome of low birthweight infants. In V.C. Kelley (Ed.), *Practice of pediatrics* (pp. 1–24). Philadelphia: Harper & Row.

Bennett, F.C. (1987). The effectiveness of early intervention for infants at increased biological risk. In M.J. Guralnick & F.C. Bennett (Eds.), *The effectiveness of early intervention for at-risk and handicapped children* (pp. 79–112). Orlando, FL: Academic Press.

Bennett, F.C. (1988). Neurodevelopmental outcome in low birthweight infants: The role of developmental intervention. In R.D. Guthrie (Ed.), *Neonatal intensive care* (pp. 221–249). New York: Churchill Livingstone.

Blackman, J.A., Lindgren, S., Hein, H., & Harper, D. (1987). Long-term surveillance of high risk children. *American Journal of Diseases of Children, 141*, 1293–1299.

Brazelton, T.B. (1973). *Neonatal Behavioral Assessment Scale.* Philadelphia: Lippincott.

Bromwich, R.M., & Parmelee, A.H. (1979). An intervention program for preterm infants. In T.M. Field (Ed.), *Infants born at risk* (pp. 389–411). New York: Spectrum.

Brown, J., LaRossa, M., Aylward, G., Davis, D., Rutherford, P., & Bakeman, R. (1980). Nursery-based intervention with prematurely born babies and their mothers: Are there effects? *Journal of Pediatrics, 97*, 487–491.

Crnic, K.A., Ragozin, A.S., Greenberg, M.T., Robinson, N.M., & Basham, R.B. (1983). Social interaction and developmental competence of preterm and full-term infants during the first year of life. *Child Development, 54*, 1199–1210.

Dunn, H.G. (Ed.). (1986). *Sequelae of low birthweight: The Vancouver Study.* (Clinics in Developmental Medicine, Nos. 95–96). Philadelphia, PA: J.B. Lippincott.

Dunn, H.G., Crichton, J., Grunau, R., McBurney, A., McCormick, A., Robertson, A., & Schulzer, M. (1980). Neurological, psychological and educational sequelae of low birthweight. *Brain and Development, 2*, 57–67.

Escalona, S.K. (1982). Babies at double hazard: Early development of infants at biologic and social risk. *Pediatrics, 70*, 670–675.

Field, T.M. (1980). Supplemental stimulation of preterm neonates. *Early Human Development, 4*, 301–314.

Field, T.M. (1983). High-risk infants "have less fun" during early interactions. *Topics in Early Childhood Special Education, 3*(1), 77–87.

Field, T.M., Widmayer, S.M., Stringer, S., & Ignatoff, E. (1980). Teenage, lower class, black mothers and their preterm infants: An intervention and developmental follow-up. *Child Development, 51*, 426–436.

Glass, P., Avery, G.B., & Siva Subramanian, K.N. (1985). Effect of bright light in the hospital nursery on the incidence of retinopathy of prematurity. *New England Journal of Medicine, 313*, 401–404.

Goldberg, S. (1977). Social competence in infancy: A model of parent–infant interaction. *Merrill-Palmer Ouarterly, 23*, 163–177.

Gorski, P.A., Hole, W.T., Leonard, C.H., & Martin, J.A. (1983). Direct computer recording of premature infants and nursery care: Distress following two interventions. *Pediatrics, 72*, 198–202.

Gottfried, A.W., & Gaiter, J.L. (Eds.). (1984). *Infant stress under intensive care: Environmental neonatology.* Baltimore: University Park Press.

Gottfried, A.W., Hodgman, J.E., & Brown, K.W. (1984). How intensive is newborn intensive care? An environmental analysis. *Pediatrics, 74*, 292–294.

Gottfried, A.W., Wallace-Lande, P., & Sherman-Brown, S. (1981). Physical and social environment of newborn infants in special care units. *Science, 214*, 637–675.

Guralnick, M.J. (1989). Recent developments in early intervention efficacy research: Implications for family involvement in P.L. 99–457. *Topics in Early Childhood Special Education, 9*(3), 1–17.

Hack, M., & Fanaroff, A.A. (1986). Changes in the delivery room care of the extremely small infant (<750 g): Effects on morbidity and outcome. *New England Journal of Medicine, 314*, 660–664.

Hack, M., Fanaroff, A.A., & Merkatz, I.R. (1979). The low birthweight infant: Evolution of a changing outlook. *New England Journal of Medicine, 301*, 1162–1165.

Hagberg, B., Hagberg, G., & Olow, I. (1984). The changing panorama of cerebral palsy in Sweden. *Acta Pediatrica Scandinavia, 73*, 433–440.

Hedlund, R. (1987). *The Transactional Family System Program*. Unpublished manuscript. University of Washington, Child Development and Mental Retardation Center, Seattle, WA.

Hunt, J.V., Cooper, B.A.B., & Tooley, W.H. (1988). Very low birth weight infants at 8 and 11 years of age: Role of neonatal illness and family status. *Pediatrics, 82*, 596–603.

Johnson-Crowley, N., & Sumner, G.A. (Eds.). (1987a). *Nursing systems toward effective parenting-preterm: A resource manual for professionals involved with preterm infants and their families*. Seattle, WA: NCAST Publications.

Johnson-Crowley, N., & Sumner, G.A. (Eds.). (1987b). *Nursing systems toward effective parenting-preterm: A home visiting protocol guide for families with preterm infants*. Seattle, WA: NCAST Publications.

Klein, N., Hack, M., Gallagher, J., & Fanaroff, A.A. (1985). Preschool performance of children with normal intelligence who were very low birthweight infants. *Pediatrics, 75*, 531–537.

Kurtzberg, D., Vaughan, H., Daum, C., Grellong, B., Albin, S., & Rotkin, L. (1979). Neurobehavioral performance of low birthweight infants at 40 weeks conceptional age: Comparison with normal full-term infants. *Developmental Medicine and Child Neurology, 21*, 590–607.

Largo, R.H., Molinari, L., Comenale-Pinto, L., Weber, M., & Duc, G. (1986). Language development of term and preterm children during the first five years of life. *Developmental Medicine and Child Neurology, 28*, 333–350.

Lasky, R.E., Tyson, J.E., Rosenfeld, C.R., Krasinski, D., Dowling, S., & Gant, N.F. (1987). Disappointing follow-up findings for indigent high-risk newborns. *American Journal of Diseases of Children, 141*, 100–105.

Lee, K., Paneth, N., Gartner, L., Pearlman, M., & Gruss, L. (1980). Neonatal mortality: An analysis of the recent improvement in the United States. *American Journal of Public Health, 70*, 15–21.

Leib, S.A., Benfield, D.G., & Guidubaldi, J. (1980). Effects of early intervention and stimulation on the preterm infant. *Pediatrics, 66*, 83–90.

Long, J.G., Lucey, J.F., & Philip, A. G. (1980). Noise and hypoxemia in the intensive care nursery. *Pediatrics, 65*, 143–145.

Long, J.G., Philip, A.G., & Lucey, J.F. (1980). Excessive handling as a cause of hypoxemia. *Pediatrics, 65*, 203–207.

Lucey, J.F. (1977). Is intensive care becoming too intensive? *Pediatrics*, *59*, 1064–1065.

Malatesta, C., Grigoryev, P., Lamb, C., Albin, M., & Culver, C. (1986). Emotion socialization and expressive development in preterm and full-term infants. *Child Development*, *57*, 316–330.

McCollum, J.A. (1984). Social interaction between parents and babies: Validation of an intervention procedure. *Child: Care, Health and Development*, *10*, 301–315.

McCormick, M.C. (1985). The contribution of low birthweight to infant mortality and childhood morbidity. *New England Journal of Medicine*, *312*, 82–90.

McCormick, M.C., Stemmler, M.M., Bernbaum, J.C., & Farran, A.C. (1986). The very low birth weight transport goes home: Impact on the family. *Journal of Developmental and Behavioral Pediatrics*, *7*(4), 217–223.

Meisels, S.J., Jones, S.N., & Stiefel, G.S. (1983). Neonatal intervention: Problem, purpose, and prospects. *Topics in Early Childhood Special Education*, *3*(1), 1–13.

Nickel, R.E., Bennett, F.C., & Lamson, F.N. (1982). School performance of children with birthweights of 1,000 grams or less. *American Journal of Diseases of Children*, *136*, 105–110.

Paneth, N., Kiely, J.L., Stein, Z., & Susser, M. (1981). Cerebral palsy and newborn care: 3. Estimated prevalence rates of cerebral palsy under differing rates of mortality and impairment of low birthweight infants. *Developmental Medicine and Child Neurology*, *23*, 801–807.

Ramey, C.T., Bryant, D.M., Sparling, J.J. & Wasik, B.H. (1984). A biosocial system perspective on environmental interventions for low birthweight infants. *Clinical Obstetrics and Gynecology*, *27*, 672–692.

Rauh, V.A. (1979). *Content of the mother–infant transaction program*. Unpublished manuscript. Columbia University, New York.

Rauh, V.A., Achenbach, T.M., Nurcombe, B., Howell, C.T., & Teti, D.M. (1988). Minimizing adverse effects of low birthweight: Four-year results of an early intervention program. *Child Development*, *59*, 544–553.

Resnick, M.B., Armstrong, S., & Carter, R.L. (1988). Developmental intervention program for high-risk premature infants: Effects on development and parent–infant interactions. *Journal of Developmental Behavioral Pediatrics*, *9*, 73–78.

Rubin, R.A., Rosenblatt, C., & Balow, B. (1973). Psychological and educational sequelae of prematurity. *Pediatrics*, *52*, 352–363.

Sameroff, A.J., & Chandler, M.J. (1975). Reproductive risk and the continuum of caretaking casualty. In F.D. Horowitz, M. Hetherington, S. Scarr-Salapatek, & G. Siegel (Eds.), *Review of child development research* (Vol. 4, pp. 187–244). Chicago: University of Chicago Press.

Scarr-Salapatek, S., & Williams, M.L. (1973). The effects of early stimulation on low birthweight infants. *Child Development*, *44*, 94–101.

TeKolste, K.A., & Bennett, F.C. (1987). The high-risk infant: Transitions in health, development, and family during the first years of life. *Journal of Perinatology*, *7*(4), 368–377.

8
Community-Based Early Childhood Service Practices

MARCI J. HANSON AND KATHRYN A. HARING

Introduction

The importance of integrated special services for infants, toddlers, and preschoolers cannot be overemphasized. Gains made during the early years of a child's life may have significant and long-term beneficial effects as the child grows (Weiner & Koppleman, 1987). An unmeasurable value of integrated early childhood special education (ECSE) services is the message they convey to children who are not disabled and their families. The presence of children with disabilities in programs serving all children communicates that this is a natural and possibly preferred model. When the first services children receive are integrated, they may be unaware that other service models (e.g., segregated schools) exist. This benefits families of both types of children in that it sets up the expectation that those with disabilities will typically be present in regular programs. Integrated services early in life prevent future problems with negative attitudes surrounding inclusion of those with disabilities in school and community settings. Parents who experience integrated service options for their very young children may be more likely to expect or request that future programs include integration. Additionally, acceptance of individual differences and understanding of differing levels of need are basic attitudes that should be taught and modeled to young children. Integrated ECSE services can demonstrate these values effectively when program staff members are trained to make adaptations to assure that children at every level cognitively and physically participate as fully as possible in activities. Integrated ECSE curricula can be designed with relative ease because infants, toddlers, and preschoolers, regardless of ability, work on the same developmental goals. For example, in a program serving those from birth to age 6 a majority of the children will need assistance and training in self-care skills, and the age-appropriateness of activities does not present problems.

Typically, services for young children with special needs encompass a wide range of community-based services, including health care and educational services, and in some cases social services as well. In most states, no one agency or discipline is charged with the responsibility for providing the range of services for this age group; rather, a host of services is available through multiple agencies, with professionals from a variety of backgrounds involved in service delivery. Further, by the nature of children's needs early in life, effective service delivery models for infants, toddlers, and preschoolers emphasize family-related, home-based services or services located near the family in the community (Hanson & Lynch, 1989).

Early childhood services today are a complex web of services that have as the focus both services to children and services to their families. This web of services is multidimensional, multiagency or interagency, and interdisciplinary in focus. A number of contemporary societal concerns or factors are only now beginning to influence this already complex web of services. These factors include changes in society such as the increased number of mothers working outside the family's home and the consequent increased need for quality child care, the changing population demographics reflecting the multicultural nature of modern society, and the increased numbers of babies who are born at significant risk due to factors such as extreme prematurity and prenatal substance exposure. Social changes such as these will continue to shape the demand for and form of early childhood services.

The early childhood service models of today have as their genesis several influential movements or sources. These include practices in early childhood education for typically developing children, special education practices and reforms, and the compensatory education movement for disadvantaged or at-risk children. Inherent in these roots are the philosophical notions that (a) children must be helped or provided a nurturing environment in which to develop in order to reach their potential, and (b) equal opportunities should be available for all children. Help or remediation typically has been defined in the form of educational services. For years this approach was translated into practice as evaluating or identifying children's needs and determining goals and services for "fixing" those needs.

Though the literature related to early childhood services is extensive, no studies have attempted to empirically verify or define comprehensive "best practices" in the field. Therefore, the purpose of this chapter is twofold: (a) to describe underlying assumptions of current best practice in the United States, and (b) to present the results of a large survey of educators designed to identify a professional consensus on best practices in early childhood services. Strategies for providing integration of preschoolers with disabilities into regular ECSE programs and child-care settings also will be described. A number of models are explained to describe philosophical and theoretical principles as well as research results guiding quality ECSE programs.

Legislative Mandate

The passage of Public Law 99–457 in 1986 in the United States increased attention on early childhood services and provided a mechanism for the expansion of service options for children from birth to age 5. This law amended Public Law 94–142, which was passed in 1975 and is better known as the Education for all Handicapped Children Act. This act guarantees a free, appropriate public education (FAPE) for all children regardless of the level of their disability. Public Law 94–142 mandated that a written individualized educational plan (IEP) be developed annually by a multidisciplinary team. Due process protections were also specified in the law. However, Public Law 94–142 mandated service to 6- through 21-year-olds only. Safeguards for young children (from birth to age 5) were not addressed until Public Law 94–142 was amended in 1986, by Public Law 99–457.

Part H of Public Law 99–457 focuses on services for children from birth to age 3 and their families. It defines the individualized family service plan (IFSP), in which goals and services for both the child and family (in areas related to the disability or service needs of the child) are identified and a plan for meeting those needs is developed. The development of the IFSP expands upon previous models in that not only the needs, but also the strengths of the child and family are identified and considered in the planning and implementation of services. Part B of Public Law 99–457 requires states receiving federal funds to serve children with handicaps from 3 through 5 years of age. The passage of this bill culminated over 15 years of research and model demonstration projects. The law has been authorized for several years and provides the following:

1. A new state grant program for handicapped infants and toddlers from birth through age 2. States that want to participate must designate a lead agency, develop a statewide plan and agreements for interagency participation, require individualized family service plans for each child and his or her family, and guarantee full services within 4 years.
2. From fiscal year 1990 on, grants may be made only to states that assure the availability of a free appropriate public education for all handicapped children ages 3 through 5. (Weiner & Koppelman, 1987, p. 11)

Numerous questions and conflicts have emerged as states grapple to understand eligibility requirements for funding under EHA. The earlier law (P.L. 94–142) required the states to educate children with disabilities in the least restrictive environment (LRE). This concept is the foundation of the normalization principle. Within this framework, persons with disabilities are expected to work, live, attend school, socialize, and access the community in as normal a way as possible. States that provided special services to preschoolers before the federal mandate were rarely required to follow LRE guidelines. Now, states will have to serve young children with disabilities or risk the loss of federal funding. It is anticipated that providing ECSE programs within least restrictive environments will become more of an issue.

Efficacy and Best Practices

Discussing the efficacy of early intervention is a popular pursuit in the early childhood special education literature (Bricker, Bailey, & Bruder, 1984; Bronfenbrenner, 1975; Casto & Mastropieri, 1986; Dunst, 1985; Simeonsson, Cooper, & Scheiner, 1982). After more than two decades of data confirmed the efficacy of early intervention, the question continued to surface (Meisels, 1985). Issues of participant selection, description of specific intervention strategies, and instrumentation still continued to confound methodological purity, thereby limiting the generalizability of early intervention research. Nevertheless, infants and young children are seen as the most vulnerable members of our society. Society has made the decision that these children and their families have a right to early intervention services. The concern now is the form these services should take.

Interest in what constitutes best practice in programs serving children under 6 years old who are disabled or at risk is evident. It is apparent that guidelines describing basic tenets to assure program quality are needed. Research to determine most effective practices has not historically preceded practice in this area (Westlake & Kaiser, 1991).

McDonnell and Hardman (1988) carefully reviewed recent literature and determined six characteristics of exemplary ECSE programs. They provided empirical and ideological support for their assertions. Briefly, the authors suggested programs be (a) integrated, (b) comprehensive, (c) normalized, (d) adaptable, (e) peer- and family-referenced, and (f) outcome-based. McDonnell and Hardman defined integration as grouping children with and without handicaps together for instructional or social activities. They further specified that service sites outside the family home be generic and that systematic contact with the nonhandicapped children be arranged. Comprehensive programs included assessment, planning, instructional programming, service coordination, and evaluation; a transdisciplinary approach; theoretically and procedurally well-defined models; and direct instruction. A normalized program is described as one that supports the parents' role, is age appropriate, promotes generalization, encourages self-initiation, and avoids artificial reinforcement or aversive techniques. Adaptable services are those that support a variety of family structures, are flexible and noncategorical; are individualized; and emphasize functionality of response as well as formative evaluations for programmatic changes. Peer- and family-referenced services tend to include parents as full partners; consider family routines when enhancing child skill development; and reference the curriculum to individual child, family, peer, and community concerns (McDonnell & Hardman, 1988).

Assumptions Underlying Models

Although the debate continues regarding the efficacy of early services (e.g., Bronfenbrenner, 1975; Casto & Mastropieri, 1986; Casto & White, 1984; Meisels, 1985; Strain, 1984; Strain & Smith, 1986), the fact remains that the United States has made a commitment to serve young children who are disabled and/or at significant risk of developmental delays. As services expand, practitioners are challenged to develop and implement effective models for a wide range of young children and their families.

Assumptions that underlie exemplary early childhood services for young children who are disabled or at risk for disability are reviewed in this section. For purposes of discussion, these assumptions are grouped according to the following areas: (a) the importance of family involvement, (b) the nature of intervention and/or curricular goals, (c) integrated service opportunities for young children and their families, and (d) interdisciplinary/interagency coordination of services with transition supports between service delivery systems.

Family Involvement

At no other point in the lifespan must family involvement be emphasized to the degree that it is in early childhood. The earliest, and in most cases the most crucial, social exchanges and learning opportunities for the child are found within the family. From birth, babies are active and socially responsive, and their learning is largely social in nature (Lewis, 1984). In the earliest years babies develop an awareness of objects and people, awareness of cause-and-effect relationships, coordination of actions, and primary social relationships or attachments to their major caregivers. These social relationship ties are linked to social-emotional development in later years (Ainsworth, 1973). As childhood progresses from infancy to toddlerhood to preschool development, the child becomes increasingly able to separate from the parent or primary caregiver and engage in interactions with peers and other individuals in the environment. This emphasis on early learning within the context of the family, particularly during infancy, is critical for service providers. Services that fail to support child–family interactions or that exclude family members from participation run the risk not only of being ineffective in facilitating the child's development but also of producing negative effects.

A recent review of the literature by Silber (1989) discussed the dimensions of family life that are important to the child's early development.

These dimensions included (a) an attentive attachment figure who is warm and responsive; (b) use of consistent disciplinary standards with appropriate parental explanation and affect; (c) an organized, stimulating environment; (d) encouragement of learning through questioning and cueing that responds to the child; (e) parent expectation of the child's competence; (f) absence of family conflict, harmonious parents, and encouraging siblings; and (g) positive relationship of the family to the outside environment, including access to community services and the extended family.

The importance of the family is recognized in the shift away from early childhood services that are exclusively child-oriented and toward more family-focused approaches (Bailey et al., 1986; Dunst; 1985). This shift is reflected in Public Law 99–457, Part H, through the options for including family services in the IFSP. The development of the IFSP is viewed as a *process* rather than a product, with the formation of partnerships with families a paramount goal.

While the degree and type of family involvement and input in the education/intervention process may change somewhat during the preschool years, the concept of family involvement must be maintained. Though preschool-age children will spend more time engaged with peers and separated from their family members, their primary learning environments remain the family and their primary learning opportunities remain social ones.

Like all families, families of young children with special needs represent an interconnected and dynamic system (Seligman & Darling, 1989). Recently, the clinical literature on family systems (e.g., Minuchin, 1974; Olson et al., 1983) has been applied to the formation of a framework for serving families of individuals with special needs (e.g., Turnbull, Summers, & Brotherson, 1983; Turnbull & Turnbull, 1986). The view of the family through family systems theory emphasizes the interrelatedness of all family members. The focus is on the entire family as it defines itself rather than on a particular member, such as the child with a disability. This focus translates into new approaches to the delivery of early childhood services. Emphasis is being placed on supporting and strengthening families through the recognition of the family's own strengths and resources (Dunst, 1985; Dunst, Trivette, & Deal, 1988), and services increasingly reflect a family-focused or family-driven system for goal setting (Bailey et al., 1986).

Educational and child-care services must be adaptable to support the wide range of needs that the families of children with disabilities, just as all families, experience. Programs must be flexible, provide a wide range of service options, and deliver services in a respectful and culturally sensitive manner (Hanson & Lynch, 1989). In addition to direct interventions and educational programs for children, early childhood services may provide information to families, family support groups and/or counseling, parent education, and assistance in activating community resources or networks. Further, as the population of the United States continues to change and reflect an even more diverse group of people, the need increases for professional personnel to become more sensitive and knowledgeable about a variety of cultures and deliver services in a manner that is respectful and supportive of this diversity (Hanson, Lynch, & Wayman, 1990). Finally, Kaiser and Hemmeter (1989) recently cautioned against a totally needs-based approach to family intervention and offered a more value-based approach as an alternative. They presented four value elements to be considered in designing family interventions. The following are four element questions to be asked in the development of family interventions:

1. Does the intervention enhance community?
2. Does the intervention strengthen the family?
3. Does the intervention enable parents to do their jobs well?
4. Does the intervention enhance individual development and protect the rights of individual family members? (Kaiser & Hemmeter, 1989, p. 78).

As the authors state, "Based on these values, an ideal intervention will be one which is community-enhancing, strengthening to families, enabling of parents, and which enhances and protects each individual member of the family" (Kaiser & Hemmeter, 1989, p. 79).

Intervention Goals

The intervention goals for young children with special needs and their families are as varied as the families themselves. However, several intervention dimensions characterize most effective practices. First, interventions must be *individualized.* Regardless of whether the focus of intervention efforts is on the child or the family or both, the goals set must be individually tailored with family input to meet the needs of that child and family, and they must be implemented in a culturally appropriate manner that strengthens and supports the family. Second, given the *social* nature of development, the child's learning will be best enhanced in a social context. For services in the early years, this translates into supporting early parent–child interactions and the child's ability to interact with the environment and communicate with others. In addition, as the child grows older, peer interactions assume more importance. Third, interventions that recognize the child as an *active* learner and involve the child in *experiential* learning appear to be most effective. Hanson and Lynch (1989) discuss the importance of creating responsive, contingent learning environments (both social and nonsocial environments) for young children who are disabled or at-risk. Fourth, though children may be referred for intervention services because of disabilities or delays in one or more areas of development, intervention goals must reflect the *interrelatedness of areas of development*.

Lewis (1984) likens the development of the child to the growth of a tree, with early development being maximally interrelated and bound like the trunk of a tree. As the child develops, areas of development, like the branches of a tree, become increasingly differentiated. Nevertheless, all areas remain integrally interlinked with one another. Thus, intervention goals must account for the relationships among developmental areas and combine developmental areas when appropriate. Fifth, historically early childhood services have emphasized developmental approaches to service delivery and curricula often have been constructed around developmental milestones. While a developmentally focused approach is necessary for the fast-changing, growth-oriented early years, the use of milestones for curricular goals must be questioned due to the uneven development often observed in developmentally delayed children under 5 years of age. In addition to being developmentally and age appropriate, selected intervention goals must also be functional for the child (Hanson & Harris, 1986). The definition of *functional goals* is highly embedded in the family's cultural and environmental context. Goal setting and implementation of services must account for cultural variability (Wayman, Lynch, & Hanson, 1991). For instance, in some families early independence from the parents may be stressed, whereas for others, prolonged dependence on adult caregivers is culturally valued. Finally, recent expansion of early childhood services to include family interventions has highlighted the importance of family-focused or family-driven services that *support and strengthen families and enable families to use their resources* (Dunst et al., 1988) and that are *consistent with the values held by families* (Kaiser & Hemmeter, 1989).

Integration and Normalization

Young children spend the majority of their time in their homes and neighborhoods, where they are cared for by parents or child-care providers and where they encounter peers and make early friendships. Families, too, build social supports and networks within their neighborhoods and local communities. Historically, children with special needs have been removed from these community activities and provided "special services" often in locations that are isolated from the mainstream of community activities.

A body of evidence shows that preschool-age children derive positive benefits from participating in structured integrated settings where both nondisabled and children with disabilities are served together. Odom and McEvoy (1988) provide a comprehensive review of the literature on integration in the early years. They discuss the rationale for integrated efforts, children's social interaction patterns, the types of interventions that promote integration, and the outcomes of integrated efforts. Though many questions related to best practices with respect to integrated services remain unanswered, the research addressed in this review does provide support for serving young children with disabilities in integrated educational environments. In a recent discussion (Strain, 1990), a number of conclusions were drawn from the data on integrated ECSE services. First, parents of children in early intervention strongly desire that their children develop friendships with same-age typical children. Second, no study that has assessed social outcomes for children has found segregated services to be superior. In fact, approximately 90% of integrated versus segregated studies found integrated services to be superior (Strain, 1990). The third point extrapolated from extant data indicates that social skills have been found to be the most critical variable in postschool adjustment. Clearly, the opportunities for developing social skills are significantly increased in integrated programs. The fourth conclusion indicates that positive and sustained social growth does not occur simply because a program is integrated. Staff of ECSE must plan carefully to facilitate frequent high-quality social interactions. The fifth point taken from Strain's (1990) discussion is the assurance that normally developing children derive positive developmental and attitudinal outcomes as a result of integrated experiences.

Although empirical evidence supports planned integration practices and legal mandates (Public Laws 94–142 and 99–457) call for the placement of children in "least restrictive environments" for educational services, the issue of integrated services for young children and their families is much broader. The concept of normalization perhaps more closely embraces this issue. Long before the family is faced with decisions regarding the preferred educational placements for the child, the family adapts to having a new family member—for purposes of this discussion, a new baby with a disability. The first "integration" issue faced is one of integrating the child into the family unit and supporting the child and family in that process (NEC*TAS, 1990). Early in the child's life integration issues may be more family-focused than child-focused and include issues such as the availability of child care and playgroups through the same resources that are provided to other families. Issues of peer interactions and integrated educational services become especially important as the child reaches the preschool years. Thus, like intervention goals, the focus of integration and normalization must be on the child within the context of the family.

Interdisciplinary/Interagency Coordination of Services With Transition Supports Between Service Delivery Systems

Most children who enter the service delivery network in the early years do so at birth or shortly thereafter, and most are first identified through the health care network. Typically, children who are born with disabilities or those who are born at significant risk for developing disabilities (e.g., due to extreme prematurity or low birthweight, prenatal trauma, or prenatal substance addiction) are screened and referred for more extensive diagnostic evaluation and subsequent referral for appropriate intervention services. A hierarchy of services should be available for children and families during the early childhood age levels (infant, toddler, preschooler) with "fluid" entrance and exit criteria. These services should run the gamut from screening, to periodic developmental assessments, to comprehensive interdisciplinary early intervention/education program services. For example, some children who are considered at-risk for developmental delay will need only periodic assessments with referral for intervention services only if delays or needs are apparent. At the other end of the continuum are those children who have identifiable needs and for which a comprehensive program is warranted that includes continuous assessment and developmental interventions. These programs may range from several hours per week to several days per week in intensity; some may be implemented in the home and others in clinics or centers. Options for family participation vary, with the ideal circumstance being a range of program options within a community so that families may select those services most appropriate for their needs (e.g., parent education, child-care center, etc.). An important dimension of this continuum of services approach is that children and families can enter and exist at the points of need. Children may enter the service delivery continuum through the system (e.g., health or education) in which they become identified. That system may then refer the family to a more appropriate service delivery system (e.g., drug and alcohol programs) or may deliver the needed services if appropriate. As children grow and change and as their needs change, the system should remain fluid enough to "graduate" them to less intensive or more appropriate services (e.g., regular preschool with no additional special services).

Realistically, this range of services can be achieved only through coordinated, interagency community efforts. Most communities do not have the resources to provide a full range of services. When various agencies collaborate (e.g., health care, education, social services, developmental disabilities, mental health, etc.), often services can be pooled or shared and a more efficient and comprehensive system can be developed (Elder & Magrab, 1980). This concept is reflected in Public Law 99–457, which calls for states "to develop and implement a statewide, comprehensive, coordinated, multidisciplinary, interagency program of early intervention services for handicapped infants and toddlers and their families" (Section 671b).

Interdisciplinary Service

The concept of an interdisciplinary team approach to service delivery was in many ways born in early intervention services because of the wide range of needs experienced by infants who are disabled or at-risk. These needs typically span several disciplines and have necessitated that professionals work closely and collaboratively together in service delivery. At the minimum, most children and families are involved with professionals from the health care and education professions. Often a variety of different professionals are involved in services for a given child and family.

Three different types of team approaches have been discussed in the literature: multidisciplinary, interdisciplinary, and transdisciplinary teams (Holm & McCartin, 1978). Each defines different mechanisms for interactions among team members and with the family. Briefly, in the *multidisciplinary* approach, each professional conducts an evaluation and makes recommendations independently. The professionals then jointly confer with the family and share their findings and recommendations. The *interdisciplinary* approach is more collaborative. Following independent evaluations, the team members typically meet as a group to form recommendations for the child and family. The *transdisciplinary* model is the most interactive and is in many respects the hybrid model. The transdisciplinary approach is characterized by shared evaluations and planning and by role release (Lyon & Lyon, 1980). In other words, through extensive in-service training, team members train one another in various aspects of their spheres of practice such that they are able to collaborate, set, and implement goals that are interlinked. For example, the speech therapist, special education teacher, and parent may meet and as a team evaluate and set goals for the child. As the teacher or parent helps the child to activate a toy or identify pictures in a book, she or he will also attempt to incorporate the speech and language facilitation techniques recommended by the speech therapist. Though the transdisciplinary model necessitates commitment by each member of the team (including the child's parents as they desire) to joint planning and training, the coordination of services is greatly enhanced.

Transitions Between Services

In the first 5 years it is possible that children who are disabled or at risk for disabilities and their families will experience up to four major transitions in the service delivery system. These include the transitions from the hospital to the home, from home to early intervention services, from early intervention services to preschool services, and from preschool to elementary school services. At each transition different potentially stressful events are encountered. For example, when the child is discharged from the hospital parents are often required to perform complex tasks, such as feeding with a gastrostomy tube. The parents usually have had to rely on the health care professionals to care for their child—even to save their child's life—and suddenly new and frightening responsibilities are thrust upon them. The transition to an intervention program in many communities requires that the parent make contact with service agencies. Parents may be faced with a series of child and family assessments, searches for appropriate services, and a myriad of interviews with professionals. Admittance to an intervention program may bring relief in the form of assistance and support, and/or it may being added responsibilities for getting the child to and from appointments and managing the family's crowded schedule. In some states entrance in preschool represents a shift to a whole new system of service delivery—the public schools. With this transition parents are faced with learning their legal rights and how to negotiate a new system. Often the one-to-one support and contact that they have experienced in an early intervention program is not available in preschool services. Finally, the move from preschool to the elementary school may increase the distance between families and services. Typically, parents are less involved in their children's educational programs in the elementary years than in the early childhood years. For some parents this distance may be welcome, whereas others may experience isolation.

A number of studies have identified these transition periods as critical events for families that may be associated with increased stress (e.g., *see* Neisworth & Fewell, 1990). Support services and planned transitions can ease this process for families. This need for thoughtful and organized transitions is underscored by the inclusion in Public Law 99–457 of planning for transition in the development of the IFSP. Though more attention has been given to developing services to enhance families' transitions in recent years (Hanline & Knowlton, 1988), current practice in most communities falls far short of the needed services in this area.

Best Practices Survey

To more adequately define best practices for programs serving young children, the authors conducted a survey of early childhood educators, early childhood special educators, and professionals serving individuals with severe disabilities. The survey was designed to determine the perceptions of these professionals on the importance of a large number of variables associated with services for young children with disabilities from birth to age 3 and those from 3 to 5 years old. Differences between priorities for infants and toddlers (from birth to age 3) and preschoolers (ages 3 to 5) were anticipated. The study attempted to delineate such differences as well as to pinpoint qualities of equal importance to both age groups. The survey covered program characteristics, environmental qualities, and administrative aspects of early intervention services. Best practices and service issues in each area are described.

A large-survey was determined to be the most appropriate methodology for establishing program characteristics that typify best practices. A review of commonly utilized quality indicators was conducted. Sources included the Vermont Best Practices Guidelines (Fox et al., 1987), the Program Quality Indicators (Meyer, 1987), and the article on best practices in early intervention by McDonnell and Hardman (1988). Fifty items were developed under the general topics of curriculum, educational setting, family concerns, and administrative and programmatic issues. Participants were asked to respond to each item twice. First, they assessed to what extent the indicator was of priority in programs serving infants and toddlers. Respondents were then asked to make the same determination for preschool-age children.

A second section of the instrument required participants to respond within a five-point range on a number of questions. The ranges were designed to assess more sensitive issues that described staff/child ratios; intensity of services; level of integration; and general philosophic leanings (child-centered versus adult-centered environment, structured versus free-play activities, functional versus developmental curriculum, etc.). Participants were also asked to respond differentially to the needs of children with mild disabilities and those at risk as opposed to children with severe disabilities. The final component of the survey requested demographic information.

The nature of services for young children with disabilities is such that expertise from many disciplines is needed. The questionnaire was sent to people representing 10 broad occupational categories:

1. Teachers/educators.
2. Paraprofessionals/teacher assistants.
3. Researchers.
4. Teacher/personnel trainers.
5. Child-care providers.
6. Program administrators.
7. Health care professionals (e.g., physicians, nurses, and nutritionists).
8. Physical/occupational therapists.
9. Speech and language specialists.
10. Social service professionals (e.g., social workers, psychologists).

In order to achieve a nationally representative large sample of individuals concerned with the issues of early childhood service provision, professional organizations were consulted. Randomly generated mailing labels on members of three groups were purchased. Because integration has been identified as a critical component of best practices (McDonnell & Hardman, 1988), a sample of 5,000 members of the National Association for the Education of Young Children (NAEYC) was sought. Members of this organization are generally concerned with serving children who are nondisabled. A representation of their assessment of the priorities for best practice was considered crucial in order to develop a true national perspective. In addition, if early childhood services are located on generic sites it is important for special educators to understand what elements are critical to staff of regular programs.

The Council of Exceptional Children's (CEC) Division of Early Childhood (DEC) was also sampled to represent the early childhood special education point of view. Three thousand DEC members were randomly selected for participation. Finally, 2,000 members of The Association for Persons with Severe Disability (TASH) were included in the study. This organization concentrates on issues surrounding people with severe disabilities of all ages. The survey results will be reported and discussed in the same order as the assumptions and models that were described previously in this chapter.

Family Involvement

In the area of family involvement all items were highly rated, especially for children from birth to age 3. A large majority of the survey items concerning family involvement were identified as features most critical to programs serving children from birth to age 3. Only one item, "The program reflects sensitivity to different cultures, ethnic groups, and family values," was determined to be a higher priority for children 3 to 5 years old. One additional item of note is pertinent to family involvement. This item of best practice was stated, "Families have a primary liaison responsible for coordinating services with all agencies with which the family is involved." It was identified as significantly more important for children from birth to age 3. Perhaps this was deemed more important for the younger group because a very young child with disabilities (or at-risk) may need intense early medical intervention. (See Bennett & Guralnick, chapter 7, this volume.) The parents encounter numerous health care professionals, therapists, and quite possibly social services professionals before the baby even leaves the hospital. A host of community agencies awaits to provide needed services after hospital release. New parents with a medically fragile infant at risk for disabilities or one who is disabled may be overwhelmed by immediate adjustment issues. This leaves minimum energy for seeking and organizing special services. A liaison knowledgeable about existing agencies and programs can serve as the primary contact with the parents.

A related yet distinctly different best practice was that a range of family services be provided including information, support, counseling, education/training, and utilization of community resources. The respondents considered this also to be more critical in programs for infants and toddlers. The message is that families, as well as children, need a wide range of service options. Additionally, families are the strongest mediating influence on child development. Therefore, if the earliest special services are instrumental in strengthening and supporting families, the child will benefit. Assuring that "families are included as a part of the team for planning and service delivery," was also judged to be of substantially more importance for children from birth to age 3. This may indicate that services for infants and toddlers and their families are viewed as somewhat inseparable, whereas preschool services do not require as much parent presence.

The following four items, all classified as being of greater priority for the birth to age 3 group, conclude our discussion of family involvement as a fundamental best practice:

1. A family needs assessment is provided that is nonintrusive, individualized, and actively involves family members.
2. There is an established system for parent/staff communication between the program and home, in addition to that required by the IFSP/IEP process.
3. Staff members are responsive to parents' needs, questions, and concerns.
4. The program supports parent-child interaction and fosters quality parent-child relationships.

Often the major goals of early intervention programs are to understand and support families; to enhance the parent–child bond; and to establish frequent, effective communication between the home and program. The role of family (especially parents) in infant/toddler programs is paramount because intervention and even transportation to and from programs is typically done either by parents with assistance from program staff or by staff with parents present.

Intervention/Curriculum Goals

As previously described, the intervention goals and curriculum utilized by an effective early intervention program should be generated by the five underlying assumptions that can be viewed as guiding principles. This best practices data can be interpreted to reflect the belief of surveyed professionals that early intervention goals and curriculum should be based on a developmental model. Far fewer items in the intervention/curriculum goals category were determined to be of higher priority for infants/toddlers than for preschoolers. Only 6 of 18 items in this category were identified as being of higher priority for infants/toddlers. Of these items several were developmentally oriented, reflecting the importance these professionals placed on a developmental model for programs serving the youngest children. The fact that fewer best practices in terms of intervention and curriculum goals were thought to be significantly more important for the infant/toddler population served may indicate that people are less clear about what is best practice in this realm for this age group.

There is one curriculum/goal-setting best practice for which no significant differences were found between age groups. Apparently, it is equally important for infants/toddlers and preschoolers that "IFSP/IEP goals and objectives include performance in natural environments, e.g., the home and a variety of other age-appropriate environments." This is seen as an important fundamental principle that does not vary across age groups.

The following are three best practices in curriculum that were identified as more important for infant/toddlers:

1. Intervention goals are developmentally appropriate.
2. Curriculum content and instructional methodology are based upon a normal developmental model.
3. Development is viewed as resulting from the interaction between the child and the environment and is seen as proceeding through sequential, hierarchical stages.

The additional items rated of significantly higher priority for this younger age group were ones that asked respondents to answer within a range; they were stated in the following manner:

1. The curriculum is based on child's __ (1 = chronological age and 5 = developmental age).
2. The curriculum for children who are significantly at risk or mildly developmentally delayed is __ (1 = based on child's interests and 5 = based on assessed needs).
3. The curriculum for children with intense special education needs is __ (1 = based on child's interests and 5 = based on assessment needs).

There was a consensus formed suggesting that a developmental basis for goals and curricula is most appropriate for intervention in the earliest years. There appears to be general agreement that children with developmental delays who are very young can benefit from activities geared to a normal developmental sequence. It appears that setting goals and designing curricula based on normative development is more important for infants/toddlers than for older children. When planning intervention for preschool-age and older children it is of greater relevance to look at chronological age (what activities and materials are age appropriate) and functionality of objectives (what will ultimately result in more independence and autonomy for the individual). Response to this set of best practices was consistent with previous findings that early intervention curricula must be based on children's interests. In many ways very young children's interests are related to their development. The development of increased levels of visual, motoric, and cognitive competence dictates how children perceive, manipulate, and interact with materials and people.

In a related item, "The curricular content is based on __" (1 = developmental sequences and 5 = task-analyzed skill sequences), raters felt that task analysis was more critical for preschool-age children. This is most likely due to the fact that children of that age group are engaged in learning more difficult and complex skills. Efforts to break tasks down into small steps in a sequence toward completion and to teach in a systematic step-by-step manner are often necessary.

There were two best practices in the curricula/goal-setting area that were rated to be slightly more significantly important for preschoolers. These items were stated as follows:

1. The child is viewed as an active learner. Opportunities are provided for active engagement with the environment through concrete and sensory experiences.
2. The curriculum focuses on the whole child across all developmental areas.

These best practice guidelines are essential and should be considered when designing early childhood special education services.

The following is a list of other best practices related to the issues discussed above and also considered to be of greater priority for preschoolers:

1. Teaching activities are task analyzed and preplanned.
2. Intervention goals are functionally appropriate for the child.
3. Social interaction and social-communicative competence are stressed.
4. Instructional objectives included in the IFSP/IEP are written with (a) specified conditions, (b) observable behaviors defined, (c) and criteria for accomplishment.
5. Generalization goals across settings and people are considered.
6. For each IFSP/IEP objective currently implemented, there is an instructional program written in a format that allows for reliable implementation by anyone delivering instruction.

It appears that respondents consider a more systematic, behavioral approach to early childhood special education to be desirable. Again, the concepts of functionality, generalization, and consistency are critical. This further reinforces the idea that learning not take place in isolation.

Integration and Normalization

As just discussed, the concepts of integration and normalization are a critical assumption underlying early intervention (for the birth to age 3 group) and early childhood special education (for the 3 to 5 age group). However, they are rarely dealt with in isolation. Therefore, there are only six best practice items that speak to these concepts specifically. The reader will notice that these concepts are pervasive and are indirectly addressed in a large number of other best practice variables. One item was considered significantly more important for infants/toddlers; this was stated: "Early education strategies are implemented primarily in the child's natural environments, e.g., home, playgroups, day care." Perhaps this item was identified as a higher priority for the younger children because it specified all of the settings where infants and toddlers are typically served. The principle of normalization (Wolfensberger, 1972) emphasizes that children with disabilities, or those at significant risk for developing them, be served where typical children of that age are served. For infants and toddlers this is the home or a day-care setting. The principle of integration detailed in the least restrictive environment requirements of Public Laws 94–142 and 99–457 stipulates that, whenever possible, at-risk children or disabled children are served with children who are developing in a typical manner. Therefore, it is strongly suggested that identified infants and toddlers receive early intervention in their homes or day-care settings, and that integration activities through playgroups including normal children be organized to enhance socialization.

The following best practices mirror the discussion above and were categorized as far more crucial for preschool-age children:

1. When direct services are provided, they are offered in integrated settings (i.e., age-appropriate regular classrooms, community settings, the child's home).
2. The interventionist facilitates play on a regular basis between children with disabilities and their peers who are nondisabled.
3. The program is located in a facility that also serves nondisabled young children.

A number of questions remain concerning how much integration is optimal and whether certain levels of disability or types of handicaps influence the positive effects of integration (Strain, 1990). A number of items were written to assess these concerns. For example, the third of these three items asks for the same information as the first item without using the word *integration*. This was done because the word *integration* may be problematic (value laden) for some respondents who basically agree with promoting interaction between children with and without disabilities but dislike that particular term. The second item refers to the fact that physical placement in proximity to normally developing children is not enough for social integration to take place. Interaction between typically and atypically developing young children usually must be structured, modeled, and promoted by staff (Kohler, Strain, Maretsky, & DeCesare, 1990).

The final normalization/integration best practices items questioned what percentage of time identified children should spend with peers who are nondisabled. These items asked respondents to rate within the 1 to 5 range and read as follows:

1. The percent of time children who are significantly at risk or mildly developmentally delayed should spend in a regular class/group placement is __ (1 = 0% and 5 = 100%).
2. The percent of time children who have intense special needs should spend in a regular class/group placement is __. (Raters responded twice to each item, once for children from birth to 3 years old, and again for children 3 to 5.)

In general, it was considered more critical for preschool-age children regardless of disability level to spend more time with peers who are nondisabled. Percentage of time in regular class/group was also slightly higher for the at-risk and mildly developmentally delayed children. These responses are consistent with other responses within the survey and are socially valid.

Interdisciplinary/Interagency Coordination of Services With Transition Supports Between Service Delivery Systems

The best practices identified as more pertinent in infant (birth to age 3) programs were as follows: (a) The program provides a communication link to other agencies serving the child and family to ensure coordinated services, and (b) A process for decision-making among agencies serving children who are at risk or disabled is demonstrated in order to eliminate overlapping and redundant services. The two items judged to be more salient in services to preschool-age (ages 3 to 5) children were as follows: (a) Funding and interagency agreements allow for flexible and coordinated service delivery options to enhance integrated opportunities, and (b) Identified age-appropriate current and future environments are analyzed to determine the activities and skills required to function in those environments. The interdisciplinary nature of early childhood special education services is considered to be equally important for infants and preschoolers. Two items found to be important but statistically nonsignificant between age groups were the following: (a) Programs incorporate staff members from several disciplines who are specialists and have training with young children and their families, and (b) A transdisciplinary or interdisciplinary model is demonstrated in interventions provided in the classroom or home.

Program Characteristics

There are certain characteristics of programs serving young children with disabilities, that are clearly different from those serving older persons. Obviously, the size of equipment and materials will be smaller, but there are other program aspects that are more subtle. However, there is little research data available on special education program characteristics for the very young. A number of survey items addressing best practices in this area were designed. Items that dealt with program characteristics defined issues surrounding (a) assessment, (b) administration, (c) staff training, (d) staff:child ratios, (e) physical plant/environmental settings, and (f) philosophy.

Two basic items were identified as best practices, but no significant differences were found between their importance by age group. Considered equally vital for infants/toddlers as well as preschoolers are the following; (a) An adequate financial base is provided for program operation, and (b) The child's environments, both social and nonsocial, are contingent and responsive to the child's needs. One possible reason that these two items obtained nonsignificant differences between age groups is that they are fundamental to any high-quality program, regardless of the ages served.

Fewer items in this category were considered to be of higher priority for infants/toddlers, again reinforcing the idea that people are less clear about best practices for this age group. One item of primary concern for infants and toddlers is the following: Adequate health and safety standards for small children are provided (i.e., childproof environment, diapering procedures, food service procedures, play materials safe and cleaned after each use, environment safe for toddlers and climbers). Thus, there appears to be a strong concern that particular attention be paid to care, safety, and sanitation procedures for this age group.

Two items concerned with properly identifying very young children in need of special services were categorized as more vital for the children from birth to 3 years old; These are as follows: (a) Screening, diagnosis, and referral services are provided, and (b) Childfind and assessment services are available, enabling staff to identify and evaluate infants and children who are at risk and disabled. Although the debate continues (White, Bush, & Casto, 1985), most early interventionists believe that the earlier in life services are provided, the more effective they will be. That belief necessitates rigorous childfind and diagnostic activities.

Results of the survey indicated the item "Basic special education and child development training is provided on an ongoing basis to caregivers and teachers serving both typically developing children and children with disabilities" to be slightly (though statistically significant) more important for the youngest group. Consideration should be given to how ongoing training in these areas can effectively be provided to these service providers.

There are two environmental issues of substantially greater importance in serving children 3 years old and under. The first is, "Homebased special education is available." This greater importance is likely because the home environment is the most natural one for very young children.

The second issue has to do with the instructional environment. Respondents were asked to rate issues on a scale of 1 to 5 (1 = The instructional environment is structured for specific activities and tasks, and 5 = The instructional environment is nonstructured for free play). They were again asked to respond separately by age group. Responses were significantly higher for the younger group. The nonstructured instructional environment was considered much more appropriate for younger children.

The issue of how many adults (staff members) are needed per child to assure best practice in serving young children at risk or disabled is yet to be determined. The survey asked respondents to answer according to the previously explained age differentiations to the following items: (a) The preferred adult:child ratio for children who are significantly at risk or mildly developmentally delayed is __ (again in a 1 to 5 range, 1 = 1:12, with consistently lower proportions down to 5 = 1:1); and (b) The preferred adult:child ratio for children with intense special needs is __ (responses in the same range). The results of both items were consistent: Younger children, regardless of disability level, require a lower adult:child ratio (more adults are needed for fewer children).

The issue of how intense special education services should be for young children is also a subject of debate (Casto & Mastropieri, 1986). Survey items designed to address this were similar in format to the ratio items. Raters were asked to identify the following: (a) The number of hours of special education services that should be provided weekly to children who are significantly at-risk or mildly developmentally delayed is __ (1 to 5 was again the range of responses, with 1 = 2 hours and 5 = 20 or more hours per week); and (b) The number of hours of special education services that should be provided weekly to children with intense special needs is __ (response required within the same range). The intensity (or amount of special education hours per week) was judged to be higher for older children (ages 3 to 5). This finding held over level of disability; older children were found to be in need of more special education services.

Results indicated that more items describing program characteristics were considered to be of higher priority for preschool-age children. A number of items concerning the environment were rated to be significantly more important for the preschoolers. These were as follows:

1. The program has a written program philosophy.
2. Toys are modified as needed for instruction possibilities (e.g., switches).
3. Learning occurs most effectively in a well-controlled, planned environment in which the early interventionists' role is to teach or shape the child's behavior.
4. The environment is cheerful, colorful, and child-oriented.

5. Specialized equipment is utilized as needed (e.g., abductor/adductor chairs, prone boards, corner chairs).
6. The physical environment (e.g., toys, materials, and room arrangement) encourages individual and interactive play for all children.

The way in which a special education program for preschoolers should operate was also more clearly defined by survey respondents. The following program characteristics were classified as significantly more essential for preschoolers than for infants and toddlers:

1. A current schedule of daily activities describing what children are doing, when, and with whom, is available and accessible within the program.
2. Evaluation of overall program operation occurs on an ongoing basis.
3. The program provides a systematic procedure for on going training, monitoring, and staff development for all staff members implementing programs.
4. Criterion-referenced assessment that provides a basis for curriculum planning is demonstrated.
5. Developmentally appropriate assessments for children are nonbiased, conducted by a trained assessor and are given in the child's native language.
6. The program meets all legal and regulatory requirements for the state and locality.

The professionals surveyed believe that preschoolers require a more structured environment than do infants and toddlers.

Conclusion

In this chapter the assumptions and models that underlie exemplary early childhood services have been examined through a discussion of the extant literature and the report of recent survey results. In some areas, practices are well defined, whereas in others research is needed to determine best practices. This discussion does not outline a standard for services but does highlight important considerations in the definition of early childhood service practices.

In keeping with the overall intent of the book, it is reasonable to conclude with suggested strategies for promoting integrated opportunities for young children. One of the unique characteristics of early intervention services is that they are not necessarily center-based. These services can be delivered in a variety of natural settings such as homes, day-care centers, or preschools. This greatly extends opportunities for interaction between disabled and normally developing children. The early interventionist should be able to organize play groups in which more able children are encouraged to provide models for language and social development. The early intervention service providers can also model their skills in this area so that other adults are more likely to provide social inclusion for children with disabilities. Special service providers should also be willing to analyze integrated environments and assist in adapting them if specific equipment or communication devices are necessary. This may include training other adults and children to understand the communication system or equipment needs of an identified child.

In established programs that are not designed specifically for children with disabilities, special service providers may have to overcome administrative or attitudinal barriers to integration and mainstreaming. They should carefully prepare the physical and emotional environment for the identified child and family. This can include talking with staff, parents, and enrolled children about disabilities in general and the benefits of integration for normally developing as well as disabled or at-risk youngsters. If necessary, prior training concerning the specific special needs of the individual to be integrated may be necessary.

Reverse mainstreaming, or the practice of bringing nondisabled children into programs primarily serving children with disabilities is also a common practice. Given the shortage of high-quality preschools, it is not difficult to identify parents willing to enroll their children in these settings. This is not the preferred integrated setting because it reinforces the concept that separate facilities for the disabled are necessary.

The use of team teaching in preschools has been an effective practice. This involves the merging of special and regular preschool classes, and staff members between the two share teaching responsibilities. This can be an excellent way to increase the skill levels and knowledge areas of special and regular teachers. With the identified shortages in trained early childhood special services personnel this could provide an opportunity for extant special educators to gain the necessary skills and knowledge needed to work with very young children. The trained special educators could share their expertise in behavior management, individualization, or direct instruction with the regular teacher.

Services need to be provided to children in normalized, community-based sites. Services should follow the child, so the child is not "pulled out" or isolated from others for special services. The integrated model requires that special service providers from all disciplines provide needed support or therapies to children in their home, day-care, or regular school settings. Clearly, more model demonstration research projects are needed to assist the ECSE field to meet individualized child needs in structures designed for groups of normally developing children. When special service providers are viewed as a supportive asset to regular staff members and care is taken to meet the needs of all children in a program, effective mainstreaming and integration can be achieved.

References

Ainsworth, M.D.S. (1973). The development of infant–mother attachment. In B. Caldwell & H. Ricciuti (Eds.), *Review of child development research* (Vol. 3, pp. 1–94). Chicago: University of Chicago Press.

Bailey, D.B., Simeonsson, R.J., Winton, P.J., Huntlngton, G.S., Comfort, M., Isbell, P., O'Donnell, P., & Helm, J.M. (1986). Family-focused intervention: A functional model for planning, implementing, and evaluating individualized family services in early intervention. *Journal of the Division for Early Childhood*, *10*, 156–171.

Bronfenbrenner, U. (1975). Is early intervention effective? In B.Z. Friedlander, G.M. Sterritt, & G.E. Kirk (Eds.), *Exceptional infant: Assessment and intervention* (Vol. 3, pp. 449–475). New York: Brunner/Mazel.

Casto, G., & Mastropieri, M.A. (1986). The efficacy of early intervention programs: A meta-analysis. *Exceptional Children*, *52*(5), 417–424.

Casto, G., & White, K. (1984). The efficacy of early intervention programs with environmentally at-risk infants. *Journal of Children in Contemporary Society*, *17*, 37–48.

Dunst, C.J. (1985). Rethinking early intervention. *Analysis and Intervention in Developmental Disabilities*, *5*, 165–201.

Dunst, C.J., Trivette, C.M., & Deal, A.G. (1988). *Enabling and empowering families*. Cambridge, MA: Brookline Books.

Elder, J.O., & Magrab, P.R. (1980). *Coordinating services to handicapped children: A handbook for interagency collaboration*. Baltimore: Paul H. Brookes.

Fox, W., Thousand, J., Williams, W., Fox, T., Towne, P., Reid, R., Conn-Powers, C., Calcagni, L. (1986). *Best educational practices '86: Educating learners with severe handicaps*. (Monograph series 6, no. 1). Burlington, VT: University of Vermont, College of Education and Social Services.

Hanline, M.F., & Knowlton, A. (1988). A collaborative model for providing support to parents during their child's transition from infant intervention to preschool special education public school programs. *Journal of Division for Early Childhood (DEC)*, *12*(2), 116–125.

Hanson, M.J., & Harris, S.R. (1986). *Teaching the young child with motor delays*. Austin TX: Pro-Ed.

Hanson, M.J., & Lynch, E.W. (1989). *Early intervention: Implementing child and family services for infants and toddlers who are at risk or disabled*. Austin, TX: Pro-Ed.

Hanson, M.J., Lynch, E.W., & Wayman, K.I. (1990). Honoring the cultural diversity of families when gathering data. *Topics in Early Childhood Special Education*, *10*(1), 112–131.

Holm. V.A., & McCartin, R.E. (1978). In K.E. Allen, V.A., Holm, & R.L. Schiefelbusch (Eds.). *Early intervention: A team approach*. (pp. 97–122). Baltimore: University Park Press.

Ralser, A.P., & Hemmeter, M.L. (1989). Value-based approaches to family intervention. *Topics in Early Childhood Special Education*, *8*(4), 72–86.

Kohler, F.W., Strain, P.A., Maretsky, S., & DeCesare, L. (1990). Promoting positive and supportive interactions between preschoolers: An analysis of group-oriented contingencies. *Journal of Early Intervention*, *14*(4), 327–331.

Lewis, M. (1984). Developmental principles and their implications for at-risk and handicapped infants. In M.J. Hanson (Ed.), *Atypical infant development* (pp. 3–24). Austin, TX: Pro-Ed.

Lyon, S., & Lyon, G. (1980). Team functioning and staff development: A role release approach to providing integrated educational services for severely handicapped students. *Journal of the Association for the Severely Handicapped*, *5*(3), 250–263.

McDonnell, A., & Hardman, M. (1988). A synthesis of "best practice" guidelines for early childhood services. *Journal of the Division for Early Childhood*, *12*(4), 328–341.

Meisels, S.J. (1985). The efficacy of early intervention: Why are we still asking the question? *Topics in Early Childhood Special Education*, *5*(2), 1–11.

Meyer, L. (1987). *Program quality indicators: A checklist of most promising practices in educational programs for students with severe disabilities*. Seattle, WA: TASH.

Minuchin, S. (1974). *Families and family therapy*. Cambridge, MA: Harvard University Press.

NEC*TAS (1990). *Resource packet: Least restrictive environment for infants, toddlers, and preschoolers*. Chapel Hill, NC: University of North Carolina, NFC*TAS.

Odom, S.L., & McEvoy, M.A. (1988). Integration of young children with handicaps and normally developing children. In S.L. Odom & M.B. Karnes (Eds.), *Early intervention for infants and children with handicaps*, (pp. 241–267). Baltimore: Paul H. Brookes.

Olson, D.H., McCubbin, H.I., Barnes, H., Larsen, A., Muxen, M., & Wilson, M. (1983). *Families: What makes them work*. Beverly Hills, CA: Sage.

Seligman, M., & Darling, R.B. (1989). *Ordinary families, special children*. New York: Guilford.

Silber, S. (1989). Family influences on early development. *Topics in Early Childhood Special Education*, *8*(4), 1–23.

Simeonsson, R.J., Cooper, D.H., & Scheiner, A.P. (1982). A review and analysis of the effectiveness of early intervention programs. *Pediatrics*, *69*, 635–651.

Strain, P.S., (1984). Efficacy research with young handicapped children: A critique of the status quo. *Journal of the Division for Early Childhood*, *9*, 4–10.

Strain, P.S. (1990). LRE for preschool children with handicaps: What we know, what we should be doing. *Journal of Early Intervention*, *14*(4), 291–296.

Strain, P.S., & Smith, B. (1986). A counter-interpretation of early intervention effects: A response to Casto and Mastropieri. *Exceptional Children*, *53*(3), 260–279.

J.T. Neisworth & R.R. Fewell. *Topics in Early Childhood Special Education*. (1990). *9*(4).

Turnbull, A.P., Summers, J.A., & Brotherson, M.J. (1984). *Working with families with disabled members: A family systems approach*. Lawrence, KS: University of Kansas, Kansas University Affiliated Facility.

Turnbull, A.P., & Turnbull, H.R. (1986). *Families, professionals, and exceptionality: A special partnership*. Columbus, OH: Charles E. Merrill.

Wayman, K.I., Lynch, E.W., & Hanson, M.J. (1991). Home-based early childhood services: Cultural sensitivity in a family systems approach. *Topics in Early Childhood Special Education*, *10*(4), 56–75.

Weiner, R., & Koppleman, J. (1987). *From birth to 5: Serving the youngest handicapped children*. Alexandria, VA: Capital Publications.

Westlake, C.R., & Kaiser, A.P. (1991). Early childhood services for children with severe disabilities: Research, values, policy, and practice. In L.H. Meyer, C.P. Peck, & L. Brown, (Eds.), *Critical issues in the lives of people with severe disabilities* (pp. 429–458.) Baltimore: Paul H. Brookes.

Wolery, M. (1989). Transitions in early childhood special education: Issues and procedures. *Focus on Exceptional Children*, *22*(2), 1–16.

Wolfensberger, W. (1972). *The Principle of Normalization in Human Services*. Toronto, Canada National Institute on Mental Retardation.

9
Integrated Services for Adolescents With Disabilities

STEPHEN RICHARDS, DAVID L. LOVETT, AND
ROBERT GAYLORD-ROSS

Introduction

Secondary education should be designed to prepare students for adult life. Choices must be made concerning the skills to be learned that will improve outcomes upon leaving school. When poor decisions are made, the potential costs to individuals and to society are staggering. Many secondary education programs use relatively ineffective instructional methodologies to teach adolescents with disabilities. In addition, the curriculum that is presented to students who require special education frequently does not address their needs. Considerable numbers of students in special services drop out of school prior to graduation. In a large national study, 44% of secondary special education students did not graduate (Wagner, 1989), compared to approximately 29% of students without disabilities. Those who do graduate are rarely prepared to succeed as adults. We believe that, given an appropriate education, most students who need special services can succeed in school and as adults in the community. In chapter 10 of this volume, the authors address methods to assist adults with disabilities following graduation. In this chapter, we will address major issues related to the secondary education level and outline strategies for use at that level to improve the lives of students after they leave school.

As will be described in chapter 10, follow-up studies of special education students indicate that a majority of individuals do not engage in productive work and continue living with their families longer than what might be expected. Students with more severe disabilities may live in segregated facilities (e.g., institutions or group homes). Many special education graduates do not receive, are ineligible for, or fail to access available services (Hasazi, Gordon, & Roe, 1985). In addition, as students they presumably did not receive adequate training in vocational or job-seeking skills (Haring & Lovett, 1990). The result of these factors is that many people with disabilities are largely unemployed or underemployed, although most express a desire to work (Rusch & Phelps,

1987). As indicated in chapter 10, many graduates of special education programs express dissatisfaction with their lives. This situation must be addressed through revisions and improvement in the special education and adult service delivery systems.

This chapter is designed to (a) examine models of and explore issues related to integration in secondary special education, (b) examine models for training vocational and community living skills, and (c) examine models of and explore issues related to transition planning and implementation of transition services.

Issues Related to Integration in Secondary Special Education

The decision of where and how to deliver services to exceptional individuals is a critical one. The model or approach employed will almost certainly affect students' integration into the school as well as integration into the community. Lerner (1985) outlined eight possible levels of service delivery for exceptional students as follows (listed from most to least restrictive):

1. Noneducational services such as welfare care and supervision.
2. Instruction in hospital or residential settings.
3. Homebound instruction.
4. Special stations or schools.
5. Full-time special class.
6. Part-time special class.
7. Regular class plus supplementary instructional services.
8. Full-time regular class.

A number of models for delivery of services have been implemented within the continuum of levels outlined by Lerner. Typically, the more severe a student's handicap, the more restrictive the placement. Some special school placements serve only students with handicaps. These placements may provide full-time special services (e.g., physical therapy, special counselors, school nurse) that may be offered on an itinerant basis in neighborhood schools. They do not, however, provide maximum opportunity for interaction with nondisabled peers. These placements have been criticized for lack of opportunity for integration into the mainstream of the school and community (Falvey, 1986). Many advocates for students with severe handicaps agree that such placements are not conducive to the acquisition of skills necessary for successful postschool adjustment (Brown, Long, Udvari-Solner, Davis et al., 1989).

Another model of service delivery is a cluster approach. Typically, in this type of placement, exceptional students are transported to a centrally located regular school campus. Similar to the special school placement, a cluster approach generally allows for the provision of special services on-site (Thomason & Arkell, 1980). Opportunities for integration are generally increased because the program is located on a regular school campus. This approach may be favorable to special school placement (Thomason & Arkell, 1980). However, large numbers of exceptional students may create an "unnatural" proportion of exceptional students in relation to the regular education students. This large number of students with disabilities may hinder opportunities for meaningful interaction between students with disabilities and those without.

Other authors have recommended that all students be served in their neighborhood or home schools (Brown, Long, Udvari-Solner, Davis et al., 1989). Services may be delivered in full-time special classes, in part-time special classes, or in regular classes with or without additional support. Brown, Long, Udvari-Solner, Davis, et al. have stressed that the educational environment should have a reasonable ratio of students with handicaps to those without handicaps; that it should be chronologically age appropriate; and that all facilities, resources, and buildings should be accessible to students with disabilities. In addition, these authors stressed that related services can and should be delivered in neighborhood schools. The lack of availability of related services in the home school should not be used as an excuse for placing students in more restrictive settings (Brown, Long, Udvari-Solner, Schwarz et al., 1989). These writers have maintained that even within neighborhood schools, special class placement is detrimental to integration.

Mainstreaming

Many educators have advocated mainstreaming to ensure a more age-appropriate, integrated, and relevant education for exceptional students. Mainstreaming may be achieved through the following strategies outlined by Hallahan and Kauffman (1988):

1. Encourage regular educators to employ effective techniques used with regular students on mainstreamed exceptional students (e.g., minimize time not allocated for instruction).
2. Use special educator teacher consultants to assist regular educators (e.g., assist in devising and implementing a behavioral program to control off-task behaviors).
3. Use prereferral teams consisting of regular and special educators to assist students before they require special education services (e.g., provide tutoring in problem areas).
4. Encourage cooperative learning among all students in regular classes (e.g., work in groups so that academically strong students model learning strategies for weaker students).
5. Use regular students as peer tutors for mainstreamed students.
6. Make attempts to change regular students' attitudes toward mainstreamed exceptional students (e.g., conduct activities to illustrate the negative impacts of prejudice and stereotyping).

Some writers have suggested, however, that there may be some reticence on the part of regular educators to teach students with challenging academic and behavioral difficulties (McKinney & Hocutt, 1988). Other writers have noted that the advantages of physical placement in regular classes of students with disabilities may be overestimated compared to the benefits of the instruction received in these settings (e.g., Bickel & Bickel, 1986; Hallahan & Kauffman, 1988). There is general agreement, however, that students should be given a chance to succeed in the regular class before being moved to more restrictive settings (as opposed to beginning in a more restrictive setting and working toward a less restrictive one).

In fact, cross-cultural research has uncovered this presumption of inclusion in other societies. For instance, Gaylord-Ross (1986) found that Italy has statutory regulations to place and retain the student with disabilities in the regular class. In Italy, the question is not whether to place the student in a regular or separate program; rather, the regular class placement is assumed, with the question of what kind of instruction and social support system is needed to maximize the quality of a student's education. In general, such "radical" integration approaches (from the U.S. perspective) give the opportunity for the student to succeed in regular settings, rather than assuming the student must prove or be ready to graduate to a nonseparate educational context.

In reference to mainstreaming of students with more severe handicaps, the concept of *full inclusion* has been developed (Brown, Long, Udvari-Solner, Schwartz et al., 1989). Advocates of this approach maintain that these types of students can receive an appropriate education while attending regular classes with nondisabled peers. Special services, including special education personnel, are available in the regular class. The curriculum and instruction for students with severe disabilities are based on individual needs and do not necessarily mirror those used with the regular students, although opportunities for appropriate learning should occur within regular class activities (Stainback & Stainback, 1988). What appears to be critical to proponents of full inclusion is that all students enjoy growing up and attending classes with their chronological, neighborhood peers. However appealing this concept may be, there is debate concerning its practicality (Brown, Long, Udvari-Solner, Schwartz et al., 1989). To date, there has not been presented in the literature a substantial broadscale data base documenting the advantages of full inclusion over other service delivery options.

The skills of the personnel involved and the needs of the students must be considered in deciding the particular strategy or strategies to employ. It is crucial that special and regular educators cooperate if mainstreaming is to be successful. Proponents of the Regular Education Initiative (REI) have reinforced this point (Reynolds, Wang, & Walberg, 1987; Wang, this volume; Will, 1986). Proponents of the movement essentially advocate greater responsibility of regular educators for the education of students with mild handicaps. In a recent survey of regular and special educators, results indicated that there was generally philosophical agreement among all educators that the education of special students should be a shared responsibility. However, they also agreed that the existing educational system would require considerable change to implement the REI (Taylor, Richards, Goldstein, & Schilit; in press). There is no solid evidence that educators nationwide are prepared to make the necessary changes to achieve this shared responsibility (Kauffman, Gerber, & Semmel, 1988). Nevertheless, the relationship between regular and special educators needs to improve. This may be accomplished through pre- and in-service training toward modifying regular curricula, classroom structure, and teaching methodologies to better accommodate students with disabilities in regular class settings (Taylor et al., in press).

Dropouts and Dropout Prevention

Despite efforts to provide services in the least restrictive environment, there remains a problem with dropout rates and dropout prevention. Although the rate for nondisabled students is certainly of concern, the rate for students with disabilities may be even more alarming, particularly for those with learning disabilities and behavioral disorders (Edgar, 1987). Cross, Darby, and D'Alonzo (1990) reviewed a number of studies and identified the following factors, which appear to predict the likelihood of dropping out: (a) low socioeconomic status, (b) a lack of reading materials and books at home, (c) educational level of the same-sex parent, (d) low school grades, and (e) teen pregnancy. Many students with disabilities encounter variables such as these that further hinder success. Edgar (1987) reported that in one study the results indicated significant numbers of students who had received special education services had neither graduated nor aged out. He noted his belief that many students with disabilities leave school before completing a program of study or before reaching the maximum age for services. However, it appeared that these students were difficult to locate, and therefore it was difficult to obtain data regarding the reasons for leaving school Whereas 29% of students who begin ninth grade do not graduate nationwide, Edgar noted that the statistics for special education were even worse. He reported findings that 42% of students who were learning disabled or behaviorally disordered dropped out of school. This compared to only 18% of the mildly mentally retarded students in the study. Similarly, students with severe handicaps had only a 12% dropout rate but experienced poor postschool outcomes. The dropout rate was only 8% for students with sensory impairments. The overall dropout rate for all special education students in the reported study was about one third. The majority of students (73%) who graduated or aged out were employed, continuing in school, receiving vocational training, or involved in some other training program. However, among those employed, only 15% were working for better than minimum wages. Conversely, 61% of students who had dropped out were involved in no activity associated with employment, further education, or training for employment.

Edgar's (1987) results clearly demonstrate that students with learning disabilities or behavioral disorders are at greater risk of dropping out than either nondisabled peers or students with other disabilities. Edgar and others (e.g., Reid, 1988) have suggested that the high dropout rates may be due to disenchantment among students with remedial approaches at the secondary level; an overemphasis on academic learning; and, in general, a curriculum that poorly prepares students for postschool life. However, isolating these students in special education classes in order to address these concerns creates a dilemma. Edgar pointed out that to remove special education students from the mainstream curriculum and the regular classroom may result in highly segregated special classes populated by male students from minority backgrounds. Cross et al. (1990) noted that while many dropout prevention programs stress self-improvement processes (e.g., tutorial and workshop sessions, social skills training), programs should provide a strong vocational component in addition to academic intervention. Although Edgar lamented the lack of clear direction for remedying the curriculum/mainstreaming (and consequently the dropout) problem, there appear to be at least some reasons for optimism. The following sections present issues concerning strategies to improve outcomes for students with disabilities.

Secondary Special Education: Guiding Practices

In chapter 6, the cooperative efforts required between special educators and other concerned personnel to produce meaningful outcomes for exceptional students were discussed. A major responsibility for overseeing the realization of these outcomes still rests, however, with special educators. Ianacone and Stodden (1987) listed six ways in which special educators have been counterproductive in teaching students to be independent and productive citizens:

1. Dependency structures (e.g., allowing communication modes to be vertical between teacher and student, leading to overreliance on expert knowledge).
2. Decision taking (e.g., not allowing or teaching students to make decisions).
3. Employment irrelevance (e.g., overemphasizing academic remediation).
4. Misguided reinforcement (e.g., maintaining unnatural reward schedules into early adulthood).

5. Self-fulfilling expectations (e.g., assuming a student is capable of only sheltered employment).
6. Focus on disability (e.g., overemphasizing weaknesses rather than strengths).

In the following sections are suggestions for remediating these counterproductive practices.

Issues Related to Curricula and Instruction

This section is divided into subsections that cover issues related to students with mild disabilities and issues related to students with more moderate to profound disabilities. Although many aspects of the educational and transition processes are similar across all special education groups, the teaching/learning strategies used with these groups may differ to some extent.

Issues Related to Students With Mild Disabilities

One of the most important curriculum issues related to educating students with mild disabilities is whether skills to be learned are derived strictly or largely from the regular curriculum. Patton, Cronin, Polloway, Hutchison, and Robinson (1989) pointed out that there are three basic curricular approaches with students with mild disabilities: (a) a remedial approach, which emphasizes basic skills and social competence; (b) a maintenance approach, which emphasizes tutorial services and learning strategies; and (c) a functional approach, which emphasizes vocational and life skills training. These same authors summarized and critiqued these approaches in Table 9.1. A remedial, or basic skills, approach may tend to lock students into the use of age-inappropriate materials and inordinate time spent on learning prerequisite skills (Reid, 1988). Reid argued that a remedial curriculum approach is probably the least desirable at the secondary level. Some have argued that to deny participation in the regular curriculum is to deny equal opportunity (Adler, 1982). Others have argued that the regular curriculum does not prepare students with disabilities for the demands of adulthood and that more of a life skills approach is desirable (Patton et al., 1989). The most critical curriculum decision would appear to hinge on whether or not the student may be reasonably expected to make a successful transition to postschool life prepared with those skills learned in the regular curriculum. Patton et al. suggested that developers of a curriculum for students with mild mental disabilities should consider that learning is lifelong, that content should be adult- and community-referenced, that content should be relevant to the students' own experiences, and that it should involve community-based instruction. However, such an approach may be less applicable to students with learning disabilities or other mild disabilities. Reid argued that a distinct curriculum for students with learning disabilities is unnecessary if not counterproductive. Certainly, any decision concerning the curriculum a student will access must be based on individual needs. There are, however, certain practices that may be useful for teaching in either a functional skills or regular curriculum that are designed to increase the likelihood of successful transitions.

Overall, the question of *what* to teach has been relatively overlooked for students with mild disabilities. Much more attention has been given to *where* (mainstreaming) and *how* (instructional strategies) issues. Content questions are far from being resolved. For example, should students with mild disabilities strictly follow the academic core curriculum of regular education? Proponents of academically based (back to basics) school reform might argue in the affirmative. Those with a functional curriculum perspective would argue for an emphasis on vocational skills, social skills, and related living skills in the curriculum. These rather powerful and contrary positions have not yet been resolved by curriculum and policy analysts.

Weisenstein and Elrod (1987) discussed eight areas of importance in teaching practices for students with mild disabilities. The following is a summary of their discussion. The first consideration is that training should be geared toward generalization. Students should be taught in a way that allows them to transfer learning from one situation into novel situations. That is, skills ought to be taught in a way that their utility is "transparent" to the student (Reid, 1988) and the skills applied in ways that are meaningful to the student (e.g., learning a strategy that promotes improved test scores and grades across several academic areas). Weisenstein and Elrod noted that teaching students to respond and perform equally well across instructors is another way to address generalization.

The second consideration is the fading of nonnatural reinforcement. Ianacone and Stodden (1987) stressed that special educators sometimes reinforce behaviors that inhibit independence (e.g., continuing to reinforce the act of having materials ready when the behavior has been learned and should be part of the student's natural repertoire), and the schedules used do not resemble natural schedules of reinforcement (Weisenstein & Elrod, 1987).

A third important consideration is that students must develop social learning. By social learning, the authors refer to critical thinking skills that will result in more effective decision making (Weisenstein & Elrod, 1987). This process might involve teaching students labeling (e.g., a bus schedule); detailing (noting specific characteristics about the bus schedule); inferring (Why is the schedule important?); predicting (When will the next bus come?); and generalizing (How can we use other bus

TABLE 9.1. Summary of curricular orientations.

General focus	Specific orientation	Features	Cautions
Remedial	Basic skills	Development/remediation of academic skills. Common at elementary level. Frequently found at secondary level as well.	Deficit-oriented. Problems in generalization. Too heavy a reliance on this orientation with secondary level students may be inappropriate, sacrificing attention to other area.
	Social skills and adjustment	Focus in on the development of social competence. Important area for integrative efforts and job success.	Programs need to be accountable for observable and meaningful change.
Maintenance	Tutorial	Commonly used at the secondary level. Focus is on helping students in their regular education classes. Has motivational benefits for students. Has political benefits—regular educators like the assistance in meeting the needs of special learners.	Emphasis is short-term objectives—little lasting value. Question of relevance to a student's future needs. Undertraining of special education teachers in certain subject areas (e.g., chemistry). Actual instructional techniques of tutoring may not require specialized training.
	Learning strategies	Learning to learn concept. Teaches students cognitive-based strategies. Appropriate for adolescent students.	May require students to read above third-grade level; have average intelligence; deal with symbolic as well as concrete learning tasks. Should not limit in-class time on functional topics. Strategies do not always generalize to other situations.

TABLE 9.1. *Continued*

General focus	Specific orientation	Features	Cautions
Functional	Vocational	Traditionally associated with programs of students with mild/moderate retardation. Direct relationship to postsecondary work environments. Motivational to students. Recent advances in supported employment are encouraging.	Not all programs are community-based. Students can get locked into a vocational track. Training skills that lack community validity. Training facilities may not have state-of-the-art equipment. Some students in other (e.g., curricular programs) diploma-track may be excluded.
	Life skills/adult outcomes	Stresses comprehensive life skills orientation. Community validity should be in evidence. Top-down perspective. Shifts focus on schooling for students who have experienced longstandig academic deficits.	Programs can be developed haphazardly (i.e., unsystematically). May need to be augmented with directive social skills training. Should be accompanied by vocational preparation.

Reprinted with permission from: Patton, J.R., Cronin, M.E., Polloway, E.A., Hutchison, D., & Robinson, G. (1989). Curricular considerations: A life skills orientation. In G.A. Robinson, J.R. Patton, E.A. Polloway, & L.R. Sargent (Eds.), *Best Practices in Mild Mental Disabilities*, pp. 21–37. Reston, VA: Council for Exceptional Children.

schedules?). These skills may enable students to better evaluate the environment and make sense of their own observations.

A fourth consideration listed by Weisenstein and Elrod (1987) is to help students become better planners and problem solvers. This might be accomplished through helping students realize how concepts may be applied across settings and situations. For example, a student might be taught the concepts of *greater than* and *less than* (Weisenstein & Elrod, 1987). He or she might then be taught how purchases can be evaluated based on greater than (e.g., one container of a product has a greater quantity than another) and less than (e.g., however, the smaller container may be less in price per ounce than the larger).

The fifth consideration is the need for prevocational skill training. Research has indicated that students with mild handicaps sometimes lose jobs because of deficits in related vocational skills that could be learned at early ages (Rusch, 1986). For example, learning to be on time and to complete work in an accurate and timely fashion are but two skills that are necessary for vocational success that may be taught prior to specific vocational skill training. These skills are not necessarily taught as specific prevocational skills because they may be incorporated into academic and social skill learning (Weisenstein & Elrod, 1987).

The sixth consideration is the teaching of cognitive behavior modification. Meichenbaum (1979) suggested the use of a strategy by which students are taught self-control by using their own speech (ultimately internally). However, the focus of this strategy eventually shifted to self-monitoring of behaviors that affect academic performance, such as paying attention (Hallahan et al., 1983; Reid, 1988). For example, a teacher might model the appropriate behavior (e.g., attending behaviors), then ensure the student understood the targeted behavior, and finally implement a system by which the student monitors his or her own behavior (e.g., recording whether or not he or she is paying attention at a given time). Hallahan et al. reported this strategy yielded improved time-on-task and improved academic performance. Lovett and Haring (1989) used similar strategies to increase the completion of daily tasks by adults with mental retardation.

The seventh consideration is closely related to cognitive behavior modification. Metacognition is an area that has received recent attention. Advocates of strategy training cite early studies and authors that indicated that students' learning problems were the direct result of approaching tasks nonstrategically or with inefficient strategies (Bauer, 1977; Borkowski & Cavanaugh, 1979). Reid (1988) has characterized metacognition as the process of learning and knowing about one's own learning and knowing. Metacognitive strategies include planning, scheduling, monitoring, revising, and evaluating one's own performance in the acquisition, storage, and retrieval of information (Reid, 1988). These strategies include but are not restricted to summarizing, rehearsal, self-questioning, reviewing, and self-testing. Researchers from the University of Kansas have developed programs for teaching such specific learning strategies, such as error monitoring and sentence writing (Deshler, Schumaker, Lenz, & Ellis, 1984a, 1984b). Palincsar and Brown (1984) outlined "reciprocal teaching," a strategy-based method for increasing the comprehension of problem readers. This method emphasizes the active participation of the student (e.g., through modeling for other students, leading class lessons) and "negotiated" learning (i.e., a process that places responsibility for learning on both teacher and student). Overall, the basic intent of metacognitive strategy training is to help students "learn to learn" and effectively apply and demonstrate their knowledge.

The final consideration listed by Weisenstein and Elrod (1987) is the training of motivational skills. The interaction of beliefs about self-efficacy with success has been demonstrated (Bandura, 1977) but not always addressed in the schools. Reinforcement programs may assist teachers in fostering motivation in students, but there is at least some evidence that students' self-perceptions or attributions contribute to levels of motivation (Borkowski, Carr, & Pressley, 1987). Butkowsky and Willows (1980) suggested that many students with learning disabilities have experienced failure and attribute that failure to internal (i.e., self-deprecating) factors. Attributional retraining has been used recently as an adjunct to metacognitive strategy training to help students overcome self-defeating attributions (Borkowski, Weyhing, & Turner, 1986). Attributional retraining involves addressing the student's beliefs about the possibilities of success and failure, what constitutes success and failure, and what individual actions contribute to success and failure (Borkowski et al., 1987). Retraining is generally conducted through discussions concerning effort and performance on actual tasks. These researchers have suggested that the learning problems of many students must be simultaneously addressed as strategy and motivation deficits (Borkowski et al., 1986).

These eight considerations may be applicable, at least in some part, to students with moderate to profound handicaps, but their use with this population may be limited in comparison to that with students with milder handicaps. Researchers and educators have suggested other strategies that may prove useful with both groups but that are typically used with populations with more severe disabilities.

Issues Related to Students With Moderate to Profound Disabilities

Wehman, Moon, Everson, Wood, and Barcus (1988) listed three major issues in providing services to students with moderate to profound handicaps. First, the curriculum used should be "functional." That is, the behaviors learned as part of the school curriculum should increase the independence of the individual student. This curriculum design might be based on an ecological approach. In this approach environments are analyzed to determine skills that are used in specific settings. Functional behaviors have been defined as behaviors that would have to be performed by someone else if not performed by the student (Brown et al., 1984). This type of training is intended to prepare students to live and work in both present and future environments (Brown et al., 1984). Therefore, a functional curriculum addresses what is both functional now as well as what is anticipated to be functional in the future. Brown et al. (1985) pointed out, however, that all goals need not be "functional" in the strictest sense. These authors suggested that goals be selected based on the following factors:

1. Are the number of environments in which the student participates increased (e.g., a recreation/leisure skill that is useful in many situations)?
2. Is the goal chronologically age appropriate (e.g., selecting clothing that emulates those of peers without disabilities)?
3. Will the student have the opportunity to practice the skill in other environments (e.g., using a microwave oven at school as well as at home)?
4. Is the skill required in adulthood (e.g., using a telephone)?
5. Is the behavior preferred by the student?
6. Is the skill preferred by the parents/guardian of the student?
7. Does the skill enhance the physical well-being of the student (e.g., therapeutic recreation skills that enhance several aspects of a student's life)?
8. Does the skill enhance the social contacts of the student (e.g., communication skills)?
9. What is the probability of acquisition of the skill (e.g., will the student learn to read at a reasonably functional level or would an essential sight vocabulary be more likely to be acquired)?
10. Does the skill enhance the student's status (e.g., learning to take orders from the public in a fast-food restaurant as opposed to learning only to bus tables)?

Brown et al. (1985) also noted that a skill should not be selected if it does not represent some credible dimension of the areas listed above, if it rarely leads to instruction in real-life environments, or if it is not meaningful to the individual student.

Some students with the most severe handicaps may be so limited in their physical capacity to acquire skills that learning truly functional behaviors may become problematic, that is, they will be dependent on others for basic care needs into the foreseeable future (Sternberg, 1988). These students may "partially participate" in functional activities contributing to their own independence at their individual levels (Baumgart et al., 1982). For example, a student with severe physical handicaps resulting from cerebral palsy may not be able to perform the functional skills needed to dress himself or herself, but may be able to partially assist through whatever movement he or she has, selecting clothing appropriate for the weather, color coordinating clothing, and so forth. Helmstetter (1990) suggested that the concept of partial participation should be extended to include passive participation. Helmstetter emphasized that while an ecological approach to curriculum development is probably appropriate for students with profound disabilities, greater dependence on technological adaptations and assessment of the communicative intent of students' behaviors should be stressed. Indeed, it is probably reasonable to assume that technological advances and further research into training strategies for use with students with profound handicaps will yield new and innovative ways to increase the individual's potential for physically performing skills that otherwise would have been thought improbable (Guess, 1983). For example, Gaylord-Ross et al. (1991) demonstrated that adults who were deaf-blind and severely disabled could work successfully in nonsheltered settings such as restaurants and corporate office buildings. Jobs often had to be redesigned to foster partial participation, and communication devices were installed to promote social exchanges (Gaylord-Ross, Lee, Johnston, & Goetz, in press). The reader may find Brown and Lehr's (1990) and Sternberg's (1988) books particularly useful in designing programs for students with profound disabilities.

A functional curriculum should include goals and objectives that prepare students for successful adjustment in school; in environments outside of school; and in environments in which they are likely to work, live, and play as adults. Typically, the functional curriculum domains include vocational/employment, residential/home living, community living, and recreation/leisure skills, with social/affect and communication/language skills emphasized across all environments.

According to Wehman et al. (1988), the integration of school goals and community needs is another aspect of curricula and instruction that should be addressed. These authors noted that the integration of students with disabilities into vocational training programs that include workers without disabilities provides opportunities to interact with nondisabled persons and to learn the standards for performance and behavior as applied to all adult workers. Second, this integration ensures that students who are job-ready may be placed or employed immediately as opposed to having to complete a training program that may be unnecessarily long and time-consuming for the individual. It should be noted that the integration of school goals and community needs also includes a recognition of community and cultural expectations that should be taken into account during school-based interventions. Finally, school/community integration should include specific goals and objectives related to community functioning and taught directly in the community.

Brown, Nietupski, and Hamre-Nietupski (1976) proposed the "criterion of ultimate functioning" as a guideline for developing instructional models. This principle is based on the idea that many students with disabilities are, by definition, likely to learn fewer skills and take more time to acquire those skills than their nondisabled counterparts. Subsequently, those skills taught ought to be meaningful and functional. That is, the criteria for selection of instructional goals and objectives should relate to those environments where the student is likely to ultimately reside and work. Falvey (1986), among others, has emphasized that given the skill transfer and generalization problems of many exceptional students, skills must be taught directly in those environments where the skills will be applied. Therefore, community-referenced instruction (as well as community-based instruction) should be an integral part of special education programs (Falvey, 1986).

Community-referenced instruction may involve both concurrent and community-based instruction. With concurrent training, students practice skills in school immediately prior to community-based instruction; for example, the student practices counting out correct change for a vending machine just prior to going to use an actual vending machine in the community (Brown et al., 1983). The time lapse between school-based and community-based instruction should be minimized. Many writers (e.g., Falvey, 1986; Wehman et al., 1988) stress that students should not be denied community-based instruction based on performance of skills taught in school (e.g., not allowing a student to work on crossing streets because he is unable to distinguish "Walk" and "Don't walk" on cards resembling street signs). Subsequently, experts recommend all students with moderate to profound handicaps (and many with milder handicaps) should receive direct instruction in the community (Brown et al., 1983; Patton et al., 1989). As a student becomes older, up to 80% or more of the student's instructional day might be spent in community-based instruction (Hill & Morton, 1988). This practice does, however, remove the student from the integrated school setting. It should be pointed out that students who are 18 or older are not with the majority of their chronological peers if they are spending most of the school day at a high school. Therefore, predominantly providing community-based instruction for these students would not appear to be inappropriate. For younger students, there should be consideration of a balance between the need for contact with chronological-age peers and the need for integration in the community at large.

There are a number of issues that school personnel should address concerning the implementation of community-based services. Falvey (1986) and Wehman et al. (1988) included the following topics as important for consideration. The first is establishment of policies governing instruction that specify procedures for emergencies, who is responsible for students' safety, what to do if a student is lost, and so forth. Second, staff should obtain informed consent from parents/guardians before instructing students in the community. Third, school districts should provide insurance for accidents/injuries. Fourth, students should be educated in their home schools (and in their home communities) to reduce transportation time. Fifth, the instruction should be consistent and ongoing as opposed to a field-trip approach to community-referenced learning. Sixth, the instruction should involve individual or small groups of students to maintain as natural a proportion as possible of people with disabilities to those without.

A number of barriers to community-based instruction have been cited (Wehman et al., 1988). These include transportation difficulties, liability concerns, personnel assignment problems, scheduling difficulties, misunderstanding of the roles of different agencies involved, and funding problems. These authors and others (Falvey, 1986; Gaylord-Ross, Forte, & Gaylord-Ross, 1986; Wehman, Wood, Everson, Marchant, & Walker, 1987) offer a variety of strategies to overcome these difficulties.

A major focus of the curriculum and instruction for many students, regardless of level of disability, should be vocational adjustment. Unquestionably, work is a major influence on the lives of most adults. Additionally, students must acquire skills related to domestic adjustment and mobility, and to recreation/leisure in the community (see chapter 10). Social skills training is also a critical area and has been discussed at length in chapter 2. Consequently, the schools and adult service providers have begun an ambitious effort to provide appropriate training to students with mild to profound disabilities through a variety of service options.

Vocational Services and Other Programs

There are two major avenues in providing vocational training through the schools. The first involves the use of services available to virtually all students (e.g., vocational assessment and vocational education). The other involves a more direct approach, in which staff members are actively involved in helping students learn specific vocational and related skills, as well as obtain and maintain employment (Gaylord-Ross, 1988). Finally, the role of parents/guardians is critical to achieving desirable vocational outcomes.

Vocational Assessment

Vocational assessment has traditionally involved a number of objectives, such as describing overt skills, making inferences about underlying abilities, predicting future performance, and suggesting strategies and curriculum for instruction (Gaylord-Ross, 1986). Meehan and Hodell (1986) noted that vocational assessment may involve the use of interviews, situational assessments, work samples, and psychometric evaluation. When standardized instruments are used, a "one-shot" assessment is probably not sufficient to determine interests and attitudes (Buschner, Watts, Siders, & Leonard, 1989), and evaluators should use periodic reassessment. Although the use of standardized instruments may provide meaningful information, some writers now advocate increased reliance on the use of work samples (Peterson, 1986). Work samples involve observing the student's performance of various tasks and evaluating the performance based on speed, accuracy, and so forth. Some writers refer to the above types of assessment as vocational evaluation (Conaway, 1987). Conaway has also recommended the use of curriculum-based vocational assessment that examines a student's work-related skills, abilities, and interests on an ongoing basis through the use of existing school resources. Porter and Stodden (1986) outlined a model for this type of assessment that relies on three levels: (a) assessment of readiness and awareness skills through prevocational courses and activities, (b) assessment activities in middle and high school vocational courses, and (c) assessment of work-related skills and behaviors in cooperative education programs. Conaway noted that this type of assessment may be useful in determining career and vocational development goals for inclusion in educational plans.

For students with moderate to profound handicaps, an important development in vocational assessment has been the use of ecological assessment strategies (Falvey, 1986). This approach directly links assessment with on-the-job instruction. The vocational assessment specialist (or other appropriate staff member) specifies the work environment (e.g., fast-food restaurant); determines the activities carried out in the environment (e.g., food preparation, cleaning tasks); delineates those skills embedded within those activities (e.g., frying, wrapping, sweeping, mopping); and task-analyzes those skills into sequential steps. The assessment specialist may then conduct a discrepancy analysis based on work samples or direct observation of the student in the specified environment. That is, the student's present abilities are compared with those required to perform the job successfully. Instructional objectives are then selected based on areas of deficits. Additionally, the specialist may examine or recommend reasonable modifications in the job or environment that may increase the likelihood of the student's success.

Overall, vocational assessment may be evolving to a more useful status. Its earlier approach stressed summative assessments to tap the individual's preferences and abilities. Such information often offered little guidance with regard to ongoing intervention. An assessment model that stresses the repeated measurement of vocational performance may enhance the reliability, validity, and utility of vocational assessment.

Participation in Vocational Education Programs

The Carl D. Perkins Vocational Education Act of 1984 mandates that vocational education funds spent in U.S. schools may be used for students with disabilities. These funds could be used to assist with vocational assessment or in the provision of transition services. The monies may also be used for students with disabilities to participate in regular vocational education programs with nondisabled peers (Rusch & Phelps, 1987). In fact, Hasazi et al. (1985) found that many special education students who participated in regular vocational classes increased their likelihood of employment after graduation. Hasazi and Clark (1988) noted that vocational education is intended to assist students to learn employment-related skills; personal skills affecting employment; positive work attitudes; technical, communication, and computational skills; skills that are both job specific and globally related to employment; and career planning skills.

Conaway (1987) emphasized that vocational educators may provide services through career exploration, career counseling, vocational instructional programs, cooperative vocational education, and supplemental instructional services. Conaway noted that career exploration is generally emphasized just prior to the secondary years. Brolin (1982) outlined a program for use with students with mild handicaps that addresses many aspects of career development from the elementary through secondary levels. Career exploration involves the investigating of various occupations for information for comparison with the student's interests and abilities (Conaway, 1987). These comparative data are used in developing an individualized education program (IEP) that addresses specific career goals and objectives. For students with more severe disabilities, career exploration frequently involves direct work experience, often at school-based sites (e.g., cafeteria) but also may be provided in the community. (See a more in-depth discussion below.) Career counseling is used to assist students in making career-related choices (Conaway, 1987). Having experienced career exploration, counseling helps students realize the variety of options available. Students may also be counseled to enroll in a vocational instructional program. A vocational instruction program typically involves three courses in a specific area: (a) theory and general information and knowledge about the selected area, (b) instruction in specific occupational skills, and (c) how knowledge may be applied in the student's academic program. Conaway also noted that related vocational skills are stressed. Cooperative vocational education may involve on-the-job experience during school. The student, school staff, and community employer enter into a cooperative agreement whereby the student attends school part-time and works part-time. This option may also be referred to as a work-study program. The student's work experience is overseen by a teacher who visits the job site and ensures the job allows for the application and further development of skills learned in school. Conaway noted that there are other programs to assist students in obtaining employment and developing on-the-job skills. Cooperative education programs are intended to link theory and practice and generally provide a more comprehensive knowledge base. Finally, Conaway noted that students may also be provided with supplemental instructional services in either mainstream or special vocational education classes. Typically, these services involve special or vocational educators training paraprofessionals to provide instruction at school- or community-based sites. Conaway summarizes her discussion by stressing that the key to successful vocational education remains the inclusion of goals and objectives in the IEP that are related to career development. Hasazi and Clark (1988) have noted, however, that even with the best school- and community-based vocational training, it is sometimes necessary to specifically train students in how to obtain and maintain employment.

Job-Seeking Curriculum

Given the complex nature of vocational training, it is apparent that students with moderate to severe disabilities should probably be assisted directly in obtaining employment. Although interviewing skills and other skills such as filling out appolications and tax forms may be taught, there may be an assumption that someone (i.e., school staff or family member) will be present to assist and ensure such tasks are completed correctly. For individuals with mild handicaps there may be an assumption that obtaining employment on their own is a reasonable expectation. Hasazi et al. (1985) found that most of the students in their study obtained employment through the "self–family–friend" network. This may indicate that students should be specifically instructed on how to use such a network (Hasazi & Clark, 1988). Students should also be instructed in how to contact potential employers, develop résumés, and maintain contact with employers (Cobb & Hasazi, 1987). Elksnin and Elksnin (1988) have recommended the use of job clubs involving a social support system among job seekers. Members are taught to access the family–friend network as well as learning more traditional means of seeking employment (e.g., advertisements). They also learn related skills to obtaining employment (e.g., interviewing skills). Elksnin and Elksnin cite results from studies indicating that job clubs have been very effective in assisting students with disabilities in obtaining employment.

Specific Vocational Training and Employment Strategies

Given the results of follow-up studies, one might conclude that most adults with disabilities never received vocational training or participated in vocational classes. However, several studies have indicated that this was not necessarily the case (e.g., Haring & Lovett, 1990; Hasazi et al., 1985). It is more likely that the vocational training was inadequate. What has become apparent is that participation in vocational training or vocational classes does not guarantee successful employment (Hasazi et al., 1985). In fact, a problem has been that vocational programs may have failed to help students acquire or apply marketable skills, or failed to help students obtain employment (Haring & Lovett, 1990). Particularly for students with moderate to mild disabilities, a direct community-based instructional approach may be necessary to assist students in obtaining and maintaining employment.

The vocational curriculum must provide students with those skills needed in the local (or anticipated) work force (Wehman, Moon, &

McCarthy, 1986). This may be addressed through two major avenues. First, surveys of local employers and job advertisements may be conducted to determine what types of workers are needed (Wehman et al., 1988). These surveys could provide information on the entry level skills required to obtain these jobs. Second, local employers and employment agencies should be encouraged and invited to participate with educators and other service providers on teams. These teams can help create a more comprehensive and locally sensitive vocational program as well as assist individual students in obtaining training and employment. This information and support should help special and vocational educators develop a specific job skills curriculum and training program to enhance employment opportunities.

Wehman et al. (1988) have listed the elements of vocational training necessary to ensure employability of students with disabilities:

1. Select appropriate school-based and community-based sites for training.
2. Determine what training activities will be conducted at each site and sequence the goals and measurable objectives embedded within those activities.
3. Formulate skill sequences and task analyses based on the goals and objectives.
4. Select instructional techniques that ensure acquisition and generalization of skills based on individual student needs.
5. Select data collection procedures to provide information relevant to student progress and to identify problem areas.
6. Teach related skills necessary to obtaining and maintaining employment.
7. Plan for phasing out of school staff supervision and phasing in of employer supervision.
8. Design school schedules to maximize community-based training.

Wehman et al. (1987) pointed out that the school instructor should also note and address aspects about the work environment that may not be explicitly stated or obvious (e.g., inappropriate social behaviors that may influence employability). These training programs may involve direct instruction at employment sites; externships; paid work prior to graduation; and, finally, job placement.

Training at Employment Sites

Direct instruction with students who are "on the job" is a commonly used strategy in many school districts. This type of training may or may not involve paid work. Students may be provided career exploration opportunities through these "externships" (Wehman et al., 1988). Externships involve rotating students through various work situations (e.g., an office, a food services business, an assembling operation, etc.) for a period of weeks at each site. These experiences allow for direct assessment of students' strengths, weaknesses, and interests. This type of information is critical for a successful student–job match as graduation approaches; the student–job match involves selecting work settings where the student's abilities and the job requirements are loosely interfaced (Wehman et al., 1987). School personnel rather than employers provide instruction and supervision. These sites may be individualized or provide training for small groups of students. Wehman et al. (1987) outlined several guidelines for vocational training in or in preparation for paid work placements:

1. Identify potential employers who may allow training and ultimately employment of students in their businesses; adult service providers may assist in this process, and a needs assessment of the local job market may be helpful.
2. Provide daily training at these community-based work sites.
3. After a placement is established, stress improvement in the student's production and work quality; increasing a student's stamina and endurance also should be emphasized until the student is capable of working the expected number of hours if employed.
4. Develop a file of job placements that serves as both a reference source for school personnel as well as a vocational training/employment history for the student.

Following these steps, the student should be ready for paid work experience.

Paid Work Experience

Studies have indicated that students who experience paid work during their school careers are more likely to obtain competitive employment following graduation (Hasazi et al., 1985). Hasazi et al. found that after-school and summer jobs were significantly related to obtaining competitive employment following graduation. These findings illuminate two concerns. First, special and vocational educators need to provide opportunities for students to experience paid work during their school careers. Second, families and friends of students with disabilities, as well as students themselves, should be concerned with obtaining employment outside the school.

Hasazi and Clark (1988) listed a number of benefits obtained from paid work experiences. First, paid work provides obvious natural incentives for being employed. Even for students with severe disabilities who may not fully understand concepts of wages and money, arrangements can be made to ensure that students enjoy reinforcement directly attributable to their employment and earnings. Second, paid work experience typically is acquired in integrated settings. These settings provide students opportunities to interact with others and learn critical social skills related to maintaining good relationships with co-workers and supervisors. Third, paid work provides students with opportunities to meet the real-life demands of employment and to experience natural consequences for behaviors (e.g., loss of pay or job for excessive absences or calling in sick). This experience provides school personnel with an opportunity to evaluate student performance and identify problem areas that may not be evident in less demanding simulated work. Fourth, paid work (assuming the experiences are generally successful) demonstrates to families, employers, and the community that individuals with disabilities are productive and reliable workers. Finally, paid work provides opportunities for students to learn skills that may be useful in other jobs in the future or skills that serve as a foundation for advancement.

As a final option, the student may be placed in a "permanent" employment situation prior to graduation (Wehman et al., 1987). Wehman et al. stressed that successful job placement involves (a) continuous and effective communication among school staff, parents, and employers; (b) the previously mentioned student–job match; (c) the presentation of the student as a capable worker; and (d) a commitment by all service providers to ensure ongoing support prior to and after graduation.

This model of providing paid work experiences while students are still in school hinges upon adequate training for the staff. Many special education teachers and paraprofessionals may not be very familiar with the strategies listed above. Therefore, school districts and universities have begun training educators who provide services and instruction to the on-the-job student. In addition to school personnel and employers, the importance of the role of parents in the education of students with disabilities is obvious. As has been previously cited, the role of family members may be critical in students' obtaining employment.

The Career Ladder Program (CLP) (Siegel, 1988) offers an example of a longitudinal transition program for youth with mild disabilities. The students engage in paid work experiences during the secondary years. They also participate in career education activities such as career awareness, social skills training, and job clubs. Subsequent to graduation, they receive postsecondary counseling to further their employment. Such postschool vocational support appears critical to enhancing employment outcomes.

Parent/Guardian Issues

It is essential that parents understand and emphasize the importance of work to their children. Moon and Beale (1988) offered several guidelines for parents to assist in preparing students for work. At the elementary level, these included the following:

1. Familiarizing themselves with state and federal regulations concerning education for students with disabilities.

2. Working with local schools to ensure that vocational training is part of the curriculum.
3. Assigning specific duties for the student to perform at home and paying the student a small allowance based on successful completion of chores.
4. Finding out about school and community vocational programs that have successfully trained students with disabilities to obtain and maintain employment.
5. Creating opportunities for the student to learn about workers and different aspects of the jobs.
6. Emphasizing personal appearance, fitness, coordination, and stamina.
7. Building good social and communication skills.

At the middle school level, Moon and Beale (1988) recommended (a) actively supporting the school's efforts to provide community-intensive instruction, (b) ensuring the student's IEP includes goals and objectives related to specific vocational training in a variety of potential vocations, (c) finding out what type and to what extent job training is available, (d) establishing communications with local rehabilitation and other adult service agencies about available services and job opportunities, (e) finding work for the student outside the home during periods when the student is out of school, and (f) providing opportunities for the student to enjoy community leisure and social activities. Additionally, parents should continue to emphasize responsibilities in the home, personal appearance, and physical fitness.

As the student enters high school, Moon and Beale (1984) recommend (a) ensuring that specific job training is included in the IEP, (b) ensuring that a transition team is formulated that includes relevant personnel from both the school and community, (c) encouraging school staff to find and assist the student in obtaining and maintaining employment including on-the-job training, (d) making plans with adult service agencies to provide continuing training and/or support following graduation.

As is evident in Moon and Beale's (1988) recommendations, the overall process of planning and programming for a smooth transition from school to work and adult life is critical if appropriate outcomes are to be achieved. Special educators have realized that even though functional and vocational skills may have been taught and acquired in natural environments, students may still fail to achieve successful vocational and community adjustment. Adults with disabilities may require differing degrees of, and even lifelong, support following graduation from high school. This realization has led educators, adult service providers, students, and families to join in a collaborative and cooperative effort to ensure successful transitions.

Transition

Although the concept of transition has recently been expanded to include services provided on a lifelong basis from birth to death, here we will focus on the concept of transition from high school to work and post-school life. Will (1984) stated that transition includes the high school years, graduation, postschool placement, and the initial years of employment. Transition services include secondary education programs that prepare students to work and live in their home communities and adult service programs that meet the needs of individuals with handicaps and provide support in work and life in home communities; together they form a process involving cooperative and comprehensive planning. The model of transition developed by the Office of Special Education and Rehabilitation Services (Will, 1984) includes the provision of services that may be generic (e.g., assistance in signing up for Scholastic Aptitude Tests for college admission); time-limited (e.g., vocational rehabilitation funding of initial job training and placement); or ongoing (e.g., supported employment services funded through a variety of agencies).

Current Transition Services

The concept of transition has been supported over the years by several legislative mandates. Rusch and Phelps (1987) provided a historical overview of legislative efforts to increase vocational and ultimately transition opportunities for individuals with disabilities. A summary of their overview follows. The first vocational rehabilitation act was enacted in 1918 to assist veterans of World War I and blind individuals. The first vocational education legislation was enacted in 1917, but it made no provision for individuals with disabilities. Amendments in 1943 to the Vocational Rehabilitation Act of 1918 provided serivices to individuals with mental disabilities. Work-study classes were created beginning in the 1950s that focused on employment for students in high school. The 1960s marked an era of growth in services to persons with disabilities. The Civil Rights Act of 1964 was critical in eliminating discrimination in federally funded programs. These guarantees were extended to people with disabilities through legislative and court actions during the next two decades. Amendments to the Vocational Education Act set aside 10% of funds for students with disabilities. The Carl D. Perkins Vocational Education Act of 1984 expanded services to increase the likelihood of successful transitions for disadvantaged students as well as those with disabilities. The Rehabilitation Act of 1973 ensured increased services for people with more severe disabilities, including nondiscrimination in hiring and mandated public access for individuals with disabilities. Finally, the provision of educational services mandated under Public Law 94–142 established programs intended to better prepare students with disabilities to be productive citizens in the mainstream of society.

Section 626 of U.S. Public Law 98–199, entitled "Secondary Education and Transitional Services for Handicapped Youth," was enacted to strengthen education, training, and related services to assist students with disabilities in making successful transitions from school to postsecondary education, employment, or other adult services (Rusch & Phelps, 1987). This law and provisions of Public Law 99–457 were clearly intended to stimulate the transition planning and programming process across the country. Incentives were provided for starting programs and demonstration projects. However, the prevalence of transition services is still less than what one might deem desirable.

Benz and Halpern (1987) reported in one statewide study that although a majority of school administrators felt that transition services were very important, an equal percentage felt the services provided were inadequate. The most widely used mechanisms were informal written agreements with vocational education, community service agencies, and vocational rehabilitation. Only 19% of the districts in the study offered placement assistance, and 15% of the districts had no mechanisms in place to coordinate transition services. A majority of teachers in the study reported dissatisfaction with the levels of communication and parental involvement. Only slightly more than one third of the districts obtained and used follow-up data on graduates to assist in evaluating follow-up services, and only 15% of these districts had formalized the process. Perhaps it is not surprising, then, that over one third of the parents surveyed expressed "don't know" to questions related to expectations for their son's or daughter's level of employment. Almost half, however, expected their child to be competitively employed 10 years after graduation. More than one half expected their child to be living at home the first year after school, but almost two thirds expected the student to be living independently at the end of 10 years. The results of this study indicate that services are neither evenly nor widely implemented in at least that state. While many parents were uncertain about their children's future, clearly there was some expectation for growth in both employability and ability to adapt and live in the community. These expectations, coupled with the general dissatisfaction expressed by both administrators and teachers, suggest that a greater effort is needed to improve both the quantitative and qualitative scope of transition services (Benz & Halpern, 1987). Indeed, Wehman et al. (1989) found that the provision of systematic transition services yielded vocational/postschool benefits to students with measured IQs ranging from 27 to 59 from both segregated and integrated school settings. Wehman et al. (1989) stressed that placement into competitive employment prior to graduation and ongoing parental participation appeared to be critical to the successful transitions in their study. They also noted, however, that longitudinal studies are required to determine how transition service delivery systems may need to be revised.

Issues Related to Transition Planning and Implementation

It appears that transition planning and implementation are critical to postschool success for youth with disabilities. It is less clear what services ought to be provided. A number of specific models exist for transition planning and programming, and a number of issues related to transition planning and implementation are generally recognized regardless of the specific model. These issues may be categorized into the following (though not mutually exclusive) areas: parent/consumer issues, interagency collaboration issues, and individual transitioning issues.

Parent/Consumer Issues

Parents and students are obviously the people most affected by the success or failure of transition programs. It is paramount, therefore, that parents and students participate in the transition process to the fullest extent possible. Turnbull and Turnbull (1988) suggested several areas where families and schools may improve efforts to increase vocational opportunities and the chance of successful transitions: First, students and families should be encouraged to increase personal decision making. The need to exert control in one's life is universal. Participation in the development of IEPs and individualized transition plans (ITPs) is one excellent way to increase the opportunities for personal decision making. Second, families should be encouraged to brainstorm about and plan for the future. Students and parents should be provided with formal opportunities to discuss the future (e.g., during IEP meetings) and encouraged to do so informally as well. Third, parents should be encouraged to help their son or daughter develop friendships with nondisabled peers. By providing integrated educational settings, the schools may encourage and enhance this possibility. Such friendships may not only help the student with a disability learn how to interact more appropriately, but may also encourage individuals with no handicaps to accept and even advocate the inclusion of people with disabilities in community and work environments. Families should assist members with disabilities in learning responsibility and acquiring work skills through performing chores around the home as well as through after-school or summer employment. As noted previously, summer and after-school employment may be the most significant variable in successful vocational adjustment following graduation (Hasazi et al., 1985). Finally, Turnbull and Turnbull noted that as assistive technology advances, parents and students will need support in learning to acquire and use the technology. Schools and other service providers should be instrumental not only in developing this technology but also in increasing its affordability and availability.

Wehman et al. (1988) listed several responsibilities that parents and families can assume in the actual transition process. These included (a) attending ITP meetings; (b) providing input to the team concerning the family's and student's needs and what responsibilities family members are willing to assume; (c) advocating for an ITP that ensures community integration and decreases the student's dependence on the family and adult service providers; (d) focusing the team's planning on family and student needs; (e) requesting information about services, programs, and issues that the family will need to address or contact (e.g., vocational rehabilitation, financial planning, recreation/leisure opportunities); and (f) providing additional training in the home and community that complements school-based interventions. Professionals must be aware of and sensitive to the family's needs and desires. However, transition team members must be prepared to provide the best possible services regardless of the level of parental involvement (Wehman et al., 1988).

Interagency Collaboration Issues

Hasazi and Clark (1988) noted that local interagency agreements are one excellent mechanism for promoting cooperation among schools and adult service providers. Participants in these agreements might include personnel from special and vocational education, vocational rehabilitation, developmental disabilities councils or services, and employment and training agencies. Such agreements, according to Hasazi and Clark, should specify (a) what services are provided by each agency; (b) a means for identifying local needs both in terms of what services are needed as well as to what extent; (c) provisions for developing a plan to meet those needs; (d) ways to identify, locate, and contact individuals who may need services; (e) provisions for across-agency in-services to enhance understanding of each agency's roles and responsibilities; and (f) a means for measuring, evaluating, and modifying services provided under the agreement. Hasazi and Clark also stressed that participants in local agreements should consider how more generic service agencies such as community colleges and state employment services might become involved in the agreement.

Wehman et al. (1988) also stressed the importance of state-level interagency agreements. These authors noted that it may be necessary for service providers to reexamine or restate their agency's mission in providing services to clients on a statewide level. The various agencies involved should identify a common mission and then enter into formal interagency collaboration. Staff and resources should be committed to the transition process, and written agency agendas should reflect this commitment. Wehman et al. (1988) went on to stress that management personnel should schedule interaction between agency representatives, make a list of activities and timelines for completing the activities, and identify expected outcomes. A statewide team could gather useful information for developing budgets and allocating resources.

Peters, Templeman, and Brostrom (1987) emphasized that local "ownership" and the empowerment of local transition team members to formulate policy appeared to be critical to successful transition programming. State-level agreements may serve as a stimulus to prompt local cooperation and collaboration. The authors stressed that although plans developed at different localities shared salient characteristics, each also had unique aspects peculiar to that locale that appeared to increase the likelihood of the plan being implemented.

Finally, Johnson, Bruininks, and Thurlow (1987) identified four strategies necessary for successful interagency collaboration at all levels: (a) ensuring policy goals were consistent at all levels, (b) implementing effective management strategies to interpret and express policy goals and objectives through proven models for organizing and coordinating services, (c) ensuring reliable and valid data are gathered for use in decision making, and (d) systematically evaluating participant outcomes as well as costs and benefits of the programs.

Individual Transitioning Issues

At the heart of the transition process is the individual transition team and the individualized transition program. Most authorities agree that transition planning for the individual should begin no later than entry into high school (i.e., at least 4 years before leaving school) but may begin much earlier. Typically, the more severe a person's disability or the problems that must be overcome to achieve successful postschool integration, the earlier a transition team should be formulated. Wehman et al. (1988) identified the following steps in developing and implementing a successful transition process: organize individual transition plan (ITP) teams, hold initial ITP meetings, implement the ITP, update the ITP annually, and hold an "exit" meeting.

The Individual Transition Team

The individual transition team is formulated to develop and implement an individual transition plan. Initially, the team should identify all youth in need of transition services. As noted, this process should begin when a student enters high school at the latest, but the plan may be formulated sooner. During the initial stages of transition planning, special education staff, family members, and the student may be the only participants. However, before the student leaves school, personnel from vocational education and outside agencies may also be included on the individual transition team. Typically, school personnel will assume the role of transition coordinator at the team's inception. That is, a special education teacher will initiate contact with appropriate personnel and the family and student to inform them of the team's purpose. Ultimately, however, the parent/guardian or even the student himself or herself should assume the role of transition coordinator (Wehman et al., 1987). The initial transition team meeting and subsequent meetings may be conducted in conjunction with the annual IEP meeting. According to Wehman et al. (1988), annual meetings are probably sufficient until the final year of school, when the team may need to meet as often as bimonthly to ensure that goals and objectives are met. These authors stressed that a final "exit" meeting should be held to ensure that the transition of responsibility from school to adult service personnel is smooth, timely, and does not result in an interruption or delay in services.

The Individualized Transition Plan

The individualized transition plan (ITP) typically specifies, as does the IEP, present levels of performance, goals, objectives, timelines, and responsible persons. However, some differences exist between the IEP and ITP. Gillet (1987) suggested that the following components be included in an ITP:

1. Competencies needed for independent living, personal/social adjustment, and vocational success.
2. Behaviors most important for independent living and competitive employment.
3. Services required prior to graduation.
4. Prioritization of activities required to achieve the desired outcomes.
5. Options for employment and future residence.
6. Services required following graduation.
7. Names of persons, businesses, and agencies that cooperate in the plan.
8. Timelines for the completion of service provisions.

Wehman et al. (1988) also stressed that only those weaknesses that interfere with successful postschool adjustment ought to be addressed as part of the ITP (e.g., not being able to add and subtract may be a weakness but may not be critical to postschool success).

Wehman, Moon, and McCarthy (1986) noted that ITP objectives are delineated as either educational or administrative. That is, objectives may be related to employment or community living adjustment or to objectives to be carried out by school or agency personnel or by parents/guardians (e.g., conducting an assessment of necessary skills in the preferred residential option).

Conclusions

One of the main purposes of education at the secondary level is to provide students with the knowledge and skills they need to succeed as adults. Unfortunately, many students with disabilities drop out and/or fail to learn the necessary skills to participate successfully in community life (Will, 1984). It is imperative that educators develop instructional methods and curricula to help meet the needs of these individuals after they leave school.

The methods used and the skills selected for instruction should be based on the individual needs, abilities, and interests of the student. It is important to teach skills that will improve social interaction and be useful in future environments. To accomplish this goal, the curricula should be both community-referenced and community-based. It is extremely important that while in secondary education programs students with disabilities have the opportunity to interact and receive instruction with their nondisabled peers. These opportunities will enhance the prospects for successful community participation as adults.

Employment is of major importance to almost every adult. Vocational training is an essential component of the education of adolescents with disabilities. This training should focus not only on specific jobs but also on job-seeking and work-related skills that will be useful in obtaining and retaining a variety of employment options.

The support of parents and families is essential to the success of students in secondary education and during the transition to adult life. Educators should encourage parents and families to be active participants in the educational process. In addition, it is critical that educators work with employers and adult service personnel to ensure that the educational services students receive are designed to help them achieve success as adults.

The secondary education years are the culmination of the efforts of many people and agencies. Certainly those people desire that students enjoy the best possible outcomes in return for the years of effort. For some individuals who are labeled as disabled, a good education and well-planned transition will result in integration into the mainstream in such a way that they are no longer labeled. They will be largely self-sufficient. For others, their need for support will be lifelong. It is imperative that their needs are met in a systematic and responsible fashion. Issues regarding the lives of adults with disabilities in integrated settings and guidelines for the provision of appropriate services are discussed in chapter 10.

References

Adler, M.J. (1982). *The Paideia proposal: An educational manifesto*. New York: Macmillan.

Bandura, A. (1977). Self-efficacy: Toward a unifying theory of behavioral change. *Psychological Review*, *84*, 191–215.

Bauer, R.H. (1977). Memory processes in children with learning disabilities: Evidence for deficient rehearsal. *Journal of Experimental Child Psychology*, *24*, 415–430.

Baumgart, D., Brown, L, Pumpian, I., Nisbet, J., Ford, A., Seet, M., Messina, R., & Schroeder, J. (1982). Principle of partial participation and individualized adaptations in educational programs for severely handicapped students. *Journal of the Association for the Severely Handicapped*, *7*, 17–27.

Benz, M.R., & Halpern, A.S. (1987). Transition services for secondary students with mild disabilities: A statewide perspective. *Exceptional Children*, *53*, 507–514.

Bickel, W.E., & Bickel, D.D. (1986). Effective schools, classrooms, and instruction: Implications for special education. *Exceptional Children*, *52*, 489–500.

Borkowski, J.G., Carr, M., & Pressley, M. (1987). "Spontaneous" strategy use: Perspectives from metacognitive theory. *Intelligence*, *11*, 61–75.

Borkowski, J.G., & Cavanaugh, J.C. (1979). Maintenance and generalization of skills and strategies by the retarded. In N.R. Ellis (Ed.), *Handbook of mental deficiency: Psychological theory and research* (2nd ed., pp. 569–618). Hillsdale, NJ: Erlbaum.

Borkwoski, J.G., Weyhing, R.S., & Turner, L.A. (1986). Attributional retraining and the teaching of strategies. *Exceptional Children*, *53*, 130–137.

Brolin, D.E. (1982). *Vocational preparation of persons with handicaps*. Columbus, OH: Charles E. Merrill.

Brown, F., & Lehr, D. (1990). *Persons with profound disabilities: Issues and practices*. Baltimore: Paul H. Brookes.

Brown, L., Long, E., Udvari-Solner, A., Davis, L., VanDeventer, P., Ahlgren, C., Johnson, F., Gruenewald, L., & Jorgensen, J. (1989). The home school: Why students with severe intellectual disabilities must attend the schools of their brothers, sisters, friends, and neighbors. *Journal of the Association for Persons With Severe Handicaps*, *14*, 1–17.

Brown, L., Long, E., Udvari-Solner, A., Schwarz, P., VanDeventer, P., Ahlgren, C., Johnson, F., Gruenewald, L., & Jorgensen, J. (1989). Should students with severe intellectual disabilities be based in regular or in special education classrooms in home schools? *Journal of the Association for Persons With Severe Handicaps*, *14*, 8–12.

Brown, L., Nietupski, J., & Hamre-Nietupski, S. (1976). Criterion of ultimate functioning. In M.A. Thomas (Ed.), *Hey! Don't forget about me!* (pp. 2–15). Reston, VA: Council for Exceptional Children.

Brown, L., Nisbet, J., Ford, A., Sweet, M., Shiraga, B., York, J., & Loomis, R. (1983). *The critical need for nonschool instruction in educational programs for severely handicapped students*. Madison, WI: University of Wisconsin and Madison Metropolitan School District.

Brown, L., Shiraga, B., Rogan, P., York, J., Zanella, K., McCarthy, E., Loomis, R., & VanDeventer, P. (1985). *The "why" question in educational programs for students who are severely intellectually disabled*. Madison, WI: University of Wisconsin and Madison Metropolitan School District.

Brown, L., Sweet, M., Shiraga, B., York, J., Zanella, K., & Rogan, P. (1984). *Functional skills in programs for students with severe handicaps*. Madison, WI: University of Wisconsin and Madison Metropolitan School District.

Buschner, P.C., Watts, M.B., Siders, J.A., & Leonard, R.L. (1989). Career interest inventories: A need for analysis. *Career Development for Exceptional Individuals*, *12*, 129–137.

Butkowsky, I.S., & Willows, D.M. (1980). Cognitive motivational characteristics of children with varying reading ability: Evidence for learned helplessness in poor readers. *Journal of Educational Psychology*, *72*, 408–422.

Cobb, B., & Hasazi, S.B. (1986). School-aged transition services: Options for adolescents with mild handicaps. *Career Development for Exceptional Individuals*, *10*, 15–23.

Conaway, C. (1987). Transition: A vocational education perspective. In R.N. Ianacone & R.H. Stodden (Eds.), *Transition issues and directions* (pp. 120–124). Reston, VA: Council for Exceptional Children.

Cross, T., Darby, B., & D'Alonzo, B.J. (1990). School drop out prevention: A multifaceted program for the improvement of adolescent employability, academic achievement, and personal identity. *Career Development and Exception Individuals*, *13*, 83–94.

Deshler, D.D., Schumaker, J.B., Lenz, B.K., & Ellis, E. (1984a). Academic and cognitive interventions for LD adolescents: Part I. *Journal of Learning Disabilities*, *17*, 108–117.

Deshler, D.D., Schumaker, J.B., Lenz, B.K., & Ellis, E. (1984b). Academic and cognitive interventions for LD adolescents: Part II. *Journal of Learning Disabilities*, *17*, 170–179.

Edgar, E. (1987). Secondary programs in special education: Are many of them justifiable? *Exceptional Children*, *53*, 555–561.

Elksnin, N., & Elksnin, L. (1988). Improving job-seeking skills of adolescents with handicaps through job clubs. *Career Development for Exceptional Individuals*, *11*, 118–125.

Falvey, M. (1986). *Community-based instruction: Instructional strategies for students with severe handicaps*. Baltimore: Paul H. Brookes.

Gaylord-Ross, C., Forte, J., & Gaylord-Ross, R. (1986). The community classroom: Technological vocational training for students with serious handicaps. *Career Development for Exceptional Individuals*, *9*, 24–33.

Gaylord-Ross, R. (1986). The role of assessment in transitional, supported employment. *Career Development for Exceptional Individuals*, *9*, 129–134.

Gaylord-Ross, R. (1987). School integration for students with mental handicaps: A cross-cultural perspective. *European Journal of Special Needs Education*, *2*(2), 4–17.

Gaylord-Ross, R. (1988). *Vocational education for persons with handicaps*. Mountain View, CA: Mayfield.

Gaylord-Ross, R., Lee, M., Johnston, S., & Goetz, L. (in press). Social-communication and co-worker training for deaf-blind youth in supported employment settings. *Behavior Modification*.

Gaylord-Ross, R., Lee, M., Johnston, S., Lynch, K., Rosenberg, B., & Goetz, L. (1991). Supported employment for youth who are deaf-blind and in transition. *Career Development for Exceptional Individuals*, *14*, 77–89.

Gillet, P.K. (1987). Transition: A special education perspective. In R.N. Ianacone & R.H. Stodden (Eds.), *Transition issues and directions* (pp. 113–119). Reston, VA: Council for Exceptional Children.

Guess, D. (1983). Some parting thoughts and reflections from the editor. *Journal of Association for Persons With Severe Handicaps*, *8*, 25–29.

Hallahan, D.P., Hall, R.J., Ianna, S.O., Kneedler, R.D., Lloyd, J.W., Loper, A.B., & Reeve, R.E. (1983). Summary of research findings at the Univeristy of

Virginia Learning Disabilities Research Institute. *Exceptional Education Quarterly*, *4*, 95–114.

Hallahan, D.P., & Kauffman, J.M. (1988). *Exceptional Children: Introduction to Special Education* (4th ed.). Englewood Cliffs, NJ: Prentice-Hall.

Haring, K., & Lovett, D. (1990). A study of the social and vocational adjustment of young adults with mental retardation. *Education and Training in Mental Retardation*, *25*, 52–61.

Hasazi, S.B., & Clark, G.M. (1988). Vocational preparation for high school students labeled mentally retarded: Employment as a graduation goal. *Mental Retardation*, *26*, 343–349.

Hasazi, S.B., Gordon, L.R., & Roe, C.A. (1985). Factors associated with the employment status of handicapped youth exiting high school from 1979–1983. *Exceptional Children*, *51*, 455–469.

Helmstetter, D. (1990). Curriculum for school-aged students: The ecological model. In F. Brown & D.H. Lehr (Eds.), *Persons with profound disabilities: Issues and practices* (pp. 239–263). Baltimore: Paul, H. Brookes.

Hill, J.W., & Morton, M.V. (1988). Transition programming: Improving vocational outcomes. In L. Sternberg (Ed.), *Educating students with severe or profound handicaps* (2nd ed., pp. 439–471). Rockville, MD: Aspen.

Ianacone, R.N., & Stodden, R.A. (1987). Transition issues and directions for individuals who are mentally retarded. In R.N. Ianacone & R.A. Stodden (Eds.), *Transition issues and directions* (pp. 1–7). Reston, VA: Council for Exceptional Children.

Johnson, D.R., Bruininks, R.H., & Thurlow, M.L. (1987). Meeting the challenge of transition service planning through improved interagency cooperation. *Exceptional Children*, *53*, 522–530.

Kauffman, J., Gerber, M., & Semmel, M. (1988). Arguable assumptions underlying the regular education intiative. *Journal of Learning Disabilities*, *21*, 6–11.

Lovett, D.L., & Haring, K.A. (1989). The effects of self-management training on the daily living of adults with mental retardation. *Education and Training in Mental Retardation*, *24*, 306–323.

Lerner, J.W. (1985). *Learning disabilities: Theories, diagnosis, and teaching strategies* (4th ed.). Boston, MA: Houghton Mifflin.

Meehan, K.A., & Hodell, S. (1986). Measuring the impact of vocational assessment activities upon program decisions. *Career Development for Exceptional Individuals*, *9*, 106–112.

Meichenbaum, D. (1979). Teaching children self-control. In B.B. Lahey & A.E. Kazdin (Eds.), *Advances in clinical child psychology* (Vol. 2, pp. 1–33). New York: Plenum.

McKinney, J.D., & Hocutt, A.M. (1988). The need for policy analysis in evaluating the regular education initiative. *Journal of Learning Disabilities*, *21*, 71–74.

Moon, M.S., & Beale, A.V. (1984). Vocational training and employment: Guidelines for parents. *Exceptional Parent*, 14, pp. 35–38.

Palincsar, A.S., & Brown, A.L. (1984). Reciprocal teaching of comprehension fostering and monitoring activities. *Cognition and Instruction*, *1*, 117–175.

Patton, J.R., Cronin, M.E., Polloway, E.A., Hutchison, D., & Robinson, G. (1989). Curricular considerations: A life skills orientation. In G.A. Robinson,

J.R. Patton, E.A. Polloway, & L.R. Sargent (Eds.), *Best practices in mild mental disabilities* (pp. 21–37). Reston, VA: Council for Exceptional Children.

Peters, J.M., Templeman, T.P., & Brostrom, G. (1987). The school and community partnership: Planning transition for students with severe handicaps. *Exceptional Children, 53*, 531–536.

Peterson, M. (1986). Work and performance sample for vocational assessment of special students: A critical review. *Career Development of Exceptional Individuals, 9*, 69–76.

Porter, M.E., & Stodden, R.A. (1986). A curriculum-based assessment procedure: Addressing the school-to-work transition needs of secondary schools. *Career Development for Exceptional Individuals, 9*, 121–128.

Reid, D.K. (1988). A cognitive developmental approach to learning disabilities. In D.K. Reid (Ed.), *Teaching the learning disabled: A cognitive developmental approach* (pp. 5–74). Needham, MA: Allyn & Bacon.

Reynolds, M.C., Wang, M.C., & Walberg, H.G. (1987). The necessary restructuring of special and regular education. *Exceptional Children, 53*, 391–398.

Rusch, F. (Ed.). (1986). *Competitive employment issues and strategies*. Baltimore: Paul H. Brookes.

Rusch, F.R., & Hughes, C. (1988). Supported employment: Promoting employee independence. *Mental Retardation, 26*, 351–355.

Rusch, F.R., & Phelps, L.A. (1987). Secondary special education and transition from school to work: A national priority. *Exceptional Children, 53*, 487–492.

Sailor, W., Gee, K., Goetz, & Graham, N. (1988). Progress in educating students with the most severe diabilities: Is there any? *Journal of the Association for Persons With Severe Handicaps, 13*, 87–99.

Siegel, S. (1988). The career ladder program: Implementing Re-ED principles in vocational settings. *Behavioral Disorders, 14*(1), 16–26.

Stainback, S., & Stainback, W. (1988). Educating students with severe disabilities. *Teaching Exceptional Children, 21*, 16–19.

Sternberg, L. (1988). *Educating Students with Profound Handicaps*. Rockville, MD: Aspen.

Taylor, R., Richards, S.B., Goldstein, P., & Schilit, J. (in press). Teaching exceptional students . . . Where? Teacher perceptions of the regular education initiative. *Teaching Exceptional Students*.

Thomason, J., & Arkell, C. (1980). Educating the severely/profoundly handicapped in the public schools: A side-by-side approach. *Exceptional Children, 47*, 114–122.

Turnbull, A.P., & Turnbull, H.R. (1988). Toward great expectations for vocational opportunities: Family–professional partnerships. *Mental Retardation, 26*, 337–342.

Wagner, M. (1989). *The transition experiences of youth with disabilities: A report from the national longitudinal transition study*. Menlo Park, CA: SRI International.

Wehman, P.H., Kregel, J., Barcus, J.M., & Schalock, R.L. (1986). Vocational transition for students with developmental disabilities. In W.E. Kiernan & J.A. Stark (Eds.), *Pathways to employment for adults with developmental disabilities* (pp. 113–127). Baltimore: Paul H. Brookes.

Wehman, P., Moon, M.S., Everson, J.M., Wood, W., & Barcus, J.M. (1988). *Transition from school to work: New challenges for youth with severe disabilities*. Baltimore: Paul H. Brookes.

Wehman, P., Moon, M.S., & McCarthy, P. (1986). Transition from school to adulthood for youth with severe handicaps. *Focus on Exceptional Children*, *18*, 1–12.

Wehman, P., Parent, W., Wood, W., Talbert, C.M., Jasper, C., Miller, S., Marchant, J., & Walker, R. (1989). From school to competitive employment for young adults with mental retardation: Transition in practice. *Career Development for Exceptional Individuals*, *12*, 97–105.

Wehman, P., Wood, W., Everson, J., Marchant, J., & Walker, R. (1987). Transition services for adolescent age individuals with severe mental retardation. In R.N. Ianacone & R.H. Stodden (Eds.), *Transition issues and directions* (pp. 49–76). Reston, VA: Council for Exceptional Children.

Weisenstein, G.R., & Elrod, G.F. (1987). Transition services for adolescent age individuals with mild mental retardation. In R.N. Ianacone & R.H. Stodden (Eds.), *Transition issues and directions* (pp. 38–48). Reston, VA: Council for Exceptional Children.

Will, M.C. (1984). *OSERS program for the transition of youth with disabilities: Bridges from school to working life*. Washington, DC: Office of Special Education and Rehabilitative Services, U.S. Department of Education.

Will, M.C. (1986). Educating children with learning problems: A shared responsibility. *Exceptional Children*, *52*, 411–415.

10
Integrated Services for Adults With Disabilities

DAVID L. LOVETT, STEPHEN RICHARDS, AND ROBERT GAYLORD-ROSS

Graduates from special education programs face an uncertain and often dismal future. Most people with disabilities are inadequately prepared for adult life and do not receive the social services they need as adults (Edgar, 1987; Haring & Lovett, 1990; Harris, 1987; Wehman, Moon, Everson, Wood, & Barcus, 1988). These conditions have contributed to a high unemployment rate and underemployment among those with jobs. Typically, people with disabilities encounter long waiting lists to enter community programs, placement in segregated vocational and residential settings, and reduced opportunities for independence. This is a costly waste of human potential. Society should ensure that special services are provided to assist adults with disabilities to become participating members of society.

This chapter is designed (a) to describe and summarize the results of follow-up research that analyzes how well students who have left special education programs adjust to adult life, (b) to examine issues related to the delivery of adult services, and (c) to explore methods to develop and improve comprehensive systems of integrated service delivery to adults with disabilities.

Although increased public concern for people with disabilities has promoted policies designed to provide better education and adult services, the outcomes, in some respects, have been discouraging. Two thirds of all adults who have disabilities are not working (Harris, 1987). The vast majority of adults with disabilities are not living independently. Their living situations are dissimilar to those of their same-age peers (Haring & Lovett, 1990; Wagner, 1989). For example, many adults with disabilities live with their parents or other family members; many others live in supervised and segregated settings with other adults who have disabilities. Generally, people with more severe disabilities live in larger and more restrictive residential environments (Bruininks, Rotegard, Lakin, & Hill, 1987).

Recreational options for adults with disabilities also may be extremely limited (Haring & Lovett, 1990; Harris, 1987). Some studies have indicated low engagement rates in recreational activities (Harris, 1987). Those activities they do engage in are often solitary, such as watching television (Dattilo & Mirenda 1987; Pierce, 1989). On the whole, adults with disabilities experience limited mobility in their communities (Haring & Lovett, 1990; Harris, 1987). Public transportation systems may be inaccessible or unavailable. In addition, many individuals with disabilities lack training in mobility. Limited transportation options and mobility restrict the employment and recreational opportunities available to these individuals. These limitations, coupled with restricted recreational options, may hamper the development of friendships and social interaction (Harris, 1987).

As the above discussion indicates, many factors should be considered in evaluating adult adjustment. It is important that vocational, residential, recreational, and transportation domains are considered in evaluating a person's satisfaction with life. These are, however, determinants for which it is difficult to set specific standards. A person's satisfaction with his or her life depends on an individual perspective. (The reader is referred to Chapter 11 of this volume for a detailed discussion of the issues surrounding life satisfaction and the quality of life.) Nevertheless, to better understand how adults with disabilities have adjusted after leaving school, it is extremely important to examine their lives in relationship to the above factors. A common method used to conduct such an examination is follow-up research.

Follow-up Research

Follow-up studies are frequently used to examine the efficacy of special education services (Wehman et al., 1988). One measure of special education efficacy is to determine how well, or how effectively, special educators prepare students to live in the adult world. Typically, specific variables, such as postschool employment and living arrangements are examined. The interest of researchers and educators in this information is reflected by the large number of follow-up studies examining the social and vocational adjustment of special education graduates (see Haring & Lovett, 1990; Siegel et al., 1990; Wehman et al., 1988).

Early studies focused on "educable" (EMR) and "trainable" (TMR) students with mental retardation. Results in these studies reflected some difference in the employment of these persons as compared to individuals without mental retardation (Baller, 1936; Fairbanks, 1933; Kennedy, 1948). Baller found that individuals with mental retardation were 30% less likely to be gainfully employed than were persons without mental retardation. In later follow-up studies (Bobroff, 1955; Carriker, 1957; Cassidy & Phelps, 1955; Dinger, 1958; Kennedy, 1962), the employment rates of EMR and TMR students ranged from 77% to 92%. Most subjects were employed in unskilled or semiskilled positions. In general, results from follow-up studies indicated that graduates who were mentally retarded had limited self-sufficiency, with earned incomes below the poverty line (Dinger, 1961; Gozali, 1972; Keim, 1979; Peterson & Smith, 1960; Saenger, 1957; Titus & Travis, 1975).

Findings from several studies of graduates with mental retardation and, more recently, those with learning disabilities (LD), indicated that a majority of disabled adults still lived at home (Coonley, et al., 1980; Gozali, 1972). There is some indication that parents who have adult offspring living at home wish them to live more independently (Haring & Lovett, 1990).

Studies about the relationship between the kind of school program attended and vocational outcomes are few and report contradictory results (Boyce & Elzey, 1978; Collister, 1975; Dearborn Public Schools, 1970; Dinger, 1973; Kernan, 1979). Authors of studies that included gender as a variable in postschool adjustment reported conflicting findings (Dinger, 1961; Peterson & Smith, 1960). More recently, other researchers found gender to be a significant factor in employment (Wehman et al., 1988; Hasazi, Gordon, & Roe, 1985). Women, however, tended to be underrepresented in the research, and those included as subjects were considerably underemployed. Overall, the results of follow-up studies indicated that people with disabilities were not very successful in adjusting to adult life (Edgar, 1987; Wehman et al., 1988). There may be, however, some methodological factors involved that influenced results and require discussion.

Methodological Limitations

Follow-up studies, in general, have several methodological limitations. These studies are expost facto analyses. That is, students have completed their schooling before the research begins. Therefore, many factors that may have influenced adult adjustment are beyond the control of the researcher. For example, the researcher could not examine the actual quality of previous educational training. In addition, the nature of special education and the very values and policies that guide it ensure that the placement of a student with disabilities is based on individual need. Educational research often includes the use of random assignment of subjects to ensure a valid examination of the relationship between training and learning. Random assignment of special education subjects into different types of programs is not possible because all students with disabilities are entitled to special services and an appropriate education. Therefore, experimental control to analyze the effects of different programs, such as no special services versus special education, is unethical.

Another problem with many follow-up studies is that they are "one-time" analyses rather than longitudinal. That is, many researchers examine the lives of people at only one point in time. Usually such surveys are conducted soon after the person has left school. This is not sufficient to assess adjustment to adult life. Evidence exists that people make increasingly successful adjustments to life as they age (Haring & Lovett, 1990). Although follow-up research should be longitudinal, such research requires much time and money and therefore is rarely conducted. One possible way to help ensure future contact with subjects and to make longitudinal researchers' efforts more efficient is to identify a minimum of two contact people who would always know how the subject can be located. The names, addresses, and phone numbers of relatives, friends, neighbors, employers, and others should be obtained during the high school years to assist in follow-up.

Many studies focus on small geographic locations. It is difficult to generalize findings from one area to another because of the differences between communities. Characteristics such as the ethnic makeup of the community, local economic factors, and population concentration are factors that should be considered when interpreting and making service delivery decisions based on results of follow-up studies.

Inadequate subject descriptions pose another problem. For example, some recent research described subjects as 60% mildly mentally retarded and 40% moderately, severely, or profoundly mentally retarded. This was neither precise nor adequately indicative of the level of mental retardation being discussed. More thorough subject descriptions would facilitate comparisons between studies. These descriptions might include not only a more complete delineation of the type and degree of disability, but also the age at which special education began; socioeconomic status of the subjects or their families; or at least a description of the local economy, type of living arrangements, and family characteristics.

Another problem is that many studies do not adequately describe the nature of the special education programs being examined. Reported characteristics in the classification of shcool programs should include the type of curricula, teaching methods, the classroom setting, and the length of time in special education. Also, the amount of time, if any, spent in regular education classes might be of interest. In many studies this type of information is not reported. It is not sufficient to rely on respondents' memories to classify school programs. Therefore, it might prove beneficial to identify potential subjects long before they leave school in order to obtain sufficient information about their school program.

In addition to the limitations previously discussed, very little follow-up research exists regarding handicapping conditions other than mental retardation. Over 90% of special education follow-up studies have been primarily concerned with subjects who had mental retardation (Mithaug, Horuichi, & Fanning, 1985). The majority of these studies have focused on persons classified as mildly mentally retarded. Additionally, the primary variable of concern has been vocational adjustment. Other variables (e.g., participation in community-based activities) should also be assessed. As noted earlier, the individual perception of satisfaction with life may involve a number of factors. A broader view of adult adjustment is necessary to truly evaluate the status of special education graduates. Questions remain for future researchers to address. Does participation in special education make students with disabilities more likely to be employed and to become participating members of the community? Do efforts to integrate individuals with handicaps in public school programs correlate with the inclusion of persons with disabilities in generic social and recreational services used by people without disabilities? Is the type or duration of a school program related to vocational or community living status? With carefully designed studies, researchers may obtain more definitive results that will assist in modifying and improving adult services.

Summary

Follow-up research, in general, has concentrated on individuals with mild mental retardation. Follow-up studies prior to 1970 reported fairly optimistic employment rates. More recent studies are less positive; subjects were, for the most part, underemployed and not living independently (Haring & Lovett, 1990). Although the results were more positive in earlier follow-up studies, it would be erroneous to draw the conclusion that special education was less effective after 1970. As noted in the discussion of the history of special education (chapter 1 of this volume) many factors have changed regarding special education services and those who receive such services.

Based on the results of follow-up research presented here, the following modifications in service delivery are recommended if youth with disabilities are to experience successful transition into adulthood:

1. Secondary special educators should improve their communication with parents, regular educators and students, community members, employers and adult service providers to ensure that students are better prepared to meet the demands of adult life.
2. Comprehensive adult community services should be developed that provide ongoing training and support to ensure that career development, social/recreational opportunities, and residential living options are as normalized as possible.
3. Parents/family members must be prepared to act as informed decision makers who demand that a variety of service options be made available; these services should provide training to individuals with disabilities that will help them succeed in less restrictive environments.

The evaluation data accumulated on the Career Ladder Program (CLP) (Siegel, Avoke, Robert, & Gaylord-Ross, in press) is an exception to the bleak picture just portrayed of follow-up data. CLP is a longitudinal transition program serving students with learning disabilities. Students participate in work experience and career education activities as early as the 10th grade. When they graduate, vocational services continue as transiton counselors job develop, job coach, and career counsel for the postschool adults.

Siegel and his colleagues (Siegel et al., in press) conducted a comprehensive longitudinal evaluation of the program by following the employment experiences of the graduates. Project participants from 1 to 4 years out of school were monitored and contrasted to a comparable normative group. That is, Wagner (1989) collected large-scale national samples of the employment experiences of a variety of disability groups. The CLP participants substantially exceeded their national cohort on a variety of measures including percentage of cohort employed, wage, and engagement in continuing education. Short of assembling randomly assigned control and experimental groups, the normative comparison approach represents a viable evaluation strategy for follow-up research.

Present and future follow-up data will provide impetus to improve service delivery. Special educators and adult service providers should modify their service delivery models based on the implications of this research. Otherwise, follow-up researchers may continue to paint a bleak picture for graduates of special education. The material in the remainder of this chapter includes strategies for implementing these service delivery modifications.

Integrated Adult Services

This section includes descriptions of issues concerning the enhancement of adult services in integrated settings. Topics include (a) deficiencies related to integration in existing service delivery systems, (b) guiding principles in the provision of integrated services, and (c) policies and procedures that foster the implementation of coordinated integrated services.

Difficult decisions may have to be made in modifying service systems to promote integration. In order to make these decisions it is first necessary to understand the existing adult service system. Adult service systems are complex and usually unique to particular locales. Because of the uniqueness of local systems, only general observations will be made. Nevertheless, these observations should have implications for many types of adult service systems.

Government Policy and Integrated Services

Primarily, departments of rehabilitation have been responsible for people with disabilities who were considered employable. These agencies provided services to people with a wide variety of disabilities. Many of these agencies were originally designed to rehabilitate adults who had recently been injured and needed retraining in order to return to work. These types of services have been called *time-limited* because training lasted only a short period, usually just a few months at most. This system was designed to encourage rehabilitation workers to close their "cases" as quickly as possible in order to serve more clients. Obviously, such a system encouraged accepting clients who required a minimum amount of training. The larger the number of clients served, the greater the funding provided to the agency. Therefore, there was an emphasis on a fast turnover of cases and on primarily serving clients with recently acquired physical disabilities who could soon return to work. Those individuals with lifelong histories of disability were generally not provided services through rehabilitation agencies. Today, individuals with mild mental disabilities, such as learning disabilities, generally have not qualified for rehabilitation services. After they leave school they are on their own. As noted previously, the result of these policies has been poor adult adjustment for many individuals with disabilities.

The Career Ladder Program (CLP) offered a partial soulution to long-term funding. CLP amalgamated federal and open-case service funds from the department of rehabilitation to provide long-term services for adults with learning disabilities. Project Work in San Diego (Pumpian, West, & Shepherd, 1988) developed an even more comprehensive package by housing its transition program for adults with learning disabilities at a community college. Participants received vocational services under the aegis of being students at the community college. Ultimately, legislation at the national level will be needed to make follow-up services for adults with learning disabilities statutory. It is estimated that the number and amount of such services will be small (based on the CLP program) but that they will go a long way in elevating employment success.

Traditionally, long-term services have been provided only to those adults with severe disabilities. Individuals receiving these services typically included people with mental retardation and/or severe physical disabilities or sensory impairments. The services received, depending on the disability, ranged from residential care in large supervised institutions to stipends provided by government agencies to help individuals live more independently. Although employment was a concern in this traditional system, many people failed to secure work. Most individuals served in this system did not achieve independence.

Typically, these services for adults with more severe forms of disabilities have been provided directly by government agencies or by organizations that receive funds from the agencies. These generally have been segregated employment and residential services. Institutions for people with mental retardation are common under these systems. As described in Chapter 1 these institutions have been designed primarily to remove individuals from the community rather than to provide training that would help them participate more fully in the community. A more innovative system would focus on "habilitation" (i.e., the teaching of skills for more independent living to individuals who have never possessed those skills and who have never been independent).

Among individuals with more severe disabilities remaining in the community, many live with family members or in group homes. Although these types of living arrangements are more integrated than institutions, they still are dissimilar to the living arrangements of most adults. Most nondisabled adults live either with their spouses, with their friends, or alone.

In addition to living arrangements, most work options for people with more severe disabilities are restrictive, segregated options such as sheltered workshops. A continuum of vocational programs has developed since the 1960s to serve people with more severe disabilities. Payne and Patton (1981) have described four steps on the continuum: activity centers, sheltered workshops, semisheltered employment, and competitive employment. Individuals are expected to progress through this continuum from more to less restrictive programs (e.g., from sheltered to competitive employment). The funds for these programs and the source of the funds differ based on the type of program and where it falls on the continuum. People with less severe disabilities are placed in regular program workshops where sheltered work is designed to prepare them for competitive employment. For example,

> Work evaluation and work adjustment in these sheltered workshops are typically funded by the state vocational rehabilitation agency and other agencies responsible for time-limited services. Consequently, the admission standards for these programs often reflect the funding agencies' emphasis on offering services to those most likely to benefit in terms of employability. (Bellamy, Rhodes, Mank, & Albin, 1988, p. 4)

Those "most likely to benefit" may be, in actuality, persons with more mild handicaps.

Individuals with more severe disabilities often are placed in work activity or day activity programs (Schalock, McGaughey, & Kiernan, 1989). Work activity programs provide training in work-related skills that are necessary for individuals to enter the workshop program. Day activity programs focus on skill training in the areas of daily living, self-care, and recreation rather than work. In the United States most states administer day activity programs through mental retardation and mental health agencies.

This continuum of services is designed to enable individuals to move from lower to higher levels of employment. However, examination of the progress from day activity programs to higher level programs indicates a movement rate of only 1% to 3% per year (Zivolich, 1984). This percentage represents virtually no movement. Rather than these placements being temporary and habilitative, most individuals remain in them for extended periods.

In lower level programs (e.g., work activity programs), earnings range from none to less than $2.00 per work day (U.S. Department of Labor, 1979). Although individuals earn very low, if any, wages, the costs of such programs has increased dramatically over the last several years. The cost for these programs in the United States has risen to almost $1 billion annually. Additionally, this figure does not include the cost of program administration within government agencies (Bellamy et al., 1988). The problems of lack of movement along the continuum, low wages, segregation, and cost escalation have led to a search for new models of service provision.

Funding Issues

One of the most complex and controversial issues regarding service provision is the appropriation of adequate funds. Funding the provision of services to adults with disabilities is no exception. In fact, because social ethics have traditionally been a basis for serving individuals with disabilities, these services may not be considered a societal priority. When funding is scarce (and it often is), services for these individuals are typically one of the first areas reduced. When funds are less restricted, provision of these services is not a high priority. People with mental retardation have been viewed as a surplus segment of the population, "a segment of the total population exceeding the number of individuals needed to fill the slots in a social organization" (Farber, 1968, p. 19). If this is true, it is justifiable to ask why and how resources should be allocated to provide services to these adults. However, recent movements have stressed the important social and economic roles people with disabilities have in our society. More in-depth philosophical and practical reasons for why these services should be provided have been discussed in detail in other chapters of this volume. Nevertheless, the distribution and quantity of funds remain fundamental issues and are often cited as reasons for the limitations in the quality and availability of adult services. Lack of funding generates limitations on services and also limitations on the integrated roles of persons with disabilities. Issues concerning funding constrains and methods to alleviate those constraints should be explored.

Substantial support, both in intensity and duration, is often necessary to assist adults with disabilities to maintain employment or to live more independently. The amount of support required is sometimes used as an excuse for limiting funding to establish or maintain integrated adult services. Many studies have indicated, however, that the financial burden on society may be reduced if people with disabilities are given this support. They become productive (and possibly taxpaying) citizens instead of remaining unemployed and in tax-dependent situations (National

Council on the Handicapped, 1986). There is a need to educate society about this reality in conjunction with a reallocation of funds to promote integrated services.

If integrated services are to exist, legislators must support policies and funding that promote the integration of people with disabilities. The financial processes at work in the provision of special services reflect the unique political characteristics of each state and local system. Despite these unique processes, some general recommendations can be made for encouraging the development and maintenance of integrated services for adults with disabilities. Whitehead (1989) has made recommendations for state and local actions to expand the employment of individuals with disabilities. These recommendations serve as the basis for the following general suggestions for developing and maintaining integrated services:

1. Policies and procedures should be established to ensure that funds are available for community services. For example, large institutions for persons with more severe disabilities have long existed. Mechanisms for funding these institutions are well established. It is difficult to enact legislation to ensure that equal funds are available for the development of community-based services. Indeed, funds may not "follow" an individual moved from an institution into the community, and this becomes an obstacle to integrated services. Procedures should encourage the allocation of funds for the provision of services in least restrictive environments. In addition, an adequately funded system is needed that supports adults with mild disabilities. Pressure from various advocacy groups should be brought to bear on politicians and bureaucrats to ensure that such systems are developed and maintained. This pressure must come from professionals, from families of people with disabilities, and from people with disabilities themselves.

2. Advocates for integrated services should participate in developing proposals for change and then monitor changes in state and federal regulations. Advocates must be constantly aware of proposed modifications in the service systems to direct change toward integrated services. Agencies and advocacy organizations may share information and work together to keep track of current legislative developments.

3. Procedures should be established to ensure that all qualified/eligible persons are enrolled and receive full benefits from national assistance programs. Financial hardships for individuals with disabilities and their families may be alleviated through these programs. In the United States, these "entitlement" programs include, but are not restricted to, Supplemental Security Income and Medicaid, which provides health care benefits.

4. Disincentives to employment ought to be eliminated. For example, in some past cases, after an individual with disabilities secured employment, health care benefits previously received from the government were in danger of termination. Steps have recently been taken in the United

States at the federal level to eliminate the possibility of reduced benefits after an individual is employed. Advocates should examine other regulations to ensure that similar disincentives are eliminated. More specifically, recent federal legislation permits workers with disabilities to make up to $500 per month without any of their Supplemental Security Income (SSI) being scrutinized. Recent legislation has also made it more straightforward to be reinstated on the SSI rolls if one has been removed because of substantial employment. Still, there needs to be further development of a user-friendly system for employees with disabilities that will enable them to become employed and have no fears that their SSI benefits will be placed in jeopardy. For example, each local SSI office should have an ombudsman or case specialist who directly and supportively communicates about such matters with employees who are disabled.

5. Procedures should be established to ensure that agencies coordinate financial support efforts. Given the limited availability of funds, it is imperative that agencies communicate and cooperate to ensure an effective and efficient delivery system. This coordination can reduce duplication of services and will assist staff in long-range planning of services. Some specific suggestions for interagency collaboration are described later in this chapter.

6. Formal cooperative agreements between agencies should be established to ensure the continuity of services when responsibility for an individual shifts from one agency to another. For example, schools and adult service agencies must agree on their respective roles and responsibilities as persons with disabilities leave school and enter adult life. Agreeing on who will oversee this transition process and on how to pay these personnel may be a major stumbling block to ensuring adequate transition services. Cooperative agreements require an understanding of the responsibilities of each agency, a willingness to cooperate, and a commitment to transcend traditional arrangements to ensure appropriate services.

The restructuring of the system for funding special services can be both complex and challenging. However, restructuring appears to be one of the more effective methods for ensuring the provision of special services. By changing the process by which funds are allocated, and by ensuring that people with disabilities receive the financial support to which they are entitled, integrated services may be developed and maintained.

Training

The vocational training of adults with disabilities for community employment has been traditionally short-term. Training typically was designed to teach a person specific skills related to a particular job. This type of training, when offered, was provided predominantly to people with mild disabilities. People with more severe disabilities typically did not receive vocational training. In addition, training rarely was provided to help individuals with disabilities in other domains of adult life such as recreation or independent living.

This traditional pattern of service provision need not continue. Many innovative models with improved training programs have been developed. For example, recent work has focused on the framework of vocational training. The components of vocational training have been delineated as attendance, social skills, job-keeping skills, job skills and job search (Siegel, Greener, Prieur, Robert, & Gaylord-Ross, 1989). The reader is referred to chapter 9 of this volume, on secondary education and transition, for a detailed discussion of these components. In addition, innovative programs in postsecondary education have been created to help adults with learning disabilities develop not only job skills but also skills in the social and independent living domains (HEATH, 1988a). Independent living centers have been established to assist adults with severe physical disabilities. Skills are taught to increase their independence, for example, skills to increase mobility in the community (HEATH, 1988b). Additionally, adult service providers are learning effective systematic training techniques used in special education to teach adults with disabilities.

Systematic Instruction

The use of systematic instruction with students has been discussed in detail in chapters 6 and 9 of this volume. The concern here is how to apply the same techniques to the training of adults with disabilities. This is particularly difficult given the fact that the staff: client ratio in adult services is usually far leaner than that in schools. However, many of the same approaches used in community-based training can be applied to adults learning work skills. Indeed, such effective training techniques may help to alleviate some of the problems associated with staff shortages. For example, the use of explicit instructions, prompts, and systematic reinforcement as well as peer tutoring and heterogeneous grouping can be extremely effective in adult programs.

Systematic instruction may be more effective when employed in natural settings (i.e., where the skills will be used). Training in these environments will likely increase the individual's awareness of particular task demands, make those tasks more meaningful, and may also promote interaction with people without disabilities. In addition, when training is undertaken in natural settings, the instructor can more easily identify skill areas that are problematic for the trainee. Thus, skills for instruction can be quickly targeted without an unnecessary focus on presumed prerequisite skills. Not only can specific skills be trained more efficiently in natural settings, but also the influence of naturally ocurring cues and consequences in these settings increases the likelihood that skills will generalize to other situations where similar cues and consequences occur.

As the performance of skills comes under the control of natural stimuli, maintenance over time is more likely.

A recent and exciting development has been in the area of making nondisabled co-workers instructors for persons with disabilities. Gaylord-Ross, Lee, Johnston, and Goetz (in press) have recruited co-workers to become social advocates for their co-workers who are disabled. That is, a co-worker advocate identifies and carries out integration strategies for the employee with disabilities. Gaylord-Ross et al. reported an array of engaging strategies that led to social behavior integration of one of two employees who were deaf-blind and severely mentally retarded.

One problem in the use of systematic instruction is the inadequate supply of adult service personnel who have specialized training in these techniques. Several programs have been developed recently to train adult service personnel in systematic instruction. Some institutions of higher education have combined the efforts of departments of rehabilitation and special education to provide this training. At San Francisco State University the departments of special education and rehabilitation have established a joint training project. One of the goals of this project is to train students to use systematic instruction in adult service settings. Many other professionals have used their expertise to train adult service personnel in these instructional techniques through workshops and in-service training. For example, the University of San Francisco has developed materials and an extensive series of workshops to teach adult service providers the techniques of systematic instruction.

Self-Management

One type of systematic instruction, training the use of self-management techniques, has shown promise with adults with disabilities. In self-management (or self-control), individuals are taught to control their own behavior. Self-management techniques include self-monitoring, self-evaluation, and self-reinforcement. Self-management requires that the person first monitor, then evaluate, and finally compare his or her behavior to some standard. The individual then may reward himself or herself for good performance. For example, a person could monitor performance on the job and, if performance was satisfactory, enjoy a refreshment after work as a reward.

Many studies have shown that these techniques can be used to improve the vocational performance of people with disabilities (Liberty & Michael, 1985; Mickler, 1984). Self-management techniques also have been used with adults with mental retardation to improve completion of daily activities, such as housekeeping, shopping, and appointments (Lovett & Haring, 1989). In addition to the possibility of improving the self-directed performance of persons with mental handicaps, self-management techniques also may help establish long-term maintenance and generalization of desired skills (Cole, Gardner, & Karan, 1983; Mank & Horner, 1987).

Park and Gaylord-Ross (1989) demonstrated the promise of self-management techniques in the workplace. Three employees with mental retardation were trained in social problem solving strategies. That is, they learned to decode social situations, generate alternatives for their solution, select and enact a solution, and self-evaluate its effectiveness. The training successfully generalized to actual social interactions with co-workers. Park et al. (1990) successfully replicated this self-management problem-solving procedure with employees who were mentally retarded and with those who had learning disabilities.

Supported Employment

Supported employment is one of the most exciting innovations in service provision for adults with disabilities, especially for those with more severe disabilities. Supported employment is a service model designed to enable individuals with more severe disabilities to work in integrated settings (Bellamy et al., 1988; Wehman & Moon, 1988). Unlike models in which extensive training is required prior to job placement, the supported employment model emphasizes placing the individual in a job and providing the support needed to successfully maintain the individual in that position. A supported employment specialist provides job placement, job-site training, and continuous follow-along services. The employment specialist should have a strong background in systematic instruction. A thorough understanding of the job requirements and the local community are equally important.

There are three major features of supported employment programs. First, they provide meaningful work for which the individual is paid. Second, they take place in integrated settings where the individual can interact with nondisabled co-workers. Third, they provide intensive and long-lasting support to meet the needs of the individual and ensure success on the job. The supported employment model is designed to meet individual needs rather than needs of facilities and bureaucracies. Greater emphasis is placed on the choices of the family and the consumer, as opposed to choices made by agency personnel. This is an extension of the movement toward individualization, integration, and independence for persons with disabilities in the community.

The majority of people (65%) served in supported employment programs are in individual placements (Wehman, 1990). In this type of placement no other person with disabilities from the same program works at the site. Other supported employment approaches employ small groups (or enclaves) in a single integrated setting or use mobile crews that move from one community site to another. Most people who are in supported employment programs work 20 hours or more per week and many are served by the vocational rehabilitation system (Wehman, 1990). Although, the number of people served in these programs is growing, it is small when compared to the number of people served by traditional rehabilitation and day programs.

Although the supported employment model is relatively new, it has received substantial support. The federal government has recently implemented policy and funding initiatives to foster the development of supported employment opportunities in every state. There has been substantial growth in the number of individuals served by supported employment programs and in the total number of these programs (Wehman, 1990). Most of these programs, however, serve people with mild and moderate mental retardation, although there has been some movement to serve people with other disabilities such as long-term mental illness, physical disabilities, and sensory impairments. Although supported employment was initially designed to serve people with severe disabilities, less than 10% of those served by these programs have severe or profound mental retardation (Wehman, 1990).

The implementation of supported employment services has important implications for both professionals and programs. Because individuals are placed directly into the community, the service provider is identified less with a facility or building and more as an integral part of the community. The operation may be perceived more as a business and less as a social service. This is a result of a greater number of program staff members working directly with the consumer at the employment site. As noted, this staff may require extra training in direct service and job development. Because the client is placed and trained immediately on a real job, the outcomes of employment (real wages, increased community participation) are clearly focused and quickly realized. In addition, the consumer assumes greater responsibility for making choices about employment. This increased choice making requires personnel to relinquish some control in decision making. The staff's role shifts toward assisting families and consumers in making choices. The implementation of supported employment services is a great opportunity to transform service agencies into community-based operations with stronger links to the regular labor market, rehabilitation services, employers, and consumers and their families.

Increasing Integrated Employment Opportunities

The growing participation of the business community bodes well for the employment of adults with disabilities. In the past, employers were the receptors of social service efforts to place persons with disabilities into jobs. This strategy for placement will undoubtedly continue. Yet the new and exciting notion of a "corporate initiative" has made businesses the leaders in the employment process. That is, some businesses are setting ambitious targets for the employment of persons with disabilities. For example, Pizza Hut hopes to have an employee with disabilities working on every shift of every Pizza Hut throughout the nation. The company has also provided resources for training and adapting the workplace for employees with disabilities. Most notably, the Marriot Foundation for Persons with Disabilities has invested substantial sums of money in funding job coaches, counselors, and related vocational personnel in order to facilitate the transition of youth with disabilities to adult employment. Clearly, when businesses begin funding as well as hiring persons with disabilities, the whole employment process will accelerate and become even more cost-effective.

There are some specific areas of competence for adult service providers in the vocational domain that are worthy of mention here. Basically, personnel in adult service programs that focus on employment of people with disabilities should possess knowledge in the following areas:

1. Client assessment,
2. Adaptive devices,
3. Development of individualized program plans,
4. Community support systems,
5. Local labor market analysis and labor unions,
6. Job development,
7. Job analysis.

Integrated Vocational Services in a Changing Society

To determine the most effective structure of integrated employment services is a difficult task. This is especially true considering the changing face of our postindustrial society. One change already in process in the economic realm of industrialized nations is the increasingly smaller proportion of young adults in the labor force. The reduced number of younger workers probably will force employers to seek additional sources of labor. One of these sources may be people with disabilities. Also, new technologies may enable people with physical and mental disabilities to perform jobs unavailable to them in the past. These devices may increase people's capabilities and therefore increase opportunities for integration.

Another primary societal change that has already begun in the United States and other industrialized countries is a shift toward a more service-oriented economy (Bluestone, 1989). If existing trends continue, four out of five new jobs in the American labor market will be in the service sector. Because employment in the service sector often involves work with the public, individuals with disabilities should learn to interact appropriately with a wide variety of people. In turn, this will necessitate that members of the public have a greater awareness of the capabilities of people with disabilities. Thus, special service professionals not only must educate people with disabilities but must also help educate the entire populace. It is only through this combination of efforts that comprehensive integrated adult services can be successful.

Postsecondary Education

Some of the most innovative models of service provision to adults with disabilities have been created in the area of postsecondary education. Many of these model programs provide services to adults with mild disabilities (e.g., learning disabilities, sensory impairments). These educational programs are usually designed to help students succeed in future environments. These future environments include settings where potential employment or additional education is received. At postsecondary sites, (e.g., community colleges, vocational/technical schools) adults with disabilities receive instruction on the same campuses as their nondisabled peers. This provides the opportunity for increased interaction.

Over the years, there has been an increase in the number of students with disabilities who attend institutions of higher education (Nelson & Lignugaris/Kraft, 1989). A number of support programs have been developed to serve students with learning disabilities on college campuses (Mangrum & Strichart, 1983). For example, officials at 106 California community colleges reported that 7,982 students were receiving services through learning disability programs (Ostertag, Baker, Howard, & Best, 1982). These programs have developed for several reasons (Nelson & Lignugaris/Kraft, 1989). First, federal legislation promoted access to postsecondary programs for people with disabilities. Second, the development of services at the college level represents an extension of services provided in schools prior to high school graduation. Third, national and local organizations have advocated that college and university personnel develop programs on college campuses to assist students with disabilities. Finally, many colleges face declining student enrollments. Students with learning disabilities represent a source of new enrollments.

Nelson and Lignugaris/Kraft (1989) identified factors influencing the provision of postsecondary services to students with disabilities. The mission of the school appears to impact the types of services made available. Community (or 2-year) colleges provide opportunities ranging from preparation for the general equivalency diploma (GED), to noncredit special-interest courses, to vocational training courses. In contrast, traditional 4-year colleges offer students academic training in a range of specific fields.

Program emphasis also influences program objectives. The principal objective of some programs is to provide basic-skills remediation. Typically, 4-year institutions place less emphasis on remedial training than do community colleges. For example, at some community colleges a central feature is remediation of basic skills through peer tutoring. Other programs provide support to students to increase success in regular courses. For example, students may be provided tutoring, access to tape-recorded textbooks, and assistance from vocational rehabilitation services. Some programs provide both remediation of skill deficits and support services (Nelson & Lignugaris/Kraft, 1989).

The services offered by a particular institution also vary according to service goal priorities. "Institutions for which the development of learning strategies and basic skills remediation are a priority provide considerably more services for their students with learning disabilities and are also more likely to employ LD specialists to deliver those services than institutions focused on" increasing access to regular courses (Bursuch, Rose, Cowen, & Yahaya, 1989, p. 244). Bursuch et al. found that peer tutoring was a widespread practice, although tutors apparently were selected for their abilities in specific content areas rather than for any mastery of effective instructional techniques for use with students with learning disabilities. Funding allocations may influence how services are delivered. For example, the funds available to a program might determine whether tutors are specialists in the field of learning disabilities or peer tutors, and whether a program provides individual or group counseling (Nelson & Lignugaris/Kraft, 1989).

Unfortunately, research that might help in the design of postsecondary programs for students with learning disabilities is limited. Research is needed to determine measures for use in identifying adults with learning disabilities. Such research may lead to establishing guidelines concerning student eligibility for LD programs. In addition, research is needed to identify what types and the scope of services presently provided to students with disabilities. In particular, information on course accommodations acceptable to faculty in community colleges and universities would be useful for career counselors in secondary schools and for academic advisors in universities. This information would be especially helpful for secondary-level special educators in developing student transition plans. Transition goals can then be developed to better prepare students to access postsecondary services.

There is a need for a comprehensive data base concerning promising trends in postsecondary service delivery. Research that describes the demands made on students in postsecondary education environments would be helpful in designing instructional plans to meet those demands. For example, research on environmental demands has provided a basis for the development of intervention strategies for high school students with learning disabilities (Anderson-Inman, Walker, & Purcell, 1984; Schumaker & Deshler, 1984). Similar analyses in postsecondary schools would provide a foundation for improving instruction in those environments (Nelson & Lignugaris/Kraft, 1989). Research also should be conducted examining the effects of individual program components on student outcomes. Follow-up studies on the adjustment of individuals after they leave postsecondary programs could provide valuable data on the effectiveness of services. Bursuch et al. (1989) found that few colleges collect data on graduation rates of students with learning disabilities. This is disturbing. Data should be gathered not only on graduation rates but also on postgraduation vocational and life adjustment. Information gathered in these studies could then be used to assist in the design of future programs.

It should be noted that not all postsecondary programs focus on adults with mild disabilities. Several new programs on postsecondary campuses provide training to adults with severe disabilities. For example, at Butte College in California, adults with developmental disabilities take classes in functional reading, arithmetic, and other useful skills. In addition, the college provides vocational training classes to these students (HEATH, 1988c). Such innovative programs give adults with severe disabilities the opportunity to receive postsecondary education services with their non-disabled peers.

Integrated Residential Services

As the review of follow-up research revealed, persons with disabilities have difficulty in the residential domain. Without residential environments designed to promote the interaction of people with and without disabilities, the entire concept of integration is in jeopardy. Currently, there is a movement to improve the residential options available to adults with disabilities. The traditional residential approach focuses on fitting people into existing programs. More innovative models emphasize the person and develop supports and housing around the individual (Racino & Walker, 1988).

As in the vocational sector, a continuum of services exists in the residential domain. A variety of residential settings, from traditional institutions to individual living arrangements, may be available. This continuum is designed for individuals to move from more restrictive to less restrictive settings as their skills improve. However, Taylor (1988) has identified problems inherent in this continuum. These problems include a confusion between the intensity of services and the restrictiveness of the setting (i.e., the viewpoint that the more restrictive the setting, the greater the intensity of services). It is possible, however, to provide intense services in less restrictive environments. More restrictive environments typically have been seen as preparatory for living in less restrictive settings. However, the demands of these various settings are so different that life in more restrictive placements rarely helps people develop the skills required to live in less restrictive environments. In addition, although movement along the continuum is slow, at best, moving from one environment to another may limit stability and the development of enduring relationships.

There are several issues related to providing community residential services. One is the number of people with disabilities served in a single setting. Many innovative service systems have moved toward the placement of one to three people in a single site. These small numbers allow more individualized support and enable the staff to concentrate on the individual rather than on a group.

There has also been a move toward heterogeneity in a single setting (i.e., having people with different disabilities living together). This arrangement allows people with disabilities to use their skills to help others with disabilities. For example, a person with mental retardation might help a roommate with severe cerebral palsy to complete some cleaning tasks in the home. Such arrangements might reduce demands on staff. An additional possibility would be to have a nondisabled person live in the same house and assist person(s) with disabilities in exchange for lower rents or other compensation.

Another developing change is the division between the provision of support and the home environment. Traditionally, the type of home one was allowed to live in depended on the type of support one needed. A more innovative approach is to separate supports from the living situation. Individuals receive the support they need no matter where they live. The agency providing the support need not be the agency owning or leasing the residence. This can give greater control to the individual and family in choosing a location and type of housing. This greater control can build on and strengthen previous community ties already developed. For example, people might be able to remain in their own neighborhoods rather than moving to another location. The cost of providing integrated residential settings may be of concern. However, as discussed earlier, with changes in funding mechanisms, money could be redirected from more restricted environments toward ones that are more integrated and that promote independence.

Provision of individualized housing requires knowledge of personal characteristics to address the needs of each individual. Supports can be developed or altered that match the person's particular needs. Obviously, such support needs to be flexible as circumstances and the needs of the person change. This includes not only the intensity of support but also the type and delivery of the support services (Racino & Walker, 1988).

Recent research results indicate that people with mental disabilities can learn a variety of domestic skills (Martin, 1988). The type of individualized living arrangements discussed here may make it easier to learn skills in natural contexts. There may no longer be a need for "artificial" programming time, because individualized training can be integrated into regular routines and contexts. Training in integrated residential settings may promote the generalization and maintenance of domestic skills and therefore help increase independence.

Community Skills

One important aspect of integration is access to community resources. To access these resources people with disabilities must have the ability to move from place to place. Training may be necessary in the areas of pedestrian skills and the use of public transportation. Research results indicate that, with systematic instruction, people with mental disabilities can learn various complex mobility skills (Martin, 1988). The management of money is also an important aspect for accessing community resources. In addition to the ability of basic computation, money management includes skills in banking and purchasing. Through the development of banking skills people may gain more control and have more responsibility over the use of their money. They can make decisions about savings, expenditures, and other budgetary concerns. Adults with disabilities also should learn purchasing skills to increase their independence. These skills may include purchases at stores (e.g., grocery stores, pharmacies) and restaurants. In addition, access to recreational activities (e.g., movies, sports events) may be increased if people have the skills to make purchases independently.

Recreation and Leisure

Leisure and recreation are important parts of human life. Recreational experiences can be very meaningful and can be opportunities for social interaction. These opportunities have not always been available for people with disabilities. Recently, emphasis has been placed on the value of recreation for persons with disabilities (Fine, 1989).

Many individuals with disabilities have large amounts of leisure time (Pierce, 1989). In a survey of adults with disabilities, Harris (1987) found them to be extremely isolated and engaged in few community activities. More than one half of those surveyed stated that their disability prevented them from attending cultural or sports events or seeing friends as often as they would like. In addition, only one third were active in community groups, compared to 60% of nondisabled persons. Those with more severe disabilities engaged in fewer activities.

Specific instruction on leisure skills can help alleviate these problems. Leisure skill training should be provided throughout the school years. This training should focus not only on acquisition but also on the self-initiation or self-direction in the use of leisure skills. The reader is referred to Chapter 6 of this volume for a discussion of recreational and community skills curricula and training.

Interagency Collaboration

Throughout the discussion of integrated adult services there has been an emphasis on coordination and collaboration among agencies. Lifelong integrated services require such collaboration. Through cooperation, the system becomes stronger, more efficient, and more responsive to the needs of individuals. Interagency teams should be established at the state and local levels to develop and maintain lines of communication. These teams should include consumers, parents, employers, and adult service providers, as well as representatives from developmental disabilities and mental health agencies, public schools, postsecondary institutions, and vocational rehabilitation. Interagency collaboration may be mandated through legislation or achieved through formal agreements. Whatever the arrangement, it is important that all involved realize the benefits that can be gained through this cooperation. Some of these benefits are listed below.

1. The duplication of services can be prevented. Each agency can help ensure that the services provided are unique to that agency. Limited resources can then be used in a more efficient manner.

2. Better communication will likely increase opportunities to provide continuity of services between agencies related or dependent on one another. For example, as an adult with mental retardation becomes more successful on the job and the need for support services is reduced, responsibility for that individual's case may move from one agency to another. With effective communication, smooth transitions of responsibility are more likely.

3. As interagency communication improves, gaps in services may be identified and steps taken to rectify problem areas. For example, many agencies use their own jargon and operate through unique procedures. Better communication between agencies may prevent misunderstandings and serve to focus attention on areas of true need.

There are many strategies that can be employed to foster collaboration. These include agreeing on common goals, clarifying values, securing outside consultation, using peer trainers, identifying resources, and involving consumers in decision making. The reader is referred to the book *Building the Collaborative Community* by Schindler-Rainman and Lippitt (1980) for a detailed discussion of these strategies.

Self-Advocacy

Much of the material presented in this chapter has focused on the increased independence of individuals with disabilities. Communicating one's views is part of being independent. Advocacy has been defined as the representation of the rights and interests of oneself or others in an effort to bring about change to eliminate barriers to meet identified needs. Representing one's own rights and interests and speaking on one's own behalf is called self-advocacy (Payne & Patton, 1981).

There are several goals of self-advocacy:

1. The enhancement of the rights and responsibilities of the individual.
2. The development of the ability to make choices, which requires that the individual have two or more options (e.g., jobs or living arrangements) from which a choice can be made.
3. An increase in the individual's participation in planning services (e.g., in the development of an individualized transition plan or an individualized program plan).
4. The enhancement of opportunities for taking reasonable risks with support from peer self-help groups (e.g., entering into a new living situation or starting a new job).
5. Identification of gaps and duplications in service delivery (e.g., when there is a delay in transferring a person's "case" from one agency to another, or when identical training is provided by different agencies).
6. The establishment of procedures for the identification of most-needed services by the consumer (e.g., ensuring that youths leaving school have a voice in selecting services that are necessary for them to secure employment or other goals as adults).
7. The development of consumers to become vocal advocates for themselves with assistance from other people with disabilities; self-advocacy can be a difficult process and individuals need to learn from others who have previously participated in the process.

The goals of self-advocacy can be divided into the three domains discussed throughout this chapter: employment, residential living, and community skills. To achieve a degree of self-advocacy in these areas requires that the individual participate in planning personal goals. It also requires that people in similar circumstances develop and share information. This will help determine what services are available, inform service providers about expectations and perceived problems, and build a broad base of support among consumers and the community.

Consumers can directly influence service providers by serving on the board of directors of existing organizations or by starting their own organization to provide services. They can use political pressure to influence the entire service delivery system to appropriate or redistribute funds to support programs that provide opportunities for choice and integration. Finally, self-advocacy can strengthen one's own resolve by working with others who have similar concerns. One organization, People First, is a group of individuals with disabilities that has organized on local and national levels. The members have identified common needs and have joined together to enhance their political power.

There has been one experimental area that tangentially bears upon self-advocacy. Within the notion of self-management (see above), persons with disabilities have been taught to self-recruit feedback from their employers or significant others. For example, Mank and Horner (1987) taught workers with moderate and severe disabilities to monitor their own job performance. When they reached a criterion level of work, they approached their supervisors to obtain reinforcement. Thus, the employees gained better control of their work environment through this self-recruitment process. One could imagine how self-recruitment of other services and reinforcers could be trained and used by adults with disabilities.

There are some areas of concern regarding self-advocacy that must be acknowledged. First, by banding together as a force, self-advocates may isolate themselves from people without disabilities. Self-advocates must be aware of this possibility and ensure that they communicate and cooperate with nondisabled people. Second, there is a danger that self-advocates will rely on their advisors to the point that the advisors direct the actions of the self-advocates. Both advisors and consumers should be trained to ensure there is true self-advocacy. Finally, many professionals and organizations created to help people with disabilities believe they know what is best for consumers. They may be inclined to keep control of the system. It can be a threat to this viewpoint and to the accompanying sense of power to allow self-direction for people with disabilities. Professionals and advocates should learn that people with disabilities have feelings and beliefs about what is in their own best interests.

Systems Change

With the long history of institutionalization and segregation under traditional service systems, established political and economic forces sometimes serve to obstruct the conversion to more consumer-oriented integrated systems. For example, because many institutions for persons with mental retardation have been built in small communities, away from large metropolitan areas, they have become major economic factors in these localities. To reduce or eliminate these facilities could have a major impact on the economies of these communities (e.g., an increase in unemployment). In addition to localized economic impacts, proposed changes in service delivery to adults with disabilities will affect large bureaucracies that have been created to oversee service provision. These bureaucracies may attempt to prevent change unless it is perceived that the change is beneficial to the bureaucrats. This may lead to opposition from those political forces that have a stake in the status quo.

Traditionally, systems tend to maintain themselves against forces of change, leaving us to question whether this situation can be altered. We believe there are several methods that can be employed to bring about change. (The reader is referred to the section on systems change in Chapter 1 of this volume and the section on interagency collaboration in this chapter.) At one level, state and national government policies and legislation may be used to encourage local systems to change. At the local level, planning teams with a wide variety of community representation can be created to coordinate change efforts. At both of these levels, businesses may be provided with information concerning the capabilities of people with disabilities. Incentives may also be provided to businesses to involve them in integrated services.

Change in service provision also may mean change in staff roles and responsibilities. Therefore, ongoing technical assistance that facilitates the development and continuation of integrated services should be provided. This assistance should include specific information about implementing policies and procedures designed to promote integrated services. Such training should ensure that all concerned parties have access to the same information and that there is a cohesive approach to the provision of services. Consumers may also need help to understand and access the service delivery system.

After the delivery system is modified and operating, it is important to develop a data collection and analysis system to evaluate its effectiveness. This system could be designed to provide information regarding the type of existing services, the level of integration being achieved, and the number and characteristics of individuals receiving services. This information could not only be used for securing and distributing funds, but also could be disseminated to service providers to inform them of the systemwide progress made. Such information could also help identify additional local needs for services. Recommendations for policy modifications to improve integrated services may also be formulated using this data. A more elaborate discussion of data collection systems for the analysis of adult service provision can be found in Zivolich, Rosenberg, and DeCilla (1988).

As noted in Chapter 1 of this volume, one of the most effective and durable methods of ensuring systems change is to educate staff working in the existing system with regard to how to improve that system. It may be necessary for staff members to change not only their roles and responsibilities but also their perspective on people with disabilities. When staff members perceive people with disabilities as capable adults, professionals may be more likely to become effective change agents. This method may serve as an internal means for the improvement of adult services. It should be noted, however, that this method refers to ongoing, intensive education, not simply "1-day workshops" (Schindler-Rainman & Lippitt, 1980).

Conclusions

Throughout this chapter there has been an emphasis on special services for adults with disabilities that provide training and support community integration. The adult service personnel responsible for this training and support include vocational, recreational, and residential trainers; teachers in postsecondary education; and counselors in vocational rehabilitation. Although there are some specific skills needed by each of the above personnel groups, some general areas of competence for all groups can be identified:

1. A basic knowledge of the abilities and needs of adults with disabilities.
2. A basic understanding of the underlying philosophy, history, and development of special services.
3. A knowledge of the roles and responsibilities of relevant adult service agencies.
4. A knowledge of different service models (e.g., what supported employment is and how it can be used to help people with severe disabilities achieve competitive employment).
5. An understanding of how the private sector operates and how to work with businesses to promote employment and support.
6. An ability to use systematic instruction and behavior management to teach social, vocational, home and community living, self-management skills, and so forth.
7. An ability to work closely and communicate with consumers, families, employers, schools, and other adult service providers.

Several conclusions can be drawn from the material presented in this chapter: (a) There is a general failure of adults with disabilities to succeed in the adult world; (b) adult service systems should be more responsive to the needs of the individual and his or her family; (c) the provision of integrated services can help people with disabilities be more productive and thus benefit the community; (d) for integrated services to be realized, changes in economic, political, and bureaucratic policies will be required, along with a willingness on the part of personnel to carry out those policies; (e) one method to achieve integration is through the implementation of a system of incentives and disincentives; and (f) researchers should explore outcomes, efficiency, and collaboration to enhance integrated services.

A move toward integrated adult services requires the elimination of social, economic, and administrative barriers to community integration. It requires the design of services and supports to encourage rather than discourage involvement in community life and to cultivate rather than impede relationships between people with and without disabilities. There is no doubt that the concept and implementation of integrated services pose a challenge to those who work in the field of special services, a challenge to the families of persons with disabilities, and most of all, a challenge to individuals with disabilities themselves. We must be prepared to meet these challenges and make the most of this opportunity to ensure that adults with disabilities have the opportunities they deserve and the choices that are their right.

References

Anderson-Inman, L., Walker, H.M., & Purcell, J. (1984). Promoting the transfer of skills across settings: Transenvironmental programming for handicapped students in the mainstream. In W.L. Heward, T.E. Heron, D.S. Hill, & J. Trap-Porter (Eds.), *Focus on behavior analysis in education* (pp. 18–37). Columbus, OH: Charles E. Merrill.

Baller, W.R. (1936). A study of the present social status of a group of adults who when they were in elementary school were classified as mentally deficient. *Genetic Psychology Monographs*, *18*, 165–244.

Bellamy, G.T., Rhodes, L.E., Mank, D.M., & Albin, J.M. (1988). *Supported employment a community implementation guide*. Baltimore: Paul H. Brookes.

Bluestone, B. (1989). Employment prospects for persons with disabilities. In W.E. Kiernan & R.L. Schalock (Eds.), *Economics, industry, and disability*. Baltimore: Paul H. Brookes.

Bobroff, A. (1955). Economic adjustment of 121 adults, formerly students in classes for mental retardates. *American Journal of Mental Deficiency*, *60*, 525–535.

Boyce, D.A., & Elzey, F.F. (1978). *A study of the vocational adequacy of former special education students following high school graduation*. Sacramento, CA: California State Department of Education.

Bruiniks, R.H., Rotegard, L.L., Lakin, K.C., & Hill, B.K. (1987). Epidemiology of mental retardation and trends in residential services in the United States. In S. Landesman & P. Vietze (Eds.), *Living environments and mental retardation*. Washington, DC: American Association on Mental Retardation.

Bursuch, B., Rose, E., Cowen, S., & Yahaya, M. (1989). Nationwide survey of postsecondary education services for students with learning disabilities. *Exceptional Children*, *56*(3), 236–245.

Carriker, W.R. (1957). *A comparison of postschool adjustment of a Connecticut community revisited: A study of the social adjustment of a group of mentally deficient adults in 1948 and 1960*. Washington, DC: Department of Health, Education, and Welfare, Office of Vocational Rehabilitation.

Cassidy, V.M., & Phelps, H.R. (1955). *Postschool adjustment of slow learning children*. Columbus, OH: Ohio State University, Bureau of Special and Adult Education.

Cole, C., Gardner, W., & Karan, O. (1983). *Self-management training of mentally retarded adults with chronic conduct difficulties*. Madison, WI: University of Wisconsin.

Collister, L. (1975). *A comparison of the long-range benefits of graduation from special vs. mainstream school for mildly mentally handicapped students*. Seattle, WA: Seattle Public Schools, Department of Planning, Research, and Evaluation.

Coonley, K., Klopenstein, R.E., Sitlington, P., Wild, M.L., & Wright, E. (1980). *A fifteen year follow-up study of the North Kansas City Public Schools Work Study graduates 1966–1980*. (ERIC Document Report Service No. ED 196 211)

Datillo, J., & Mirenda, P. (1987). An application of a leisure preference assessment protocol for persons with severe handicaps. *Journal of the Association for Persons With Severe Handicaps*, *12*, 306–311.

Dearborn Public Schools, Michigan. (1970). *A follow-up and comparison of graduates from types of high school programs for the mentally handicapped: Final report*. Washington, DC: Office of Education, Department of Health, Education, and Welfare.

Dinger, J.D. (1958). *Post-school adjustment of former special education pupils with implications for curriculum revision*. Unpublished doctoral dissertation, University Park, PA: Pennsylvania State University, Department of Education.

Dinger, J.D. (1961). Former educable retarded pupils. *Exceptional Children*, *27*, 353–360.

Dinger, J.D. (1973). *A follow-up study of the post school employment success of graduates from four high school special education programs in the midwestern intermediate Unit IV in Pennsylvania for the school years 1969–1970: A final report*. Harrisburg, PA: Pennsylvania Department of Education.

Edgar, E. (1987). Secondary programs in special education: Are many of them justifiable? *Exceptional Children*, *53*, 555–561.

Fairbanks, R. (1933). The subnormal child seventeen years after. *Mental Hygiene*, *17*, 177–208.

Farber, B. (1968). *Mental retardation its social context and social consequences*. Boston: Houghton Mifflin.

Fine, A.H. (1989). The importance of recreation for adjustment in community living. *News and Notes American Association on Mental Retardation*, 2, *5*, p. 3.

Gaylord-Ross, R., Lee, M., Johnston, S., & Goetz, L. (in press). Social-communication and co-worker training for deaf-blind youth in supported employment settings. *Behavior Modification*.

Gozali, J. (1972). Perceptions of the EMR special class by former students. *Mental Retardation*, *10*, 34–35.

Haring, K.A., & Lovett, D.L. (1990). The adult adjustment of special education graduates: A follow-up study. *Journal of Special Education*, *23*, 463–477.

Harris, L. (1987). *The ICD survey II: Employing disabled Americans*. New York: Louis Harris & Associates.

Hasazi, S.B., Gordon, L.R., & Roe, C.A. (1985). Factors associated with the employment status of handicapped youth exiting high school from 1979 to 1983. *Exceptional Children*, *51*, 455–469.

HEATH. (1988a). Learning disability and college preparation. *Information from HEATH*, *8*(1), 2–3.

HEATH. (1988b). Centers for independent living and campuses benefit one another. *Information from HEATH*, *7*(3), 3.

HEATH. (1988c). New alternatives after high school for persons with severe handicaps. *Information from HEATH*, *7*(1), 2.

Kennedy, R.J.R. (1948). *The social adjustment of morons in a Connecticut city*. Wilport, CT: Commissions to Study Resources in Connecticut.

Kennedy, R.J.R. (1962). *A Connecticut community revisited: A study of the social adjustment of a group of mentally deficient adults in 1948 and 1960*. Washington,

DC: Department of Health, Education, and Welfare, Office of Vocational Rehabilitation.

Kernan, C.B. (1979). *A follow-up study of students placed in educable mentally retarded classes who graduated from programs in the Northwest Bergen Council for Special Education*. New Brunswick, NJ: Rutgers University.

Liberty, K., & Michael, L. (1985). Teaching retarded students to reinforce their own behavior: A review of process and operation in the current literature. In N. Haring (Principal Investigator), *Investigating the problem of skill generalization* (3rd. ed.). (U.S. Department of Education, Contract No. 300–82–0364). Seattle, WA: University of Washington, College of Education.

Lovett, D.L., & Haring, K.A. (1989). The effects of self-management training on the daily living of adults with mental retardation. *Education and Training in Mental Retardation*, *24*, 306–323.

Mangrum, C.T., & Strichart, S.S. (1983). College possibilities for the learning disabled: Part 1. *Learning Disabilities*, *2*(5), 57–68.

Mank, D., & Horner, R. (1987). Self-recruited feedback: A cost-effective procedure for maintaining behavior. *Research in Developmental Disabilities*, *8*, 91–112.

Martin, J. (1988). Providing training in community and domestic skills. In L.W. Heal, J.I. Haney, & A.R. Novak Amado (Eds.), *Integration of developmentally disabled individuals into the community* (2nd ed.) 169–191. Baltimore: Paul H. Brookes.

Mickler, M. (1984). Self-management skill training for EMR persons. *Journal of Special Education*, *18*(2), 143–149.

Mithaug, D.E., Horuichi, C.N., & Fanning, P.N. (1985). A report on the Colorado statewide follow-up survey of special education students. *Exceptional Children*, *51*(5), 397–404.

National Council on the Handicapped. (1986). *Toward independence*. Washington, DC: V.S. Government Printing Office.

Nelson, R., & Lignugaris/Kraft (1989). Postsecondary education for students with learning disabilities. *Exceptional Children*, *56*, 246–265.

Ostertag, B.A., Baker, R.E., Howard, R.F., & Best, L. (1982). Learning disabled programs in California community colleges. *Journal of Learning Disabilities*, *15*, 535–538.

Park, H.S., & Gaylord-Ross, R. (1989). Problem-solving social skills training in employment settings with mentally retarded youth. *Journal of Applied Behavior Analysis*, *22*, 373–380.

Park, H.S., Johnson, Tappe, P., Simon, M., Wozniak, T., & Gaylord-Ross, R. (1990). Relationship and social skill interventions for disabled youth in work settings. Unpublished manuscript, San Francisco State University, San Francisco, CA.

Payne, J.S., & Patton, J.R. (1981). *Mental retardation*. Columbus, OH: Charles E. Merrill.

Peterson, L., & Smith, L. (1960). The post-school adjustment of educable mentally retarded adults compared with that of adults of normal intelligence. *Exceptional Children*, *26*, 404–408.

Pierce, T.B. (1989). *Surveying unstructured time of adults with mental retardation in two community settings: A search for normalization*. Unpublished doctoral dissertation, University of New Mexico, Albuquerque.

Pumpian, I., West, E., & Shepard, H. (1988). Vocational education for persons with severe handicaps. In R. Gaylord-Ross (Ed.), *Vocational education for persons with handicaps* (pp. 355–386). Mountain View, CA: Mayfield.

Racino, J.A., & Walker, P. (1988). *Supporting adults with severe disabilities in the community: Selected issues in residential settings*. Syracuse, NY: Center on Human Policy.

Saenger, G. (1957). *The adjustment of severely retarded adults in the community*. Albany, NY: Interdepartmental Health Resources Board.

Schalock, R.L., McGaughey, M.J., & Kiernan, W.E. (1989). Placement into nonsheltered employment: Findings from national employment surveys. *Journal of the Association on Mental Retardation*, *94*, 80–87.

Schindler-Rainman, E., & Lippitt, R. (1980). *Building the collaborative community: Mobilizing citizens for action*. Riverside, CA: University of California Extension.

Schumaker, J.B., & Deshler, D. (1984). Setting demand variables: A major factor in program planning for the LD adolescent. *Topics in Language Disorders*, *4*(2), 22–40.

Siegel, S., Avoke, K., Robert, M., & Gaylord-Ross, R. (in press). Longitudinal postsecondary vocational services: Program and outcomes. *Journal of Vocational Rehabilitation*.

Siegel, S., Greener, K., Prieur, J., Robert, M., Gaylord-Ross, R. (1989). The community vocational training program: A transition program for youth with mild handicaps. *CDEI*, *12*(1), 49–64.

Siegel, S., Park, H., Gumpel, T., Ford, J., Tappe, P., & Gaylord-Ross, R. (1990). Research in vocational special education. In R. Gaylord-Ross (Ed.), *Issues and research in special education* (Vol. 1). New York: Teachers College Press.

Taylor, S. (1988). Caught in the continuum: A critical analysis of the principle of the least restrictive environment. *Journal of the Association for Persons with Severe Handicaps*, *13*(1), 41–53.

Titus, R.W., & Travis, J.T. (1975). Follow-up of EMR program graduates. *Mental Retardation*, *11*, 24–26.

U.S. Department of Education, Special Education Programs. (1988). *Tenth annual report to Congress on the implementation of the Education of the Handicapped Act*. Washington, DC: Author.

U.S. Department of Labor. (1979). *Study of handicapped clients in sheltered workshops*, 2. Washington, DC: Author.

Wagner, M. (1989). *The transition experiences of youth with disabilities: A report from the national longitudinal transition study*. Menlo Park, CA: SRI International.

Wehman, P. (1990). Emerging trend in the national supported employment initiative. *The Association for Persons with Severe Handicaps Newsletter*, *16*(3), 8–9.

Wehman, P., & Moon, S. (1988). *Vocational rehabilitation and supported employment*. Baltimore: Paul H. Brookes.

Wehman, P., Moon, S., Everson, J., Wood, W., & Barcus, J. (1988). *Transition from school to work: New challenges for youth with severe disabilities*. Baltimore: Paul H. Brookes.

Whitehead, C. (1989). Influencing employment through federal and state policy. In W.E. Kiernan & R.L. Schalock (Eds.), *Economics, industry, and disability* (pp. 27–36). Baltimore: Paul H. Brookes.

Zivolich, S. (1984). *Regional Center of Orange County survey of day activity programs and developmental centers*. Unpublished manuscript, Regional Center of Orange County, Anaheim, CA.

Zivolich, S., Rosenberg, W., & DeCilla, N. (1988). *Reliability training for integrated work and community integration outcome system*. Sacramento, CA: Association of Regional Center Agencies.

11
Integrating Elders With Disabilities Into the Community: A Time of Dichotomy

THOMAS B. PIERCE, JR.

Wendell's Story

Wendell is 64 years old and lives in a group home for people with mental retardation. At the age of 7, after the death of his parents, Wendell was institutionalized, partly because none of Wendell's relatives were able to care for him and partly because he was unable to keep up with his peers at school. Wendell worked at the institution in the laundry and later on the institution farm. In the late 1960s he was one of the first people to be released from the institution to a community-based group home. For the past 15 years he has lived in the same group home and has been employed in several jobs, including both sheltered and competitive settings. Most recently, Wendell was employed at the post office as a custodian and part-time mail sorter. Because of his age and his failing health, Wendell must retire from his position. The group home has a policy that all clients must have a day placement. Although there is one adult activity center in his town, the waiting list is at least 1 year long before any hope for placement is possible. The staff members of the group home are also concerned about Wendell's deteriorating health and their inability to provide the required monitoring of his health.

Wendell's social worker has actively sought a placement at the same institution from which he was released 15 years ago, this time, however, on the new geriatric unit. One other placement option is the state home for the indigent aged.

Wendell has expressed his dissatisfaction with both of these options: He wants to stay in his home. The group home points to the day placement rule as the reason for finding an alternative placement, as well as the fact that all of Wendell's housemates are at least 25 years his junior.

Wendell's life, or at least his living arrangements, have come full circle. Wendell's story mirrors the history of the disability field. All of the immediate choices open to Wendell present a no-win situation. Should he return to the institution, suggesting that his placement in the community was just a parole? Should he go to the "old-age home," where he may become isolated and neglected due to his disability? Should he stay at the group home with people a generation younger than he, in hopes that the agency will change its mind?

These are examples of some of the difficult questions facing elders with disabilities. This chapter will report on the current research and on services that are available to both the generic population of the elderly (nondisabled) and people who are disabled and elderly. This chapter explores the difficult questions surrounding how to genuinely integrate elders with disabilities and the effects on an individual's life satisfaction. The chapter will also provide information on the general population of the elderly and how this group presents its own challenges to integrating elders with disabilities in the community.

For the purposes of this chapter the term *elders with disabilities* assumes that individuals were disabled prior to reaching the age of 21. Because the majority of the research has centered on elders with mental retardation, the term *disabilities* assumes mental retardation unless otherwise stated. The term *elderly*, or *generic elderly*, refers to those people in the general population who by virtue of a chronological age were categorized as elderly. The elderly may in fact represent individuals who have become disabled due to health problems but were not labeled as disabled during the developmental period.

Growing Old in America

What Is Old?

Perhaps no other question is more appropriate for this chapter than at what point one is considered old. The criteria for answering such a question can have innumerable permutations. Age is the typical criterion used for determining who is elderly. The Social Security Administration uses the age of 65 (Seltzer & Krauss, 1987); others, such as the American Association of Retired Persons (AARP, 1988a), classify the elderly as young-old (65+) and the old-old (80+). In the disability literature the elderly have included individuals whose age is as low as 40 (Dy, Strain, Fullerton, & Stowitschek, 1981) and as high as 75 (Puccio, Janicki, Otis, & Rettig, 1983). Seltzer and Krauss (1987), in their extensive work on elders with disabilities, have used the age of 55 to determine inclusion as elderly. Whatever the age distinction, such a cutoff is used primarily for collection and analyses of data rather than for marking a significant developmental milestone.

Who Is Elderly?

The elderly represent the fastest growing segment of the population both in the United States (U.S. Bureau of the Census, 1987) and worldwide (U.S. Senate Special Committee on Aging, 1988). Much of this growth can be explained by advances in medical technology and in living conditions (Brody & Ruff, 1986; Sison & Cotten, 1989). However, this growth has also brought with it social and political concerns about services, economics, and ethics for people who are elderly.

For example, one in five Americans is 55 or older, with one in eight 65 or older; and by the year 2010, 25% of the U.S. population will be over 55 years old (AARP, 1988b). In 1986, 12.4% (3.5 million) of America's elderly, those over the age of 65, lived in poverty (AARP, 1988b). More than 10,000 persons over the age of 60 commit suicide each year, representing 23% of all suicides (Miller, 1979). For those over the age of 65, 15% to 25% will have significant symptoms of mental illness (White House Conference on Aging, 1981), and up to 86% of the elderly will have one or more chronic conditions (Brody & Ruff, 1986). One half of all people over the age of 65 will spend some time in a nursing home, at an annual cost of at least $25,000 per person (AARP, 1988b).

Certainly, the data presented do not suggest that all elderly live in poverty or in nursing homes. There are those elderly who are able to live comfortably because of pensions and other retirement and investment income. There are also individuals who are elderly who may escape the devastating effects of a prolonged illness and the need for long-term care. Because this chapter primarily focuses on elders with disabilities, specifically those with mental retardation, it should be noted that this group may not have available to them many of these economic luxuries and therefore may be at greater risk for many of the more difficult sides to aging.

These data are presented to demonstrate some of the difficulties faced by the generic elderly in America. When the issue of disability is added, the challenges faced by professionals working in gerontology become nearly overwhelming. How will elders with disabilities be able to compete for limited and expensive community services, and avail themselves of limited generic service delivery in an already overburdened system? How will people with disabilities be able to receive services and become part of the general population, when the general population presents such a bleak picture for its "normal" members? Certainly one answer is to fully integrate people with disabilities from birth. If integrating people with disabilities begins at age 65, little hope can be expected for their access to generic services and participation in the community. Therefore, the critical importance that is placed on integration, or normalization, during the developmental and early adult period becomes the groundwork for how elders with disabilities will be able to genuinely participate in an integrated society.

Elders With Disabilities

Historical Roots

The history of the field of elders with disabilities is fairly recent. People with disabilities have begun to live longer, in part because of an enlightened society with respect to pre- and postnatal care, and in part because of medical advancement in care and treatment of people with disabilities (Lubin & Kiely, 1985). For example, those people with Down syndrome typically once had shorter life spans than the general population, yet today they are living much longer than previously expected (Eyman, Call, & White, 1989).

One of the most cited historical essays on aging and people with disabilities was delivered by Gunnar Dybwad (1962). Dybwad addressed the "new phenomenon" of community placements for adults and the aged. Even though his essay is now almost 30 years old, the relevance of its policy implications to the disability field continue today. For example, Dybwad discussed the absence of family support for aging people with disabilities, the long waiting lists for services, and the need for recreational and leisure programs, all of which continue to be problems that remain unaddressed today.

Although some early research into the phenomena of aging and mental retardation was done during the 1940s and 1950s, concentrating on managing the elderly with disabilities in institutions (Bair & Leland, 1959) as well as on mental decline as age increases (Kaplan, 1943), the phenomenon of elders with disabilities was simply not an issue. It has only been within the past decade that serious study has occurred of the issues surrounding elders with disabilities (Janicki & Wisniewski, 1985; Seltzer & Krauss, 1987). Current books used by the gerontology profession typically include a chapter on aging and disabilities (e.g., Brody & Ruff, 1987; Cotten & Spirrison, 1986; Gaitz, Niederhe, & Wilson, 1985). Professional societies in both mental retardation and gerontology have dedicated special issues of their respective journals to the issues surrounding aging and disabilities (*Educational Gerontology*, 1988; *Journal of Applied Gerontology*, 1989; *Mental Retardation*, 1988).

Demographics of Elders With Disabilities

One of the most comprehensive documents prepared on elders with disabilities has been the National Survey of Programs Serving Elderly Mentally Retarded Persons (Seltzer & Krauss, 1987). The authors collected information from 327 community and institutional facilities across the country with respect to services available and services offered to people with disabilities.

To determine the number of people who are elderly with disabilities, chronological age becomes a factor. The national survey included those programs serving people 55 years and older. Extrapolating data from the U.S. Census Bureau, Seltzer and Krauss (1987) estimated that "the number of persons with mental retardation aged 55 and over ranges from 1,417,320 (based on a 3% mental retardation prevalence rate) to 472,440 (based on a 1% prevalence rate)" (p. 13). Others (Jacobson, Sutton, & Janicki, 1985), however, have suggested that considerable variation exists in the actual number of elders with disabilities.

Jacobson et al. (1985) reviewed the available literature on demographics of elders with disabilities and found that estimates ranged from 1.5% to 21.3%. Again, the differences in the criteria for inclusion (i.e., age cutoff) varied, from beginning at 40 through 59. The one thing that seems apparent from these age differences to determine membership is that there is virtually little consensus or conceptual clarity on specifically who constitutes the elderly with disabilities. In the years to come, a common denominator is warranted by which an accurate estimate can be made of how many elders with disabilities there are and whom this number includes.

Community Services for Elders With Disabilities

The recent emphasis to develop services in integrated environments has supported the idea that such services enhance the quality of life of individuals (Edgerton, 1990). This section presents several current approaches to service delivery in the community for elders with disabilities, as well as how these services fall within a continuum of services available to the generic elderly. A large portion of this section will also discuss the pitfalls and dangers associated with *quality of life* both as a term and in its subsequent use. The following section on quality of life makes the case for abandoning the shorthand attempt to justify current approaches to serving people with disabilities in community settings.

Community Options

Elders with disabilities have services similar to those typically available to both the general elderly and the population of people with disabilities. These services and living arrangements typically include community residential care (i.e., ICF/MR group homes, foster care, and independent apartments); residential institutions (i.e., nursing homes, institutions for people with disabilities); and independent living not provided for by an agency. Each of these settings has available generic services in which participation is possible (i.e., senior centers, adult day care, medical services). Agency-based service providers come from three groups: age-specific disability, mixed-age disability, and generic elderly (Seltzer & Krauss, 1987).

Residential Options

Table 11.1 presents an extensive list of services available to the generic elderly with respect to the functioning level of the individual and the restrictiveness of the setting. The following discussion briefly outlines the major types of community residential options that are available to adults with disabilities. Although there may be great variation within these settings, there are general distinctions between the types of services available in them.

TABLE 11.1 A classification of services for older persons.

Degree of impairment	Focus of service delivery: Community-based	Home-based	Congregate-residential and institution-based
Minimal	Adult education Senior centers Voluntary organizations Congregate dining programs Individual and family information and referral, advice, and counseling	Home repair services Home equity conversion Share-A-Home Transportation Telephone reassurance	Retirement communities Senior housing Congregate-residential housing with meals
Moderate	Multipurpose senior centers Community mental health centers Outpatient health services Case management systems (social/health maintenance organizations, etc.)	Foster family care Homemaker Meals-on-Wheels Case management for family caregivers and elderly impaired members	Group homes Sheltered residential facilities Board-and-care (domiciliary care) facilities Respite care
Severe	Medical day care Psychiatric day care Alzheimer family groups	Home health care Protective services Hospice care at home	Acute hospitals Mental hospitals Intermediate (health-related) nursing facilities Skilled nursing facilities Hospice care in a facility

Tobin, S. S. (1985). The function, form, and future of formal services. In C. M. Gaitz, G. Niederehe, & N. L. Wilson (Eds.), *Aging 2000: Our health care destiny*. Vol. z: Psychosocial and policy issues (p. 197). New York: Springer-Verlag.

Intermediate Care Facilities for Persons With Mental Retardation (ICF/MR)

In 1971, the Medicaid amendments provided reimbursements to states to provide smaller living arrangements in local communities rather than the larger state-supported institutions (Pierce, Luckasson, & Smith, 1990). Residents in intermediate care facilities for persons with mental retardation (ICF/MR homes) must meet specific entry requirements based on their need for specialized medical, nursing, or therapeutic services. ICF/MR homes can range in size from small-group homes to large mini-institutions (Taylor, 1987). In order for these residences to qualify for federal and state funds, they must meet licensing requirements.

Group Homes

Typically, group homes are small houses or apartments within residential communities. Frequently these homes are designed for people with functionally independent living skills, such as mobility, self-help, and communication. Licensing of these homes varies by state and by certifying agency. Staff often live in the group home.

Foster Homes

The foster home option typically provides the young child or elder with disabilities a family situation in which the individual lives as a member of the family. (Janicki, Jacobson, Zigman, & Lubin, 1987). The family receives a financial stipend for temporarily accepting children or elders with disabilities into their home. Recruiting families has been difficult, in part because the stipend to families is often minimal (Taylor, Racino, Knoll, & Lutfiyya, 1987). Foster family arrangements vary greatly as to the quality of services provided and their lack of regulated supervision by appropriate state agencies (Stroud & Sutton, 1988).

Independent Apartments

These living arrangements represent the vast majority of living arrangements for the generic elderly (Stroud & Sutton, 1988) but represent a much smaller percentage for those with mental retardation (Janicki et al., 1987). For the generic elderly supervision may be unwarranted, or it may be done by family members (Brody, 1986). Supervision of adults with disabilities living independently is often accomplished by case managers and varies between states. A major distinction in these settings is that there are those individuals with disabilities who live in apartments that are supervised by an agency or case manager, and there are those individuals with disabilities who live independently and who are unknown to the services delivery system. One of the difficulties in determining how many or how effective these living arrangements are is that these individuals may not be known to case managers.

Nonresidential Services

Fundamental to any discussion on services for elders with disabilities is a brief mention of a basic difference in the focus between those who advocate for the generic elderly and those who advocate for people with disabilities. While the generic aging community seeks and has created programs of a categorical nature, the disability field has fought for more noncategorical programs within the mainstream (Ossofsky, 1988) This fundamental difference may be the one single roadblock for mutual partnerships and understanding. Until each group is able to identify the criteria for quality services, as well as membership, all else may be moot. But there seems to be some movement toward integrating people with disabilities into the categorical programs offered to the generic elderly. As the field of gerontology begins to accommodate elders with disabilities into their service delivery system, it is important to understand the types of generic services offered.

Senior Citizen Centers

The national survey (Seltzer & Krauss, 1987) found that 60% of elders with disabilities living in community residential programs participated in senior citizen centers. This survey also revealed that 52% of the general elderly consumers were not receptive to the elders with disabilities. Staff members in senior citizen centers typically have little training in serving people with disabilities. The services provided in these centers emphasize leisure and recreational activities, arts and crafts, and socialization skills (Janicki, Otis, Puccio, Rettig, & Jacobson, 1985).

Successful integration is not simply accomplished by participating in services offered to nondisabled peers. Additionally, if a person with disabilities has not had an adequate training in leisure and recreation skills (Pierce, 1989), does such an approach seem warranted when the individual has become elderly? Whether or not senior citizen centers provide integrated services depends on the definition of integration. If integration is viewed as utilizing patterns of chronological peers, then senior citizen centers may be a viable option for elders with disabilities. If integration is viewed as having a role that is valued by society (Wolfensberger, 1983), then the negative role that the generic elderly are oftentimes assigned raises questions about utilizing senior citizen centers.

Support Networks

Much of the literature investigating service delivery systems for elders with disabilities has concentrated on developing and enhancing support networks. Elders with disabilities rarely have the availability of advocates who are specifically knowledgeable in both gerontology and disability (Calkins & Kultgen, 1987). Equally important is the loss of a group of advocates who have been steadfast throughout the lives of people with disabilities: parents.

It is simply a fact of life that parents usually do not outlive their children. For people with disabilities this has not always been the case. People with disabilities are, for the first time, beginning to outlive their parents, or becoming a part of a two-generation geriatric family (Ansello, 1988). As people with disabilities age, the lifelong commitment given to them by their parents may no longer be available (Walz, Harper, & Wilson, 1986). Brody (1986) found that between 75% and 80% of the resources needed to support the elderly in the community came from family members, primarily daughters and daughters-in-law. These same family supports may not be available to most individuals with disabilities. Therefore, utilizing the more formalized public sector supports offered to the generic elderly may be one of the few options opened to elders with disabilities. VanZandt and Cannon-Nifoussi (1989) have described these support systems to include (a) *formal community support* (large communities), such as visiting nurses, Meals on Wheels, senior citizen centers, and social service departments; and (b) *formal community support* (small communities), such as the use of local pharmacists, doctors, ministers, and attorneys.

Again, it must be emphasized that successful use of such support networks can only be achieved if there has been a foundation laid for utilizing them. If individuals have not been genuinely integrated throughout their life span, little integration can be anticipated once they become elderly.

Utilization of Services by the Elderly

For the population of elderly who require economic, social, and medical assistance, becoming old can be extremely difficult. There seems to be a great injustice done to people who are elderly, most of whom have worked all of their adult lives and many of whom may be living in poverty and in environments that may not guarantee personal safety.

Elderly people with disabilities appear to share many of the same challenges faced by the elderly poor. Experiences that are faced in nursing homes have been reported as especially discriminatory for individuals who have little means of support other than social security, Medicaid, or Medicare (Special Committee on Aging, 1984). Ironically, in the U.S. Senate's special committee report on aging (1984), titled *Discrimination Against the Poor and Disabled in Nursing Homes*, virtually no testimony was given on the disabled population.

Interaction With the Nondisabled

Elders with disabilities have been able to participate in generic service programs available to the general elderly population (Seltzer & Krauss, 1987), yet they may not be accepted by nondisabled elderly peers. In Colorado, Roberto and Nelson (1989) surveyed both agencies serving those with developmental disabilities ($N = 45$) and agencies serving the elderly ($N = 226$). Those agencies serving primarily the generic elderly affirmed that they were willing to serve elders with disabilities provided that the elders could function independently and that the staff were trained in supervising this population. The authors further found that staff had mixed feelings about whether they believed the other clients would accept people with developmental disabilities. The general acceptance of people with disabilities into the generic system was also found by Seltzer and Krauss (1987), who reported in the national survey that staff members may be more receptive to people with disabilities than to the general consumers.

Many activities currently provided in senior citizen day activity centers reflect the images of day activity centers for those with mental retardation. The use of such centers by young adults with disabilities has been criticized as not a chronologically appropriate activity. Professionals in the disability field have worked long and hard to provide services such as meaningful employment and genuine integration in hopes of avoiding past practices that isolate individuals from their communities.

Continuum Traps

Special education professionals, parents, and consumers have a long history with the idea of a continuum of services that represents different levels of care, or different levels of restriction. The concept of the least restrictive environment (LRE) provides the opportunity to see service delivery as a continuum. The notion of becoming trapped in the continuum (Taylor, 1987) stems from professionals' inability to view the continuum to provide individualized services rather than rigid environmental options. For example, group homes represent a more restrictive setting than independent apartments. The field of gerontology has a similar method for determining placement alternatives. No matter how much caution is used to assure individualization within the continuum based on a person's needs, often the continuum is seen as a vertical axis in which down (more restrictive) is synonymous with bad.

Seltzer and her colleagues (1988) surveyed 373 elderly programs in Massachusetts representing eight different service models. Among this sample they found 4.2% of clients were elders with disabilities with the largest proportion served in adult day health programs or foster care programs. Seltzer and her colleagues concluded that in Massachusetts active referral and collaboration between aging services and mental retardation agencies has demonstrated the beginnings of integration of elders with disabilities into the generic service system. Although elders with disabilities in this study were partaking in generic services, the services that represent the least restrictive environments, that is, in-home services such as housekeeping, meal preparation and social support, were offered to less than 1% of people with mental retardation. Such a finding underscores that elders with mental retardation are utilizing or are referred to agencies at the more restrictive end of the service continuum.

Jones, White, Ulicny, and Matthews (1988) support this concept of underutilization in less restrictive settings. Jones et al. found that individuals with cognitive disabilities (mental retardation, mental illness, head injuries, or cognitive deficits associated with aging) were not being proportionally served in independent living centers. When independent living center directors were surveyed, respondents reported that they believed people with disabilities were already being served by other agencies.

The continuum trap emphasizes how people can fit into the existing system rather than how the system can accommodate the needs of the individual. If those with disabilities are seen as disabled first, they will have a much more difficult time convincing others of their need of and right to generic services.

Quality of Life in Community Living Arrangements

The term *quality of life* and the attempts to measure such a phenomenon are critical when planning integrated services for elders with disabilities. Much of the following is a review of quality of life literature for people with disabilities. Little information, research, or data are available on the quality of the lives of elders with disabilities, though current services use quality of life as a justification.

Researchers have for the past 10 years grappled with identifying the key components of measuring quality of life, or personal life satisfaction (Edgerton, 1990), of people with disabilities living in the community (Landesman, 1987a, 1987b). We seem to know quality when we see it, but agreement on what quality of life is has been lacking (Blunden, 1988). Various definitions of quality of life have been offered for people without disabilities (Flannagan, 1978) as well as for those with disabilities (Blunden, 1988; Keith, Schalock & Hoffman, 1986; Landesman, 1987). Though little quantitative data exist on the specific elements representing quality (Putnam, Werder, & Schleien, 1985), most definitions suggest that the quality of an individual's life is dependent on a host of factors.

One indicator of quality of life is an individual's social well-being, which includes community presence, personal relationships, ability to make choices, competence, and respect (Blunden, 1988). Blunden offered that the social well-being of an individual living in the community may be particularly important in any discussion on quality of life because of the basic human need for social contact.

Approaches to Measuring Quality of Life

Several methods to evaluate, certify, and accredit programs are currently being used in community living arrangements. The minimal standards approach usually consists of licensing inspections on such areas as safety, sanitation, and fire regulations. Accreditation standards, such as those given by the nationally recognized Commission on Accreditation of Rehabilitation Facilities (CARF, 1989) or the Accreditation Council on Services for People with Developmental Disabilities (ACDD, 1988), provide agencies with typically higher and more specific programmatic competencies on which accreditation is granted.

These standards, however, are limited by the shortness of visits of surveyors to inspect an agency (usually two or three days) and may not reach the subtlety or sensitivity that a more in-depth review could obtain. For example, the ACDD has standards requiring an individual to be involved in the decisions made in his or her individual habilitation plan (IHP), as well as a standard requiring individuals to have available to them the opportunity to express preferences. These standards, however, measure an agency's ability to meet the standards rather than how these standards fit into the day-to-day opportunities to express preferences for residents.

In an attempt to operationalize the pragmatic implementation of normalization, Wolfensberger and his colleagues have developed the Program Analysis of Service System (PASS, Wolfensberger & Glenn, 1975) and the Program Analysis of Service Systems: Implementation of Normalization Goals (PASSING, Wolfensberger & Thomas, 1983). Agencies are rated on PASS or PASSING on physical and social integration as well as on specific normalization related activities such as age appropriateness, agency ideology, and model coherency. A similar limitation exists with this type of evaluation method. It provides a short, on-site visit and may again miss some of the subtleties for practical application of standards. Perhaps a more descriptive approach of day-to-day implementation of standards during the normal rhythm of the day might yield a more realistic perspective on the quality of the program and its subsequent effects on individuals (Pierce, 1989).

Unlike the accreditation standards approach of ACDD, CARF, PASS or PASSING, several evaluation tools exist purporting to assess an individual's quality of life. These instruments vary based on the particular quality of life variable being assessed. For example, interviews to determine an individual's personal satisfaction with his or her community placement have been frequently used (Baker & Intagliata, 1982; Heal &

Chadsey-Rusch, 1985; Keith, et al., 1986; Seltzer, 1981). In addition to the interview format, employment satisfaction scales (Mank, Rhodes, & Bellamy, 1986) and instruments to evaluate satisfaction with an individual's total community experience incorporating both the residential and employment components (Schalock & Keith, 1984) have been reported.

Although the quest to operationalize the phrase *quality of life* (Keith et al., 1986) has been undertaken, the use of the term continues with little clarity. Keith et al. developed a questionnaire to measure an individual's quality of life. This 28-item instrument was given to 450 individuals with mental retardation living in community residences in Nebraska. Quality of life was measured across three categories: environmental control, community involvement, and social relations. The questionnaire relied on verbal responses, therefore excluding people without a formal language system. (The authors suggested that for individuals who are not verbal that two staff people independently assess the client and then take the average score.) Respondents answered each area with a "usually, sometimes, or seldom/never" option. Individual scores were then divided into an index of low, moderate, or high quality of life. The authors found a positive correlation between people with higher IQ scores and higher quality of life scores.

An instrument to assess and quantify quality of life must be interpreted with caution. Quality of life scores may directly relate to the agency's view of opportunities offered to individuals rather than to individual preferences. Yet such a score may reflect negatively on the individual rather than on the agency. For example, what meaningful interpretation can be made for the person with a low quality of life score and low IQ? Will services differ? Will the individual be assigned to a different stratum within society? Will such information provide a rationale for getting caught in a continuum trap?

Luckasson (1990) has urged that the term *quality of life* be abandoned; she suggested that quantification of the term "will lead to a certain tolerance, or even preference, for the phrase and result in its increased use as a shorthand justification for denial of rights to people with disabilities" (p. 211). In both a historical and pragmatic context, Luckasson's warning against acceptance of such a term raises important cautionary implications. Conclusions about quality of life have been based on results from self-report measures (Edgerton & Langness, 1978); questionnaires (Keith et al., 1986); and staff surveys of their charges' quality of life (Bersani & Salon, 1988; Kishi, Teelucksingh, Zollers, Park-Lee, & Meyer, 1988). These instruments have gained acceptance as a quasi legitimization of evaluating quality of life. These instruments, however, have severe limitations. Edgerton's (1990) longitudinal group had mild disabilities. Keith et al. (1986) sampled individuals who need literacy skills, multiple choice discrimination ability, and language skills to complete the questionnaire. Others (Bersani & Salon, 1988; Kishi et al.,

1988) have relied on staff to answer questions of how much quality people for whom they were responsible had in their lives.

If these instruments, or their subsequent variations, become accepted methods for assessing quality of life, then Luckasson's (1990) warnings take on greater significance. The implications of such a dilemma become heartbreakingly clear. The lives of people will be assessed by test scores. Elders with disabilities may become conveniently pigeonholed and categorized. Test scores will then be obtainable for an individual's intelligence, adaptive behavior, maladaptive behavior, and employability—and even for the global quality of his or her life.

Others, however, have suggested that quality of life is not related to intelligence or functioning level but is very individual, especially for people with severe disabilities (Brown, Diller, Gordon, Fordyce, & Jacobs, 1984). Brown et al. have reported that quality of life for people with severe disabilities may include variables such as mobility, appearance, or physical condition of the living arrangement. Baumgart et al. (1982) have developed a strategy calling for "partial participation" in all chronologically age-appropriate activities. They suggest that people with severe handicaps should be instructed and incorporated in all areas of programming and leisure activities. Consequently, quality of life is enhanced by participation in these activities. The paradox for elders with disabilities, with respect to partial participation, is directly related to those activities in which their nondisabled peers participate. Is the goal of integration to adjoin the activities in which the generic elderly participate, or should the goal be to ensure that scrutiny is placed on all activities that are planned for and carried out by agencies?

Although definitions and methodologies vary in determining an individual's quality of life, most include some reference to community participation as a key indicator for quality (Blunden, 1988; Keith et al., 1986; Knoll & Ford, 1987). Even though Keith et al. have operationalized a definition of quality of life, Baumgart and her colleagues (1982) more closely approximate the critical aspects expounded on in the principle of normalization.

Quality of Life and Community Adaptation

The research on participation in the community has sometimes abandoned a definition of quality of life and instead sought to investigate outcome measures of various aspects of individuals' living in community living arrangements. These outcome measures include (a) deinstitutionalization effects; (b) demographic variables, including level of retardation; or (c) leisure and recreation training and participation.

Deinstitutionalization Effects

After the closures of residential institutions and the movement to channel funds into community facilities, many researchers followed these deinstitutionalized individuals to evaluate how they adapted to their communities (Conroy, 1985; Conroy & Bradley, 1985; Gollay, 1976; Mallory & Herrick, 1986; Pagel & Whitling, 1978; Willer & Intagliata, 1981). Most of these and similar studies have reported that the process of deinstitutionalization is evaluated by outcome measures of individuals transferred to community living arrangements. These authors have suggested that some individuals make it in the community and some do not, and to develop indicators of success or failure is almost futile (Emerson, 1985). One of the most salient points that has come out of the deinstitutionalization adaptation studies is that evaluating such transfers is extremely difficult and must be planned a priori (Conroy & Bradley, 1985). Mallory and Herrick (1986) succinctly summarize many of the investigations as follows: "We can say that 'deinstitutionalization' has occurred successfully, but the broader goal of full social integration, referred to as 'communitization,' has not been fully achieved" (p. 202).

Demographic Variables

Researchers have investigated specific observation designs to identify whether a relationship between certain demographic variables and community placement could be made. This research took a more single-variable approach to investigating community placement. For example, community adaptation and the effects of family attitudes (Wehman & Schleien, 1980); age or level of retardation (Gollay, Freedman, Wyngaarden, & Kurtz, 1978); placement alternatives (Bjaanes, Butler, & Kelly, 1981); and personal choice and autonomy (Voeltz, Wuerch, & Wilcox, 1982) have all been examined. Although each of these research efforts reported some significant changes or differences in their intervention or survey, none has been able to fully assess any relationship these variables have to an individual's successful participation in the local community. These research attempts demonstrate the difficulty researchers face in studying community living arrangements. There are difficulties not only in methodology (Butterfield, 1985, 1987) but also in the conclusions that one can draw due to methodological flaws (Emerson, 1985), including nonrandom samples, selection of samples, and unclear replication procedures.

Leisure and Recreation

Recently, the effect of leisure and recreation skills on an individual's quality of life has received attention (Aveno, 1987a, 1987b; Datillo & Rusch, 1985; Falvey, 1989; Jeffree & Cheseldine, 1984; Nietupski,

Hamre-Nietupski, & Ayres, 1984; Putnam et al., 1985; Wehman & Schleien, 1980). Leisure and recreation skills have been studied because of their relationship to the principle of normalization (Putnam et al., 1985), as well as the need for maintaining appropriate interactions within the community (Falvey, 1989). It is during this time in the community when leisure skills can enhance meaningful social interactions.

Retirement and aging might give rise to notions of recreation and leisure. Retirement may be seen as a time to enjoy those things that were difficult to complete or begin while employed. For elders with disabilities, developing genuine leisure skills will need to be a lifelong process, rather than one that begins at the age of 55. In a review of 17 data-based task-analyzed leisure and recreational skills of people with disabilities, irrespective of severity, Nietupski et al. (1984) found that existing curricula need expansion and empirical verification. Nietupski et al. specifically suggested that current curricula have limitations in addressing training skills within the natural environment and reflect an inadequate knowledge base of the leisure activities of nondisabled peers. Matthews (1982), however, interestingly found that the differences in the time spent in leisure and recreation between those with and without diabilities were not significant.

One of the difficulties reported in studying leisure and recreation skills in the community is the vast heterogeneity existing among facilities (Butler & Bjaanes, 1977). For example, among elderly populations intermediate care facilities (ICFs), skilled nursing facilities (SNFs), and nursing homes are but some of the many residential options. The ability to adequately control experimental variables, curricula, and intervention strategies is limited and prevents interpretations to populations outside of these segregated facilities. However, the principle of normalization makes no mention of an individual's functioning level or quality of life in its definition. It simply suggests that the means utilized are normative to the culture (O'Brien, 1980).

Living in segregation may never be normal in this society. Different housing styles may promote the indirect segregation from the community. A recent study in rural Manitoba, Canada, described differences between time spent in activities and housing style (Chornoboy & Harvey, 1988). Individuals lived in five different facility types:

1. Foster homes: private homes where one to four persons lived as a part of a family.
2. Familial homes: private homes where the individual lived with a parent or sibling.
3. Senior citizen homes: congregate residences for the elderly.
4. Independent homes: community homes usually shared with another person with mental retardation.
5. Group homes: community homes of six or more with on-site supervision.

The time that individuals spent in activities (typically leisure or recreation) was measured by clients responding (yes or no) as to whether they participated in an activity presented on a picture card. The authors found time spent in activities was significantly influenced by the facility type. Individuals living in senior citizen homes were reported to spend significantly more time in activities (M = 93.5 per week), followed by group homes (M = 47.9 per week), familial homes (M = 44.0 per week), independent homes (M = 41.2 per week), and foster homes (M = 35.9 per week). When these activities were categorized into sedentary or active, residents in the senior citizen homes spent significantly more time per week in sedentary activities, followed by those in familial homes. Therefore, although an individual spends more time in activities, these activities may be passive.

Time studies such as this emphasize the differences between a person's residence and the activities in which he or she engages. The results of such studies demonstrate that mere placement in the community does not necessarily provide significant impetus for integrated and normalized activities (Pierce, Luckasson, & Smith, 1990). In addition, time studies are a unique method of delving into the day-to-day activities of individuals in their residences.

Thus, merely providing elders with disabilities adequate leisure or recreation training does not necessarily facilitate integration or participation in the community. Integration, normalization, communitization, or whatever the term does not mean that mere placement, or mere skill acquisition promotes quality. Some researchers, for example, have found that living in the community, irrespective of what skills an individual has, may be just as isolating as living in an institution (Pierce, 1989; Taylor, et al., 1987).

Controversies in Measuring Quality of Life

Recently there has been an emphasis on investigating the variable of choice making when evaluating a person's quality of life and personal autonomy (O'Brien, 1980). The abilities of elders with disabilities to choose their own activities (O'Brien, 1980) and leisure skills (Dattilo & Mirenda, 1987; Dattilo & Rusch, 1985) are critical variables in achieving independence. Shevin and Klein (1984) have defined choice making as "the act of an individual's selection of a preferred alternative from among several familiar options" (p. 160). The implication of this definition suggests that critical skills are necessary before choice making can occur. These skills include having the opportunity to express preferences, having familiarity with a menu of options, and living with the choices one makes.

Although the investigation into choice making has recently become a popular method for evaluating integrated patterns for people with disabilities, little empirically based information currently exists on the actual implementation of choice making in unstructured situations. Moreover, information on choice making for people with severe disabilities is particularly lacking (Guess, Benson, & Siegel-Causey, 1985).

The limited amount of research that does exist on actual choice-making skills has demonstrated that people with disabilities, even those with severe disabilities, can be trained and can have success in making choices (Dattilo & Mirenda, 1987; Guess et al., 1985), however the opportunity to make genuine choices has also been questioned (Pierce et al., 1990). The reality of individuals spending inordinate amounts of time passively waiting, or watching television, until the staff directs the next activity has been discussed as the norm rather than the exception (Dattilo & Rusch, 1985; Pierce, 1989).

Researchers have been successful in developing approaches to encourage choice making (Dattilo & Mirenda, 1987; Wuerch & Voeltz, 1982); however, the practical implementation of such choice-making training may not be utilized outside the experimenter's purview. One possible outcome for this lack of genuine opportunity to make choices in day-to-day activities may be the continuing stigmatization and social devaluation of people with disabilities (O'Brien, 1980). This may be particularly true for elders with disabilities. Moreover, the restriction to make choices will stifle the opportunity to experience the culturally valued patterns of this society toward independence.

Perhaps the most often cited investigations of how people with disabilities adapt to their communities have been the works of Edgerton and his associates (Edgerton, 1967, 1988; Edgerton & Bercovici, 1976; Edgerton, Bollinger, & Herr, 1984; Edgerton & Langness, 1978). These works represented a departure from the more clinical intervention model of behavior change, to a more sociological (Bogdan, 1986) and qualitative approach (Bercovici, 1981; 1983; Taylor & Bogdan, 1984). Edgerton and his colleagues have made a significant contribution to understanding the life span and growth of people with mental retardation. For 30 years, Edgerton has examined how previously institutionalized persons with mental retardation have adapted to their communities. Of the original 48 individuals, 16 were available for his latest follow-up (Edgerton, 1988). These individuals continue to grow, to contribute to, and to participate in their communities. None have needed a more restrictive setting, all have participated in meaningful relationships in which they gave and received, and all but one have had a long-term sexual relationship.

Edgerton has concluded that even those adults with mild to moderate mental retardation who currently reside in restrictive settings can adapt to community settings. Such adaption to community living can become difficult the longer the person is in a restrictive setting. "When many older persons with mental retardation are offered opportunities to live more independently, they decline the offer, preferring their restricted and routine lives to the unknowns of a new life" (Edgerton, 1988, p. 335).

This sad commentary about the resistance of moving to a less restrictive setting may bolster those who support this option as a legitimate and informed choice. For those who might argue that an individual should be able to choose the setting in which he or she wants to live, extreme caution should be used: First and foremost, was the individual given a free and informed choice at the time of placement? For example, an abused child who "chooses" to live with the abusive parent rather than go into foster care certainly cannot be considered to be making a free and informed choice. Did this child have the choice to be abused or not be abused from the beginning? As long as there exists a continuum of services that provide more desirable services at one end and less desirable at the other, genuine choices regarding service options cannot be legitimately made.

Edgerton has encouraged those in the research community to assume a more naturalistic approach when studying the phenomenon of quality of life. Three principles have been suggested as integral components in the methodology used for measuring people in their natural surroundings: (a) The interaction of the individual should be seen and measured in the natural surrounding; (b) the observation should be seen not only through the eyes of the observer but also through the eyes of the participant; and (c) the surveyor should blend into the natural setting rather than intrude upon it (Edgerton & Langness, 1974).

Edgerton (1990) has concluded that people with mental retardation should have

> Access to housing, health care, recreational, activities, dignified employment, and everything else that an enlightened society can provide for its citizens. But we must never forget that all a society should do is provide options; however well-meaning, it should not impose standards. (Edgerton, 1990, p. 158)

Implications for Future Research

With this lengthy explanation a research agenda can be developed to avoid justification of community and generic services based on the erroneous assumption that such services represent quality. For example, how does the issue to choose one's activities and residence become influenced by age? Can people who are elderly have some autonomy with respect to the activities and services from which they can choose? The other assumption inherent in any discussion on quality of life, suggests a more basic question: Do the services available to the elderly in the general population represent integrated services? If not, should such services be sought for, and by, elders with disabilities?

Program Models

As was previously discussed, there is fundamental disagreement between the gerontology and disability fields with respect to the program models in which people who are elderly and those elderly with disabilities will participate (Ossofsky, 1988). As gerontology seeks categorical programs (those specifically for the elderly), disability professionals seek more mainstreamed generic programs. The following briefly describes examples of some of the program models currently available for elders with disabilities.

Disability-Specific Models

Disability-specific programs are specifically designed for elders with disabilities. A prime example of this program style is the ACCESS Project (Stroud & Sutton, 1988). The ACCESS Project is a joint venture of the University of Akron and the Kennedy Foundation. The project's purpose is to provide assistance and teach community skills to elders with disabilities over the age of 60. Using volunteers, and some paid staff, known as Kennedy Friends, ACCESS staff spend 1 day per week in the community with their charges. This weekly outing is spent in an activity of the consumer's choice. Additional support is provided for housing, employment, various therapies, and guardianship services. The project continues to gather data of the effectiveness of its program and the services delivered. Although consumers may be involved in the community, they are individually served to meet their needs. Because this program is only for those with developmental disabilities, the program is disability-centered, and those it serves may therefore lack genuine integration with those who are their chronological peers.

Collaborative Models

Collaborative models are those in which elders with disabilities are integrated into the generic services offered to the elderly. Typically, these programs emphasize a team approach to developing categorical services (for those with mental retardation) within the domain of aging. The collaborative model has been successfully used in rural communities (Cotten & Spirrison, 1988), where services typically are less available that in urban areas. However, data on specific collaborative models are not available. Although many have called for the the fields of gerontology and disabilities to begin collaboration (Hawkins & Eklund, 1989; Janicki, 1988), such models are only beginning. It will be of interest to determine whether elders with disabilities can be integrated into the generic system and still have their unique needs met. Collaborative models should not be watered-down versions of the existing system.

Summary of Service and Quality of Life

The issues presented in this chapter have made a case to investigate not what elders in the typical population do, but how a research agenda might adequately begin to develop genuine services for people who are elderly, irrespective of disability. The issues are clouded, the focus is unclear, but several points can be made. If the typical senior citizen center provides leisure and arts and crafts activities for its consumers, are these the activities that should also be provided and advocated for elders with disabilities? It seems tragic to return people with disabilities to an environment that many professionals and advocates fought to abolish. Is segregation by age much different than segregation by intelligence? Equally tragic is to have elders with disabilities restricted from participating in a genuine and fulfilling period of retirement. Think back to Wendell's story: Is it now acceptable to return him to an institution because of his age and because of the presence of a geriatric ward?

Is there a time when segregated environments are acceptable, based on an individual's age, or is the time ripe for developing and attacking the problems faced for the elderly, both with and without disabilities? Though it is easily said, and sometimes difficult to imagine, we will all be elderly. We may not all become disabled, but the services currently available to the elderly will certainly be the services of tomorrow unless the disability field leads the way in developing appropriate programs and service delivery methods to share with the general population.

Few fields of study have the extensive types of experiences and history of the disability area. The history of segregation, torture, isolation, and despair is evident. Arts and crafts, idle hours spent in meaningless activities, and the long battles to eradicate such injustices cannot be forgotten. A return for elders with disabilities to such an existence, in the guise of integration, seems at best a tragedy.

Creative problem solving is warranted. The field of disabilities has much to share, and it must realize the critical need to exchange information with the field of gerontology. We may not have the answers, but we certainly know the questions. Increasing collaboration and integration between state units on aging and state developmental disabilities agencies has been provided for in both the Older Americans Act (Public Law 100–175) and the Developmental Disabilities Act (Public Law 100–146). Determining whether or not generic services are being used by those with disabilities has, however, been limited, due in part to problems with the reliability of data and research validity (Seltzer, Krauss, Litchfield, & Modlish, 1989). For example, Krauss (1988) reported that less than one half of elders with mental retardation are known to state agencies.

The generic service delivery system for the elderly is growing rapidly (Brody & Ruff, 1986). The economics of limited financial resources is a harsh reality for all service providers. Providing services to the greatest number may exclude those in greatest need. Providing services to those in greatest need may create restrictive models in which those seeking minimal assistance (the greatest majority) will become trapped in a continuum that may not meet their needs.

Elders with disabilities will become integrated into the generic service system only when the generic services system can integrate itself into the society. When this happens, genuine relationships can develop (Dossa, 1990). For people with disabilities to be viewed as providing a reciprocal, rather than a parasitic relationship to their community, integration must begin far before they enter their senior years. Reciprocity begins when those with disabilities are "perceived not as 'individuals' requiring care and assistance but as whole persons mutually connected with others in a sharing relationship" (Dossa, 1990, p. 317).

References

Accreditation Council on Services for People With Developmental Disabilities. (1988). *The standards manual*. Landover, MD: Author.

American Association of Retired Persons. (1988a). *Aging in America: Trends and projections*. Washington, DC: Author.

American Association of Retired Persons. (1988b). *Aging in America: Issue guide*. Washington, DC: Author.

Ansello, E.F. (1988). The intersecting of aging and disabilities. *Educational Gerontology*, *14*, 351–363.

Aveno, A. (1987a). A survey of leisure activities engaged in by adults who are severely retarded living in different residence and community types. *Education and Training in Mental Retardation*, *22*, 121–127.

Aveno, A. (1987b). A survey of activities engaged in and skills most needed by adults in community residences. *Journal of the Association for Persons With Severe Handicaps*, *12*, 125–130.

Bair, H.U., & Leland, H. (1959). Management of the geriatric mentally retarded patient. *Hospital and Community Psychiatry*, *10*(5), 9–12.

Baker, F., & Intagliata, J. (1982). Quality of life in the evaluation of community support services. *Evaluation and Program Planning*, *5*, 69–79.

Baumgart, D., Brown, L., Pumpian, I., Nisbet, J., Ford, A., Sweet, M., Messina, R., & Schroeder, J. (1982). Principle of partial participation and individualized adaptions in educational programs for severely handicapped students. *Journal of the Association for Persons With Severe Handicaps*, *7*, 17–27.

Bercovici, S.M. (1981). Qualitative methods and cultural perspectives in the study of deintitutionalization. In R.H. Bruininks, C.E. Meyers, & K.C. Lakin (Eds.), *Deinstitutionalization and community adjustment of mentally retarded people* (pp. 133–144). Washington, DC: American Association on Mental Deficiency.

Bercovici, S.M. (1983). *Barriers to normalization: The restrictive management of retarded persons*. Baltimore: University Park Press.

Bersani, H., & Salon, R. (1988). *Personal integration inventory*. Syracuse, NY: Syracuse University, Research and Training Center on Community Integration, Center on Human Policy.

Bjaanes, A.T., Butler, E.W., & Kelly, B.R. (1981). Placement type and client functional levels as factors in provision of services aimed at increasing adjustment. In R.H. Bruininks, C.E. Meyers, & K.C. Lakin (Eds.), *Deinstitutionalization and community adjustment of mentally retarded people* (pp. 337–350). Washington, DC: American Association on Mental Deficiency.

Blunden, R. (1988). Programmatic features of quality services. In J.P. Janicki, M.W. Krauss, & M.M. Seltzer (Eds.), *Community residences for persons with developmental disabilities: Here to stay* (pp. 117–121). Baltimore: Paul H. Brookes.

Bogdan, R. (1986). The sociology of special education. In R.J. Morris & B. Blatt (Eds.), *Special education: Research and trends* (pp. 344–359). New York: Pergamon.

Brody, E.M. (1986). Informal support systems in the rehabilitation of the disabled elderly. In S.J. Brody & G.E. Ruff (Eds.), *Aging and rehabilitation: Advances in the state of the art* (pp. 87–103). New York: Springer-Verlag.

Brody, S.J., & Ruff, G.E. (Eds.). (1986). *Aging and rehabilitation: Advances in the state of the art* New York: Springer-Verlag.

Brown, M., Diller, L., Gordon, W.A., Fordyce, W.E., & Jacobs, D.F. (1984). Rehabilitation indicators and program evaluation. *Rehabilitation Psychology*, *29*, 21–35.

Butler, E.W., & Bjaanes, A.T. (1977). A typology of community care facilities and differential normalization outcomes. In P. Mittler (Ed.), *Research to practice in mental retardation: Care and intervention* (pp. 337–347). Baltimore: University Park Press.

Butterfield, E. (1985). The consequences of bias studies of living arrangements for the mentally retarded adult. In D. Bricker & J. Filler (Eds.), *Severe mental retardation: From theory to practice* (pp. 245–263). Reston, VA: Council for Exceptional Children.

Butterfield, E. (1987). Why and how to study the influence of living arrangements. In S. Landesman & P. Vietze (Eds.), *Living environments and mental retardation* (pp. 43–59). Washington, DC: American Association on Mental Retardation.

Calkins, C.F., & Kultgen, P. (1987). Enhancing the life chances and social support networks for older persons with developmental disabilities. In S.F. Gilson, T.L. Goldsbury, & E.H. Faulkner (Eds.), *Three populations of primary focus* (pp. 131–136). Omaha, NE: University of Nebraska Medical Center, Department of Psychiatry.

Chornoboy, E.G., & Harvey, C.D.H. (1988). Relationship between the housing facility type of aging persons who are developmentally disabled. *Education and Training of the Mentally Retarded*, *23*(2), 147–153.

Commission on Accreditation of Rehabilitation Facilities. (1989). *Standards manual for organizations serving people with disabilities*. Tuscon, AZ: Author.

Conroy, J.W. (1985). Reactions to deinstitutionalization among parents of mentally retarded persons. In R.H. Bruininks & K.C. Lakin (Eds.), *Living and learning in the least restrictive environment* (pp. 141–152). Baltimore: Paul H. Brookes.

Conroy, J.W., & Bradley, V.J. (1985). *The Pennhurst longitudinal study: A report after five years of research and analysis*. Philadelphia: Temple University Developmental Disabilities Center.

Cotten, P.D., & Spirrison, C.L. (1986). The elderly mentally retarded (developmentally disabled) population: A challenge for the service delivery system. In S.J. Brody & G.E. Ruff (Eds.), *Aging and rehabilitation: Advances in the state of the art* (pp. 159–187). New York: Springer-Verlag.

Cotten, P.D., & Spirrison, C.L. (1988). Development of services for elderly persons with mental retardation in a rural state. *Mental Retardation*, *26*, 187–190.

Datillo, J., & Mirenda, P. (1987). An application of a leisure preference assessment protocol for persons with severe handicaps. *Journal of the Association for Persons With Severe Handicaps*, *12*, 306–311.

Datillo, J., & Rusch, F.R. (1985). Effects of choice on leisure participation for persons with severe handicaps. *Journal of the Association for Persons With Severe Handicaps*, *10*, 194–199.

Dossa, P.A. (1990). Toward social system theory: Implications for older people with developmental disabilities and service delivery. *International Journal of Aging and Human Development*, *30*, 303–319.

Dy, E.B., Strain, P.S., Fullerton, A., & Stowitschek, J. (1981). Training institutionalized, elderly mentally retarded persons as intervention agents for socially isolated peers. *Analysis and Intervention in Developmental Disabilities*, *1*, 199–215.

Dybwad, G. (1962). Administrative and legislative problems in the care of the adult and aged mental retardate. *American Journal of Mental Deficiency*, *66*, 716–722.

Edgerton, R.B. (1967). *The cloak of competence*. Berkley: University of California Press.

Edgerton, R.B. (1990). Quality of life from a longitudinal research perspective. In R.L. Schalock (Ed.), *Quality of life: Perspectives and issues*. Washington, DC: American Association on Mental Retardation Monograph Series.

Edgerton, R.B., & Bercovici, S.M. (1976). The cloak of competence: Years later. *American Journal of Mental Deficiency*, *80*, 485–497.

Edgerton, R.B., Bollinger, M., & Herr, B. (1984). The cloak of competence: After two decades. *American Journal of Mental Retardation*, *88*, 345–351

Edgerton, R.B., & Langness, L.L. (1978). Observing mentally retarded persons in community settings: An anthropological perspective. In G.P. Sackett (Ed.), *Observing behavior* (Vol. 1). Baltimore: University Park Press.

Emerson, E.B. (1985). Evaluating the impact of deinstitutionalization on the lives of mentally retarded people. *American Journal on Mental Deficiency*, *90*, 277–288.

Eyman, R.K., Call, T.L., & White, J.F. (1989). Mortality of elderly mentally retarded persons in California. *Journal of Applied Gerontology*, *8*, 203–215.

Falvey, M. (1989). *Community-based curriculum: Instructional strategies for students with severe handicaps* (2nd ed.). Baltimore: Paul H. Brookes.

Flannagan, J.C. (1978). A research approach to improving our quality of life. *American Psychologist*, *33*, 138–147.

Gaitz, C.M., Niederhe, G., & Wilson, N.L. (Eds.). (1985). *Aging 2000: Our health care destiny: Vol. 2. Psychosocial and policy issues*. New York: Springer-Verlag.

Gollay, E. (1976). *A study of community adjustment of deinstitutionalized mentally retarded persons* (Vol. 3). Cambridge, MA: Abt Associates.

Gollay, E., Freedman, R., Wyngaarden, M., & Kurtz, N.R. (1978). *Coming back: The community experiences of deinstitutionalized mentally retarded people*. Cambridge, MA: Abt Associates.

Guess, D., Benson, A., & Siegel-Causey, E. (1985). Behavioral control and education of severely handicapped students: Who's doing what to whom? And why? In D. Bricker & J. Filler (Eds.), *Severe mental retardation: From theory to practice* (pp. 230–244). Reston, VA: Council for Exceptional Children.

Hawkins, B.A., & Eklund, S.J. (1989). Aging and developmental disabilities: Interagency planning for an emerging population. *Journal of Applied Gerontology*, *8*, 168–174.

Heal, L.W., & Chadsey-Rusch, J. (1985). The lifestyles satisfaction scales (LSS): Assessing individuals' satisfaction with residence, community setting, and associated services. *Applied Research in Mental Retardation*, *6*, 475–490.

Jacobson, J.W., Sutton, M.S., & Janicki, M.P. (1985). Demography and characteristics of aging and aged mentally retarded persons. In M.P. Janicki & H.M. Wisniewski (Eds.), *Aging and developmental disabilities: Issues and approaches* (pp. 115–142). Baltimore: Paul H. Brookes.

Janicki, M.P. (1988). Aging and mental retardation. *Mental Retardation*, *26*, 177–180.

Janicki, M.P., & Jacobson, J.W., Zigman, W.B., & Lubin, R.A. (1987). Group homes as alternative care settings: System issues and implications. In S. Landesman & P. Vietze (Eds.), *Living environments and mental retardation* (pp. 173–194). Washington, DC: American Association on Mental Retardation.

Janicki, M.P., Otis, J.P., Puccio, P.S., Rettig, J.S., & Jacobson, J.W. (1985). Service needs among older developmentally disabled persons. In M.P. Janicki & H.M. Wisniewski (Eds.), *Aging and developmental disabilities: Issues and approaches* (pp. 289–304). Baltimore: Paul H. Brookes.

Janicki, M.P., & Wisniewski, H.M. (Eds.). (1985). *Aging and developmental disabilities: Issues and approaches* (pp. 115–142). Baltimore: Paul H. Brookes.

Jeffree, D., & Cheseldine, S.E. (1984). Programmed leisure intervention and the interaction of severely mentally retarded adolescents: A pilot study. *American Journal of Mental Retardation*, *88*, 619–624.

Jones, M.L., White, G.L., Ulicny, G.R., & Matthews, R.M. (1988). A survey of service by independent living centers to people with cognitive disabilities. *Rehabilitation Counselling Bulletin*, *31*, 244–248.

Kaplan, O.J. (1943). Mental decline in order morons. *American Journal of Mental Retardation*, *47*, 277–285.

Keith, K.D., Schalock, R.L., & Hoffman, K. (1986). *Quality of life: Measurement and programmatic implications*. Lincoln, NE: Region V Mental Retardation Services.

Kishi, G., Teelucksingh, M., Zollers, N., Park-Lee, S., & Meyer, L. (1988). Daily decision making in community residences: A social comparison of adults with and without mental retardation. *American Journal on Mental retardation*, *92*, 430–435.

Knoll, J., & Ford, A. (1987). Beyond caregiving: A reconceptualization of the role of the residential service provider. In S.J. Taylor, D. Biklen, & J. Knoll

(Eds.), *Community integration for people with severe disabilities* (pp. 129–146). New York: Columbia Teachers Press.

Krauss, M.W. (1988). Long-term care issues in mental retardation. In J. Kavanaugh (Ed.), *Understanding mental retardation: Research accomplishments and new frontiers*. Baltimore: Paul H. Brookes.

Landesman, S. (1987a). Quality of life and personal life satisfaction: Definition and measurement issues. *Mental Retardation*, *24*, 141–143.

Landesman, S. (1987b). The changing structure and function of institutions: A search for optimal group home care. In S. Landesman & P. Vietze (Eds.), *Living environments and mental retardation* (pp. 79–126). Washington, DC: American Association on Mental Retardation.

Lubin, R.A., & Kiely, M. (1985). Epidemiology of aging in developmental disabilities. In M.P. Janicki & H.M. Wisniewski (Eds.), *Aging and developmental disabilities: Issues and approaches* (pp. 95–113). Baltimore: Paul H. Brookes.

Luckasson, R. (1990). A lawyer's perspective on "quality of life." In R.L. Schalock (Ed.), *Quality of life: Perspectives and issues* (pp. 211–214). Washington, DC: American Association on Mental Retardation Monograph Series.

Mallory, B., & Herrick, S.C. (1986). *Ramps are not enough: The movement of children with mental retardation from institutional to community-based care*, Durham, NH: University of New Hampshire.

Mank, D.M., Rhodes, L.E., & Bellamy, G.T. (1986). Four supported employment alternatives. In W.E. Kiernan & J.A. Stark (Eds.), *Pathways to employment for adults with developmental disabilities* (pp. 139–153). Baltimore: Paul H. Brookes.

Matthews, P. (1982) Some recreation preferences of the mentally retarded. *Therapeutic Recreation Journal*, *16*, 42–47.

Miller, M. (1979). *Suicide after sixty: The final alternative*. New York: Springer-Verlag.

Nietupski, J., Hamre-Nietupski, S., & Ayres, B. (1984). Review of task analytic leisure skill training efforts: Practitioner implications and future research needs. *Journal of the Association of Persons With Severe Handicaps*, *9*, 88–97.

O'Brien, J. (1980). *The principle of normalization: A foundation for effective services*. Atlanta, GA: Georgia Advocacy Office.

Ossofsky, J. (1988). Connecting the networks: Aging and lifelong disabilities. *Educational Gerontology*, *14*, 389–397.

Pagel, S.E., & Whitling, C.A. (1978). Readmissions to a state hospital for mentally retarded persons: Reasons for community failure. *Mental Retardation*, *16*, 164–166.

Pierce, T.B. (1989). *Surveying unstructured time of adults with mental retardation in two community settings: A search for normalization*. Unpublished doctoral dissertation, University of New Mexico, Albuquerque, NM.

Pierce, T.B., Luckasson, R., & Smith, D.D. (1990). Surveying unstructured time of adults with mental retardation in two community settings: A search for normalization. *Exceptionality*, *1*, 123–134.

Puccio, P.S., Janicki, M.P., Otis, J.P., & Rettig, J. (1983). *Report of the committee on aging and developmental disabilities*. Albany, NY: New York State Office of Mental Retardation and Developmental Disabilities.

Putnam, J.W., Werder, J.K., & Schleien, S.J. (1985). Leisure and recreation services for handicapped persons. In K.C. Lakin & R.H. Bruininks (Eds.), *Strategies for achieving community integration of developmentally disabled citizens* (pp. 253–274). Baltimore: Paul H. Brookes.

Roberto, K.A., & Nelson, R.E. (1989). The developmentally disabled elderly: Concerns of special providers. *Journal of Applied Gerontology*, *8*, 175–182.

Schalock, R.L., & Keith, K.D. (1984). *DD clients and staff variables influencing outcome of service delivery: Present and future models*. Lincoln, NE: Nebraska Department of Health/Division of Developmental Disabilities.

Seltzer, G.B. (1981). Community residential adjustment: The relationship among environment, performance, and satisfaction. *American Journal of Mental Deficiency*, *85*, 624–630.

Seltzer, M.M. (1988). Long-term care issues in mental retardation. In J. Kavanagh (Ed.), *Understanding mental retardation: Research accomplishments and new frontiers*. Baltimore: Paul H. Brookes.

Seltzer, M.M., & Krauss, M.W. (1987). *Aging and mental retardation: Extending the continuum*. Washington, DC: American Association on Mental Retardation.

Seltzer, M.M., Krauss, M.W., Litchfield, L.C., & Modlish, N.J.K. (1989). Utilization of aging network services by elderly persons with mental retardation. *The Gerontologist*, *29*, 234–238.

Shevin, M., & Klein, N.K. (1984). The importance of choice-making skills for students with severe disabilities. *Journal of the Association for Persons With Severe Handicaps*, *9*, 159–166.

Sison, G.P., & Cotten, P.D. (1989). The elderly mentally retarded person: Current perspectives and future directions. *The Journal of Applied Gerontology*, *8*(2), 151–167.

Special Committee on Aging. (1984). *Discrimination against the poor and disabled in nursing homes*. Washington, DC: U.S. Government Printing Office.

Stroud, M., & Sutton, E. (1988). *Expanding options for older adults with developmental disabilities: A practical guide to achieving community access*. Baltimore: Paul H. Brookes.

Taylor, S.J. (1987). Continuum traps. In S.J. Taylor, D. Biklen, & J. Knoll (Eds.), *Community integration for people with severe disabilities* (pp. 25–35) New York: Teachers College Press.

Taylor, S.J., & Bogdan, R. (1984). *Introduction to qualitative research methods: The search for meanings* (2nd ed.). New York: John Wiley.

Taylor, S.J., Racino, J., Knoll, J., & Lutfiyya, Z. (1987). In S. J. Taylor, D. Biklen, & J. Knoll (Eds.), *Community integration for people with severe disabilities* (pp. 36–63). New York: Teachers College Press.

Tobin, S.S. (1985). The function, form, and future of formal services. In C.M. Gaitz, G. Niederehe, & N.L. Wilson (Eds.), *Aging 2000: Our health care destiny. Vol. 2: Psychosocial and polciy issues* (pp. 191–200) New York: Springer-Verlag.

U.S. Bureau of the Census. (1987). Estimates of the population of the United States, by age, sex, and race: 1980–1986. (*Current population reports*, Series P-25, No. 1000). Washington, DC: U.S. Government Printing Office.

U.S. Senate Special Committee on Aging. (1988). *Aging America: Trends and projections*. Washington, DC: Author.

VanZandt, S., & Cannon-Nifoussi, B. (1989). Adult children and their aging parents. In M.J. Fine (Ed.), *The second handbook on parent education: Contemporary perspectives* (pp. 305–323). San Diego, CA: Academic.

Voeltz, L.M., Wuerch, B.B., & Wilcox, B. (1982). Leisure and recreation: Preparation for independence, integration, and self-fulfillment. In B. Wilcox & G.T. Bellamy (Eds.), *Design of high school programs for severely handicapped students*. Baltimore: Paul H. Brookes.

Walz, T., Harper, D., & Wilson, J. (1986). The aging developmentally disabled person: A review. *The Gerontologist*, *26*, 622–629.

Wehman, P., & Schleien, S. (1980). Assessment and selection of leisure skills for severely handicapped individuals. *Education and Training of the Mentally Retarded*, *15*, 50–57.

White House Conference on Aging. (1981). *Report of the technical committee on family social services and other support systems*. Washington, DC: Department of Health and Human Services.

Willer, B., & Intagliata, J. (1981). Social-environmental factors as predictors of adjustment of deinstitutionalized mentally retarded adults. *American Journal of Mental Deficiency*, *86*, 252–259.

Wolfensberger, W. (1983). Social role valorization: A proposed new term for the principle of normalization. *Mental Retardation*, *21*, 234–239.

Wolfensberger, W., & Glenn, L. (1975). *PASS 3: Program analysis of service systems: A method of quantitative evaluation of human services* (3rd ed.). Toronto: National Institute on Mental Retardation.

Wolfensberger, W., & Thomas, S. (1983) *Program analysis of service systems: Implementation of normalization goals*. Toronto: National Institute on Mental Retardation.

Wuerch, B., & Voeltz, L. (1982). *Longitudinal leisure skills for severely handicapped learners*. Baltimore: Paul H. Brookes.

12
Integration From a Parent's Perspective: Yesterday was a Long Time Ago and Tomorrow Isn't Here Yet

SUSAN LEHR

Parents of children with disabilities rarely, if ever, think in terms of life cycles. In fact, most of these parents find that getting through each day and each night can be rather daunting. Certainly, there are enough challenges to keep their attention fully occupied.

That is not to say that they do not think about the future. They do, but probably in a different way than most professionals do. Worries and concerns about their son's or daughter's future are ever present. Sometimes these worries push to the front of the parents' thinking, especially during times of crisis or disruption. At other times, parents can feel it is pointless to dwell on the future, or the future is such an unknown that they cannot conceptualize what it will be like.

What Is This Chapter and Where Will It Take You?

As I was preparing this chapter I was aware of the attention that professional researchers have directed toward studying families of children with disabilities. Numerous studies have been conducted that attempt to explain the various dynamics that come into play when a child with a disability becomes part of a family (Bruininks & Lakin, 1985; Dybwad, 1990; Krauss, Simeonsson, & Ramey, 1990; Singer & Irvin, 1989). I am not a researcher, at least not in that sense. I am a parent, and I have been asked to write this chapter from that perspective. Rather than reviewing the literature and trying to make sense of it, I invite you to do that. Because I am a parent of a son with a disability, and because over the years I have had the privilege of knowing many other parents, I want to use this valuable space to tell you what we know, what we experience, what our issues are, and what we want you to know about us. I certainly do not presume to speak for all parents, but for those who have willingly shared their stories with me. I want to share their stories and their words with you because these truly reflect who we are and how we think about our children. Since we are a rather proud lot, though, I have used pseudonyms and, in some cases, I have paraphrased the actual words. Nonetheless, these stories are just as real as the parents and their son or daughter. The issues that these stories raise are also real. We hope they will cause you to think and act in new ways.

This chapter is divided loosely into three areas. It begins with a section headed The Search, which describes some of the experiences parents have initially as they learn about their child's disability. Following this is a section about experiences with schools and the educational sector in general. The third section, Are We Transitioning Yet?, discusses some of the issues that parents and their maturing sons and daughters must deal with as formal schooling ends and adulthood becomes reality. The conclusion lists some lessons that parents would like professionals to understand and gives one final quote from a parent.

The Search

From the moment that a parent becomes aware or is made aware of the unique needs of his or her child, all of the routine expectations are suddenly thrown into question. Jane Clark's fifth child was born with all kinds of medical complications; Jane remembers thinking that she had no control over her baby's life. His doctors and nurses would make all the decisions that were necessary. She points to a photograph that her husband took of their week-old infant as he lay in the isolette in the intensive care unit of a large metropolitan hospital:

> Tony's tiny body was invaded with needles and tubes, each leading to complicated-looking machines that beeped, blinked, or hummed.

Surrounding Tony's crib, in the picture, was a host of nurses and doctors all clad in white, caps covering their hair, some wearing plastic gloves, some with stethoscopes clinging around their neck. Some were wearing blue nose-and-mouth guards. Barely visible, hanging on the outer periphery of this cloud of medical white stands Jane, her arms hanging limply at her sides, her face totally expressionless.

It took weeks for Jane to recognize that she did not want to remain a spectator, watching Tony's life from a distance. But she hesitated. She already had four older children, but she felt totally unprepared to take care of Tony.

> I didn't even know how to hold him because of all the tubes and needles. How was I supposed to feed him or bathe him? The nurses did all of this. I felt helpless.

Jane had no idea whether Tony would live or, if he did, what kind of life he could expect to have. Before she could worry about that, however, Jane realized that she had to discover for herself how to give Tony the loving care he needed for today. She knew then that she wanted to take Tony home. She would have to learn how to take care of Tony herself and get through tomorrow and the next day and the day after that without all of the professionals being there. She knew she could call them and ask for help, but she and her family, like so many others in similar situations, took control of their and Tony's life, one day at a time.

Jane's story is not unique. Although the details differ from family to family, the issues that parents face as they are initially confronted by their child's disability are similar (Carver & Carver, (1972); Featherstone, 1980; Simons, 1987; Turnbull & Turnbull, 1985). When parents first learn of their child's "differentness," most of them begin some type of personal journey to search for answers. The questions do not come in any predictable order.

Why me? Why my child?
What did I do to deserve this?
What will happen to me? To my child?
What should I do?
Can I do anything?
Who will help me?
Can I handle this?
Where do I go for help?
What will people think? What will they say?
Am I the only one? Is my child the only one?
What do I tell my family? My neighbors? Other people?
Can I deal with this?

These and similar questions express the helplessness that parents often feel in the beginning. With few exceptions, they feel frightened and alone. They question themselves to see if they are to blame for their child's disability. One mother said,

> I kept thinking back over every day of my pregnancy. If only I had not had those beers, maybe Josh would be normal.

Another father blamed himself for allowing his son to cross the street to retrieve the mail. One afternoon, 5-year-old Mark was hit by a car and suffered severe brain damage. The father cried,

> I should have known he was too young. It's my fault.

Sometimes, parents feel ashamed—ashamed of their child and of their own feelings of rejection, resentment, or disappointment. In some way, these parents feel they have failed their child, and they may feel the child, in a sense, has failed them by not being the "normal" child they expected. Unfortunately, some parents blame each other for their child's disability. All too often parents feel that professionals are also blaming them. It is an extremely painful time.

Unlike when a typical child is born, when a child is born handicapped, there is no traditional script that the parents or society in general knows to follow. Periodic letters to "Dear Abby" poignantly express this when letter writers ask if a sympathy card should be sent to the parents whose child was born with some disability such as Down Syndrome. These feelings of helplessness, shame, and confusion are not new.

Returning to Jane for a moment, she cautions, "It's not all doom and gloom." Another parent agrees:

> We enjoy getting to know our special kids. It doesn't take very long to sort of forget about the disability part and just see the kid. And we have fun with that.

Many families develop different ways of sharing the fun and excitement they feel as their child accomplishes milestones. They acknowledge that these milestones may not be appreciated or even understood by others outside of the family, but that does not diminish their significance within the family.

> I remember the first time Molly picked up a spoon on her own. For months and months we had been trying to get her to grasp the handle, but she just couldn't seem to do it. We had even built up the size of the handle with adhesive tape to make it easier for her, but still she just couldn't get a grip on it. Then one Sunday morning, she was sitting in her feeding table and I was getting ready to feed her. We were in a hurry because we were going to my mother's for the day. I put the spoon on the table and turned to get the applesauce. When I turned back Molly had the spoon in her hand. I cried. Molly was almost a year and half old when that happened.

Early on, parents become acutely aware of how everyone around them sees only the disability of their child, while the parent struggles to see the capability. One father complained wearily:

> I get so sick and tired of hearing what is wrong with Mathew. We know, probably better than the doctors, what Matt's problems are. But all we ever get told is, "he can't do this" or "he can't do that" or "he'll never be able to do that." How do they know what Mathew will be able to do? He is only a baby now. Who knows what lies ahead? But I do know that if I listen to these doctors I will never let Mathew try. I don't want to argue with them, but sometimes I think they are wrong. I have to believe that Mathew can progress.

Sometimes in the face of all this, it is difficult for parents to think positively and to regain a sense of hope and expectation. Many parents cannot. Their marriages and relationships suffer. They suffer. Some seek professional help—counseling or therapy. Some turn to their church or religion for answers. Some parents of children with disabilities turn to each other. Wherever they turn, they are seeking answers to their questions, and they are seeking support. They want to know what to do, and they want to know if what they are doing is right.

And so their search continues. They take their child to all sorts of professionals looking for a cause; a diagnosis; a treatment; a cure; and, of course, a look into the future.

How long will she live?
What will he be able to do?
How will we pay for all of this?
Where will we get the services he/she needs?
How do we know this is the right thing to do?
Should we get a second opinion?
Should we agree to this recommendation or not?
What will happen?
What if we don't like something?
Will there ever be an end to this?
Whom should I listen to?
What are my rights?
Where can I get more information?
Who will support me and my decisions?
What is my child eligible for?

During the early years of having a youngster with a disabling condition, parents will spend inordinant amounts of time, money, energy, and personal commitment in their search for answers to these questions and for help. They will be faced with the practical matters of taking time off from work to take their child to any number of appointments and evaluation sessions. Many mothers who work outside the home have complained that either they face losing their jobs because of the time they must spend arranging for and managing the intense care their child may need or they may be forced to quit their jobs in order to provide this care. Fathers are often confronted with similar concerns. They tell of worrying about health care benefits and insurance issues that may jeopardize financial status. They worry about being able to provide adequately for their families. They worry about dying.

Single parents must wrestle with an extraordinary list of things. One of their chief concerns is finding child care. Many parents, single or not, do not have the luxury of finding great day care. Many have to settle for whatever they can get. For many, it is almost impossible or the costs are extreme. One recently divorced father, Peter, told his story. He had just turned 20 when he and his wife divorced. She wanted nothing to do with their children and had left town with another man. Peter gained custody of Brian, aged $2\frac{1}{2}$, and Sara, 10 months old. Peter worked as a janitor at a local college. Suddenly, he was faced with finding a babysitter for his two children while he worked. Brian, who later was to be labeled as autistic, rarely slept, was not toilet trained, and spent much of his time tearing around the apartment making a shrill sound, breaking and tearing things, throwing toys, and so on. Sara, on the other hand, was a quiet baby who seemed to take everything in stride. Peter was panic-stricken. Where could he find a babysitter who could handle Brian and not neglect Sara? How was he going to afford to pay someone on his meager salary?

I was also terrified that someone would come and take Brian and Sara away from me. I was afraid that they would think I couldn't take care of them.

Peter had no idea where to turn or what to do. He knew something was different about Brian. In fact, later he recognized that Brian's difficult behavior was a major part of why his marriage had failed. After a lot of begging, a neighbor reluctantly agreed to help out temporarily, but Peter would have to pay her almost $10 per hour, plus reimburse her for anything Brian broke. Peter had no idea how he would pay for this. He also knew that finding a permanent sitter, especially for Brian, was not going to be easy. He felt totally alone and helpless.

Another problem that parents face is being fair to their other children. In Peter's case this was not a major problem initially. For parents like Jane and her husband, who already had four other children, finding a balance between caring for their son and his extraordinary health-related problems and caring for their four other children posed immense problems. Many parents express feelings of intense guilt over the amount of time they feel they have neglected or shortchanged their other children. They do the best they can, but they often feel that it is never enough and that it is never fair for anyone.

We try so hard in our family to not get caught into dwelling too much on Kim's problems. Ron and I actively remind each other not to talk about Kim's care or the current battles we are engaged in, in front of Kim's older brothers. We don't want them to think they are not as important to us as she is. But one night we were made acutely aware that we were not as successful as we thought. We all were at the supper table when our oldest son snapped at us, "Man, are you guys boring. All you ever talk about is Kimmy or Kimmy's school stuff. I'm sick of it." He stormed from the table.

It takes a lot of courage and perseverance for families in the beginning simply to manage. First, they have to face the reality that their child is different from what they had expected. Whether the disability is a developmental disability, a critical health problem, mental retardation, or a genetic or undiagnosed disability, it is emotionally devastating for the parents initially. Certainly, they are confused. In all likelihood, at various times they will also feel hurt, angry, sad, desolate, lonely, crazy, scared, and guilty. Yet they may also know joy, happiness, love, and support. They will need these.

Parents are often asked, "Have you accepted your child's disability?" It is an interesting question, and it provokes a myriad of responses. John, an adult with a physical disability, remarks,

I'm not sure that anyone ever really accepts his or her disability. In fact, I'm not even sure what that means. I do think, however, that you learn to see the disability as part of who you are or who your child is. Maybe acceptance is when you no longer see the disability as the most important or central part of who the person is.

Many parents will tell you, however, that just about the time that they think they have a handle on how to manage their lives and that of the child with a disability, something heppens to disrupt this equilibrium. For many families, sending the child off to school is one of the most disruptive of these experiences.

Enter: The School System

Ready or not, like it or not, the day comes when the child must become part of the educational system. Whether the child enters they "system" from the very beginning or because of some catastrophic accident or event, and no matter what the nature of the previous experiences for the parents, no one seems fully prepared for what happens. No experiences are exactly the same. However, the similarity among parent stories of their experiences when their child enters the "special education arena," as one parent called it, have some consistent and similar themes.

I thought I was fully prepared. I had been to numerous staffings about Katlyn during her preschool years. I had listened as doctors discussed their medical opinion of her future. I had heard social workers and psychologists recommend behavioral programs, counseling, and intensive intervention strategies to deal with Katlyn's various needs. I had agreed to a variety of therapies, OT, PT, speech, and so on, in the hopes that each of these individually and/or collectively would benefit. I thought I had heard it all. In fact, I was probably a bit smug in the knowledge that I thought I knew it all, or at least enough to be able to inform the school of Katlyn's needs and abilities. Oh, how wrong I was. I was totally unprepared for the fact that my knowledge of Katlyn was insignficant. In fact, it was meaningless in the eyes of the "professional educators" as they called themselves. I was shocked and hurt that not only were they not interested in what I had to tell them about Katlyn, they did not want to hear from me at all. They were the professionals, I was informed, and I was *just* a parent. They would call me if they needed me, thank you very much.

Perhaps this parent's experience is extreme. However, the stories that parents have shared about their experiences with having their child enter the school system certainly reflect an overall insensitivity and lack of appreciation for the knowledge and expertise that parents have.

It is not my intent to bash schools. That would be unfair. There are many parents who have had positive experiences with school personnel. Unfortunately, other parents' experiences with the educational system are less than pleasant or cooperative.

The first onslaught for parents is the initial evaluation process to determine whether the child needs special educational services. Some parents have decent experiences. Many do not. One father was outraged when the school psychologist who was attempting to determine whether his daughter should be labeled as mentally retarded asked the father about his marital and sexual relationships with his wife. What did this have to do with the evaluation of his daughter, and what bearing would it have on the program of services that she might receive? When he refused to answer, he was informed that he was denying his daughter's disability. In other cases, parents do not know about the information that is contained in their child's file, such as the results of medical, psychological, or specialized tests. Parents are unfamiliar with the professional way in which these reports have been compiled and, unless they have a sensitive professional, they may not know what these reports actually mean. When these files are sent on to the child's school, parents may feel confused because they are not sure how these will affect their child's schooling.

I felt scared when I went to the first meeting about Shawnda's program. I didn't know what to ask or say. I felt real stupid. I didn't say anything. I don't know what they wanted. Mrs. Cutter just told me I had to sign some papers and everything would be just fine. So I signed. I just wanted to get out of there.

This parent felt intimidated, scared, and ignorant. He was not quite sure what he had agreed to in terms of Shawnda's program, nor had anyone really explained it to him in a way that he could understand. Often these planning meetings are overwhelming for parents. The professionals use terminology that parents don't always understand. They hesitate to ask for an explanation because they don't want to appear stupid or poorly informed.

Many parents feel that their abilities as parents are also being questioned or judged by the professionals in these meetings. It seems as if the implication is that the child's problem was caused by or aggravated by the parents. The parents feel they are being blamed.

It's real hard to sit and listen to strangers tell you all the things that are wrong with your kid.

This parent felt hurt and angry because no one talked about what her son could do or how much he had progressed in his preschool program.

In contrast, one parent told of how she was asked to bring photographs of her son to the meeting. She was even more pleased when the chairperson of the meeting introduced everyone to her and then asked her to spend some time telling everyone about her son.

It seemed like they were really interested in Chaheem. They asked questions about him and about what he likes to do.

Perhaps one of the most difficult transitions for parents to make is when their son or daughter with a disbility leaves home. Whether the child is to go to day care, preschool, school, or work, or to live someplace else, the parents have to trust that he or she is safe, well planned for, and respected. In order to assure that this is the case, parents need and want information and honest communication. Parents want to know what is happening and whether their child is being treated well. They want to visit the program or classroom. They want to talk to the teachers and care providers. They want to know how their child is doing and what he or she is doing. Many parents want to know how they can build on what the child is learning in school by providing similar activities at home. Parents want to be able to share their ideas and insights with the staff. Parents want to be able to hear good things mixed in with the needs and the not-so-good. One father complained bitterly,

> I am so sick and tired of the teachers telling me "He had a good day" or "He had a bad day" and that's all. I want to know more than just that. I want to know what happened and when. What was he doing? What were the teachers doing? What was the plan? I want to know something other than just that good-day/bad-day crap. What does that tell me anyway?

Parents like to be invited to problem-solve and to share what they know. They like to be considered part of a team, not always the outsider.

Trust is another big issue for families. When their son or daughter is in the care of someone else for whatever reason, parents must be able to trust that that person will protect the child from harm. Unfortunately, many parents painfully share stories about the psychological, physical, and/or sexual abuse that their child has endured. They feel caught in a trap. In many cases it is really difficult to prove that the abuse occurred. This is especially the case if the child has the label of mental retardation or autism. The tendency is not to believe the child or to assume he or she was confused about what actually happened. Parents are often not believed when they complain about abuse. In fact, sometimes they are accused of being the problem. Also, the abuse may occur in a setting that is the only available placement for a child. Parents are told that if they are not happy with the services they can take their child elsewhere. What if there is no place else to go? Many parents feel they have no control in these situations.

> When one of the neighborhood children asked me why Sean's teacher shut him in the janitor's closet I was stunned. I called the principal immediately and asked for an explanation. I was even more shocked when he became angry with me for making such an accusation. He refused to investigate. He said that none of his teachers would do anything like that and even if they did he was sure they had a good reason. He said I was overreacting and that I should be grateful that Mrs. Jacobs had agreed to have Sean in her room because he was such a difficult child. None of the other teachers would take him, so I had better be careful not to upset Mrs. Jacobs. It was clearly a warning. What was I to do? I was afraid that if I complained too much there might be repercussions for Sean. It was just so awful.

Another problem that some parents face during the school years is isolation. Because their son or daughter may not be routinely included in regular out-of-school and after-school activities, parents do not have as many opportunities to make connections with other families. Many of the services and activities for youngsters with disabilities are not open to peers without disabilities, and certainly the opposite is true. If a child with a disability wants to enroll in activities out of school—such things as swimming, dance, or music classes—he or she is usually referred to special programs for handicapped children only. Not only does this limit the opportunities for social interaction between disabled and nondisabled children, but it also limits the parents' social contacts within the community. The social network of both parents and youngsters can become increasingly limited.

It is interesting to note that when schools generally hold open houses or "meet the teacher" nights, parents of students with special needs rarely attend. Some parents simply don't feel they are supposed to be there because their child is in the special education program. Others feel they are not welcome. Many don't even know that these events are for them. This is especially the case if the child is being educated within a segregated special education program. One parent whose son was in a special education class told about going to the first open house of the school year so that she could meet other parents from her son's classroom. When she arrived at the classroom door, it was locked and the lights were out. She sought out the school principal and asked where the teacher was. With a bit of embarrassment the principal explained that the teacher never came to these events because they were for the "normal" students. The teacher assumed that none of her students or their parents would show up. Although disappointed and a bit miffed by this, the parent decided to stay anyway and went about meeting other teachers and parents from the regular education program. The following year she requested that her son be placed in a regular classroom.

It is during the elementary and junior high years in school that kids generally develop their own friendships. That is, unless the child is a special education student. At least, that is what many parents will say. Either they see their other sons and daughters making friends or they are aware that this is happening for typical kids. It just does not seem to happen spontaneously for youngsters with special needs. Many parents feel they have to take an active role in helping their children develop and maintain friendships. There are lots of strategies that the parents use to accomplish this. They may have the best toys available for kids to play with as an attraction. One mother described how she and her husband designed a truly elaborate play area in the back yard that would accomodate their young son's motorized wheelchair and yet was challenging to the neighborhood youngsters as well. Then they made a point of specifically inviting kids and their parents to come play.

Because Mark rode on a separate bus and was in a separate room at school, I just knew the other kids would never get to know what a neat kid he is. Building the play area seemed to make sense to us.

Of course, not all families have the resources to do something this elaborate. A single mother helped her 12-year-old daughter make friends by offering to take care of several other elementary-age children after school while their parents worked. Her daughter enjoyed her friends and even learned some things that surprised her mother.

One day the girls were playing dress-up. We had a box full of old dresses and stuff. They got all dolled up and then raided my dresser and put on my make-up. They helped Demika get all dolled up. She had on lipstick and nailpolish and eyeshadow. She was grinning from ear to ear when she came into the kitchen to show me. It was a riot.

The friendships that are made during elementary school often last into middle and junior high school. However, if friendships have not been established early on during elementary school, it will be difficult at best to establish them later. Often parents are acutely aware that their child is socially isolated. They would love to have their child invited to birthday parties, to spend the night at a friend's house, or to play at someone's house on a weekend. Often this never happens. Even when it does, sometimes parents will get scared and say no.

When Danny was invited to his first birthday party, I think he was 6 or 7, I was afraid to let him go because I was afraid he would spoil everything. I called Joey's parents and made some lame excuse why Danny couldn't come. Secretly I was worried what would happen if Danny got upset and acted out. I was sure he would never get invited back. It just seemed easier not to let him go in the first place Fortunately, Joey's parents didn't agree with me. They explained that Joey really wanted Danny at his party. Danny was one of his best friends and he would be crushed if Danny couldn't come. It seemed I could not refuse. I think they sensed my fears because they suggested that Kara, Danny's older sister, might want to come along to help out with the games and such. It was a wonderful suggestion, and it did make me feel better. I let Danny go and he had a ball. I think Kara liked being the big sister helper too.

Are We Transitioning Yet?

During the elemetary and junior high years is when the parents really begin to think more acutely about their son or daughter's future. They begin to wonder what will happen. Where he or she will work, and what will he or she do? Where will he or she live, and with whom? What kind of support will he or she need, and how will that happen? Who will be there for them when they need it? Often family crises force parents to think about these things even when they may not want to. Crises such as the loss of a job; separation or divorce; the death of a spouse, grandparent, or other family member; illness; or financial problems—anything can cause a major upheaval, compelling families to think and plan for the future. Parents begin to face the reality that they will not live forever, and they begin to question what that may mean for their son or daughter.

As youngsters with disabilities grow older and become teenagers, it becomes increasingly more difficult for parents to arrange for their social life. Although friendships do occur, parents may have to rely more on other teens and adults to initiate and foster these opportunities. One young teenage boy labeled as severely learning disabled loved to read comic books. Practically every afternoon after school he would go to a little shop to browse through its collection of Captain Marvel, Superman, Archie, and other comics. Soon he began a collection of these. He developed a friendship with the owner of this shop. He began trading comics with other teens to whom the owner introduced him.

Another parent explained that as long as his son's older sister was around it seemed that the house was always full of teenagers:

> Not that they always included Sam when they went places, but when they were at the house they would talk with him. Once I even found the boys teaching Sam how to shoot baskets. One of the guys told me he thought it would be good for Sam to watch MTV since everyone else did. Sam seems to like having people here, but when they decide to go to a movie or something they never invite him along. It hurts to see him left behind.

This type of experience is more likely to happen when nondisabled teenagers begin to drive cars and have after-school jobs. Their social lives take on new dimensions. They begin to date, get jobs, and spend less and less time with their parents. Teens with disabilities may get jobs also, and they may learn to drive. Sometimes they go on dates. Transportation can be one stumbling block for parents if their child with a disability cannot drive or use public transportation for whatever reason. In addition, teenagers with disabilities may need other kinds of support to make all of this happen. Where will the support come from? It is almost impossible for parents to arrange.

> I decided that the only way Tomiko was going to have some teenage friends was if I set it up. I arranged for three high school boys to be his companion after school until I got home from work. One of them was to meet his school bus and bring him home each day. If all three of them wanted to do this that was okay with me too. By arranging for all three I thought there would be a better chance of someone always being there, and I thought they might feel better about this idea if they were together. My instructions to them were quite simple. They could not smoke in the house, and they were to include Tomiko in whatever they planned to do as well as do some of the things that Tomiko wanted. I paid them $5.00 per hour. How they divided up the money was up to them. Tomiko loved it. Sometimes they would watch videos, and sometimes they would bake cookies and

cakes. Sometimes they just sat around and talked. My friends thought I was taking a big risk by having three teenage boys alone in my house with Tomiko, but I trusted that they would act maturely and they do. Tomiko invited two of them to go to the state fair to go on the rides with him. He thinks of one of them as his best friend.

The bottom line for all parents is that no matter what they do or when, they simply cannot force friendships to happen. when friendships do happen, it is great. When they don't, it is sad and lonely for everyone.

Most students with special needs leave school in their late teens or early 20s. Even though they have access to education until the age of 21, and even later in some states, many students with disabilities drop out of school before graduation. Some stay on. In either case, the issues facing the parent and the student are the same—where to work, where to live, and who will make the decisions. For many parents who have appreciated the benefits their son or daughter has received as a result of Public Law 94–142, the Education for All Handicapped Children Act, the leap into the adult world is both frightening and confusing.

The first shock they receive is having to acknowledge that there is no entitlement to services as an adult.

I couldn't believe it. I mean I knew that Kia was not really entitled to services after he graduated, but I really didn't realize what that actually meant. We had planned his transition well, or at least we thought we had. He had been in a supported job training program during the last 2 years of school. We hoped that he could continue on at the hardware store where he was working. After graduation all of the supports stopped. There wasn't any agency in our town that could pick Kia up for job coaching. He did okay for awhile, then he started to flounder. My husband tried to talk to the superivisor, but we realized that they needed the support, too, and we just could not do it ourselves. They are good people and they were really trying, but Kia was not doing the job and we knew they were going to fire him. They didn't really want to; they liked him. But they needed the work done and he wasn't doing it. We had nowhere to turn. Oh, we talked to a few agencies, and they were very nice. They either said they could put Kia on the waiting list for supported employment or they could refer him for sheltered employment. We had fought long and hard for Kia to be integrated in school. Little did we know that there would be no opportunities for him when he got out. In a funny sort of way, we felt betrayed. Why hadn't anyone warned us what is was really like? Why didn't the school know? Kia sits at home now watching TV. It is such a waste.

Upon graduation, unfortunately, many students find there is a morass of eligibility criteria for entrance into different job training and work programs. Often there are long waiting lists for services, or worse yet, because of a long list of reasons a person may be denied access to services and supports. In an honest effort to prepare for the best, while acknowledging that the worst may happen, parents are encouraged by professionals to plan for the youngster's transition out of school and into the adult community. Parents find all too often, however, that the school personnel and the adult service workers, especially the vocational evaluator or placement specialist simply have not talked to each other. Transition planning is important, however, and experiences like the one described above could have been avoided if transition planning had included representatives from job training and placement agencies. With good planning and coordination, students should be able to make a smooth transition out of school and into a meaningful job with the necessary supports intact.

Indeally, transition planning should begin around the age of 12 or 13 and should include an array of practical experiences in the community. Students need to learn how to accomplish a variety of skills if they are to make it in the adult world. Besides learning how to perform different jobs, students should develop other practical skills such as meal planning, grocery shopping, using public transportation, and using community recreational activities. Additionally, students should be guided in understanding how to behave in a mature and responsible fashion while at work and in the community. This means being courteous, dressing appropriately for the activity, and learning the subtleties of informal and formal social settings. Many parents would be proud of seeing their son or daughter learning skills that would benefit them as they move around the community.

I'd love it if Janine could use money right. Once she was on a field trip with her class and she disappeared. When the teacher found her she had a whole lot of food and candy. Where did she get that? Who gave it to her? What happened? I just don't know. Janine doesn't understand about money. She just knows that other people have it. She has to know what to do when she has money.

Another parent of a 14-year-old daughter began to cry as she expressed her own guilt for not taking her daughter with her when she went shopping or on errands.

I know I should take her. I know it would be good for her. But I am afraid she will embarrass me. I know everyone is looking at us. I feel so awful. If she could behave better I think I would feel better, but I don't know how to teach her.

This parent desparately needs the school to take on the responsibility of teaching her daughter how to manage herself while in the community. In her special education classroom some of her actions do not seem out of place, but when she is out in the community these same actions seem bizarre. If she is to transition into a job in the community some day, she needs to begin now to learn some of the necessary skills and behaviors. Her mother also could benefit from seeing how this training is accomplished.

For many parents, adolescence is also a time during which they begin to realize that their son or daughter really is growing up. In a sense they feel that time is beginning to run out for them more quickly. It can be a period in their lives that is both exhilarating and frightening.

Many parents are accused of overprotecting their youngster. This is especially likely to happen as he or she reaches young adulthood. This may very well be true, but it is often for good reasons. Parents are painfully aware of the hazards in the community as their son or daughter moves into adulthood. They know there will be instances of ridicule, rejection, and solitude. They are aware that services that can offer the kind of support that parents want for their child are limited or, in some cases, nonexistent. Many parents also recognize that there is no one else who can or is willing to take over for them. They get tired. They want to relax and enjoy themselves as they reach their middle years. They had not planned to still be parenting, if you will, on a full-time basis.

One mother spoke wearily of having waited patiently for a local support service to find an apartment for her 18-year-old daughter, Leanna. Instead, Leanna was placed in a group home. It soon became apparent to everyone that this was not a good place for Leanna. She wanted to have her own apartment with a roommate, "like other girls my age." Three years passed while Leanna and her mother waited for the agency to find and apartment and roommate. Finally, they realized that it just wasn't going to happen. This agency simply did not have the resources to search for such a place and provide the necessary support even though it said it wanted to. After advertising in a local paper, Leanna's mother found her a roommate. At least for the present, the mother was able to assure that her daughter had a home. What would happen as a result of this arrangement was yet to be seen. How long the roommate would stay was another matter. Whether she would build a reasonable relationship with Leanna was a hope, a dream. This story is still being written.

"When will it end?" asked another father now in his 70s. His 50-year-old son was a resident in a group home. He had been found in the bedroom of one of the women residents sitting on her bed. The father had been called and asked to take the son home. "What am I supposed to do? What can I say?" he asked. He was resentful that the group home staff thought that his son had done something wrong and he was angry that they wanted him, the father, to correct his son.

> Every time there is something wrong, or something happens that the staff doesn't like, they send Brian home. What am I supposed to do? Where will they send him after I am gone?

This is the greatest fear that parents have. Who will be there? Who will stand up for this person as they have? Who will care? Is there anyone, anyone at all?

Conclusion

And so, where are we? In a sense, we have traversed the life cycle, if you will, of the child and his or her family. We have looked at the fears, worries, concerns, dilemmas, and frustrations of the lives of families as they trip and plod through the life cycle of their child. What have we learned? That it is sad, depressing, scary? Yes! That parents get angry, they feel hurt, they react? Of course they do! Should we then pity these poor souls? You could. Many people do. But ask yourself, What good does that do—for anyone? Rather than pity, we may learn some lessons from what parents have experienced and from their stories. Let's look at these.

Lesson 1: Parents are people, and so are their sons or daughters. They are not cases, clients, consumers, recipients of services, case managers, they enemy, or the "other." They are simply people, just like you. They have the same wants, desires, feelings, fears, and frustrations. They are human beings. Please treat them as you would want to be treated.

Lesson 2: Parents do not have all the answers, but they sure do have some. Ask us what we think, what we know. Expect us to be partners in the planning and delivery of services to our child. We want to be a part. Invite us in. Expect us to contribute, but if we cannot, for whatever reason, don't blame us. We are doing our best.

Lesson 3: We love our children. That's all. No more or no less. We, above all, love our children.

Lesson 4: Always remember and respect that our greatest allies are other parents. They understand in a way that no other person can ever appreciate. Never deny us our need and love for other parents. Often they are the greatest experts because they have been there.

Lesson 5: If we choose allies to help us achieve our goals, respect that this is not a luxury but a necessity. Sometimes we parents feel helpless or powerless. Perhaps it is only a perception, but it does feel real to us. Allow us the right to pull our own weight by enlisting allies, friends, and supporters. But don't call us weak because we do this. We know we are weak at times, but we know we can regain our strength by enlisting the support of other people who understand our values and principles.

Lesson 6: Recognize that we do believe in something. We have principles and values that guide our every decision. They may not be the ones you want us to have, or they may be in conflict with what you have been led to believe. Recognize and accept that we may differ, and then be honest in trying to work from there forward.

Lesson 7: Give us joy. Recognize our accomplishments, not with pity, but with respect. Salute the achievements of our sons and daughters. Be proud of us. Laugh with us over the funny moments (and there are a lot of these), and in so doing, recognize that our lives are not always gloom and doom. We have some very wonderful experiences, which we love to share.

Lesson 8: Please don't make assumptions about us or about our child. Get to know each of us for who we are, not who someone else expects us to be.

Lesson 9: Be honest. You don't have to be brutal, but please tell us the truth as you know it. Long after your involvement with us is over we will have to carry on with the knowledge you have given us.

Lesson 10: Listen to what we have to say and what our sons and daughters have to say before you speak on our behalf. Don't presume that you know how we think and feel until you have asked us.

If everyone who comes into contact with parents and individuals with disabilities would keep these lessons in mind many of the issues that are described above would simply melt away. It is tough being a parent of a child with a disability, but it doesn't always have to be like that. We have not necessarily chosen this responsibility, but it is ours for a lifetime. Clara Claiborne Park says it best:

> This experience we did not choose, which we would have given anything to avoid, has made us better. Through it we have learned the lesson that no one studies willingly, the hard slow lesson of Sophocles and Shakespeare—that one grows by suffering. And that too is Jessy's gift. I write now what fifteen years past I would still not have thought possible to write: that if today I were given the choice, to accept the experience, with everything that it entails, or to refuse the bitter largesse, I would have to stretch out my hands—because out of it has come, for all of us, an unimagined life. And I will not change the last word of the story. It is still love.[1]

References

Biklen, D. (1987) *Achieving the Complete School.* New York, NY: Teachers College Press.

Blatt, B. & Morris, R.J. (1984) *Perspectives in Special Education Personal Orientations*. Grenville, IL: Scott, Foresman & Co.

Bruininks, R.H. & Lakin, K.C. (1985) *Living and Learning in the Least Restrictive Environment.* Baltimore, MD: Paul H. Brookes.

Carver, J. & Carver N.E. (1972) *The Family of the Retarded Child*. Syracuse, NY: Syracuse University Press.

Dorris, M. (1989) *The Broken Cord*. New York: Harper & Row.

Dybwad, G. (1964) *Challenges in Mental Retardaton*. New York, NY: Columbia University Press.

Dybwad, R. (1990) *Perspectives on a Parent Movement*. Boston, MA: Brookline Books.

1. C. C. Park, *The Siege*, quoted in M. Dorris, *The Broken Cord*. New York: Harper & Row, 1989, p. IX.

Featherstone, H. (1980) *A Difference in the Family*. New York, NY: Penguin Books.

Katz, A.H. (1961) *Parents of the Handicapped: Self-Organized Parents' and Relatives' Groups for Teatment of Ill and Handicapped Children*. Springfield, IL: Charles C. Thomas.

Krauss, M.W., Simeonsson, R. & Ramey, S.L., (Eds.) (1990) American Journal on Mental Retardation, 94 (3) *Special Issue on Research on Families*. Albany, NY: American Association on Mental Retardation.

Lippman, L. Goldberg, I. (1973) *Right to Education—Anatomy of the Pennsylvania Case and Its Implications for Exceptional Children*. New York, NY: Teachers College Press.

Lipsky, D.K. & Gartner, A. (1989) *Beyond Separate Educations: Quality Education for All*. Baltimore, MD: Paul H. Brookes.

Scheerenberger, R.C. (1983) *A History of Mental Retardation*. Baltimore, MD: Paul H. Brookes.

Simon, R. (1987) *After the Tears—Parents Talk about Raising a Child with a Disability*. New York, NY: Harcourt Brace Jovanovich.

Turnbull, A.P. & Turnbull, H.R. III (1986) *Families, Professionals, and Exceptionality: A Special Partnership*. Columbus, OH: Charles E. Merrill.

Turnbull, H.R. III & Turnbull, A.P. (1985) *Parents Speak Out Then and Now*. Columbus, OH: Charles E. Merrill.

Vohs, J. (Ed.) (1989–90) Coalition Quarterly, 7 (1) *As the Walls Come Tumbling Down*. Boston, MA: Technical Assistance for Parent Programs (TAPP) Project.

13
Future Trends in Integrated Lifecycle Services

David L. Lovett and Kathryn A. Haring

The closing chapter of this book is an appropriate avenue for discussing the development of special services and how that development has set the stage for future expansion of those services. It is pertinent to remember that the field of special education in North America is developmentally a toddler when compared to the long history of general education. The passage of Public Law 94–142 was an attainment of a developmental milestone for special education, the beginning of efforts to serve people of *all* ability levels in the public schools. In the years since public law has mandated a free and appropriate education for all children, the field has moved forward rapidly. However, as this book has repeatedly illustrated, there is a long way to go. This final chapter is concerned with developing a vision of the future of special services.

Five major concepts are integral to a discussion of the conceptual and practical considerations of providing special services to people with disabilities throughout their lives in integrated settings:

1. Special services must become a lifelong commitment of assistance as needed.
2. Special services must be provided in integrated settings.
3. A system paradigm must be created upon which effective lifelong services in integrated settings can be built.
4. A more effective system of service delivery must be based on research and evaluation.
5. Family involvement and individual autonomy are critical to the creation of a more effective system.

This chapter will provide a discussion of these concepts based on the material presented in previous chapters of this book. From this information the reader will have a clearer understanding of the need for, and methods by which to develop, a system that provides special services throughout the life cycle in integrated settings.

As a society we have made the commitment to serve all children. We have developed principles and policies that reflect this commitment, such as a free and appropriate education in the least restrictive environment. We have developed instructional methodologies and concepts to implement these policies, for example, systematic instruction, curriculum-based assessment, functional curricula, and so forth. However, many factors that are considered new are reworkings of past efforts. Indeed, the field of education has a history of neglecting a systematic analysis of new concepts and methodologies. Frequently, the field of education tends to vacillate from one popular notion (and its implications for instruction) to another. There are often shifts in instructional approaches to teaching basic academic skills. For example, in reading instruction, a school system may shift among sight word (recognize–memorize); phonic (sound related to meaning); or total (whole) language (personal experience converted to print and relearned as a reading experience) approaches in the course of just one decade. Rather than pulling valuable ideas from each approach, one method may be abandoned in favor of a "new" approach. Unfortunately, the efficacy of any given approach or curriculum is rarely well assessed.

There is danger that we will inadequately comprehend the history of special education and repeat past mistakes. Without a historical perspective, we may make serious errors in present and future service delivery. A limited historical understanding can hinder progress. For example, when analyzing the history of special education it is easy to conclude that segregated schools and institutions were wrong. Carrying this reasoning further may lead to demands that special services be abolished and that all people with disabilities be placed into "normal" environments. On the surface, it makes good sense to merge special education funds into general funds. This would provide financial incentives to help ensure that regular educators accept and adapt to students with disabilities. However, historically, regular educators have supported the concept of excluding people with disabilities from their classrooms. There is little evidence that this basic attitude has changed. If anything, pressures on regular teachers have greatly increased with (a) the influx of non-English-speaking students; (b) limited funding; (c) the increase of two-working-parent and single-parent families; (d) a general tendency to blame schools for all of the problems of society; and (e) increased numbers of impoverished families (e.g., one fourth of children in the United States live below the poverty line). With these pressures it may prove difficult for regular educators to accept responsibility for students with disabilities. In addition, there may be too few safeguards to assure that if special education funds are subsumed into the general (regular) fund, they will be used to support students with disabilities in regular classrooms. Finally, there is no guarantee that regular schools and classrooms are high-quality environments. Indeed, recent evidence indicates that the regular education system is inadequate, overburdened, and insensitive to individual needs and that increasing numbers of students who are nondisabled are at risk for failure. History indicates that prior to federal laws that provided additional funding and mandated free and appropriate public education for all children, public schools did not adequately serve many children with disabilities (Haring, N.G., & McCormick, 1990). It becomes apparent that any call for change in the existing educational system must be based on a clear understanding of how and why the system developed. It is important to maintain and comprehend the history of special services in order to improve them and to avoid problems of the past.

The premise that a historical perspective is extremely valuable could not be more timely. Many excellent special educators support the regular education initiative (REI) (Stainback & Stainback, 1989; Lipsky & Gartner, 1989; Reynolds, Wang, & Walberg, 1987). The REI, or general education initiative (GEI), is the movement that seeks to achieve a merger of special and regular education. Proponents of the initiative believe that all students with disabilities should be educated in the regular classroom. Special educators have, at times, provided inadequate instruction and support to students with disabilities, as indicated by the high dropout rates for students with mild disabilities and the dismal findings of follow-up studies (Edgar, 1987; Haring, K. A., & Lovett, 1990). Nevertheless, a majority of students with disabilities who are in public schools would not be there without special services. Providing special services requires more resources than providing typical education services. In addition, the services that regular education has traditionally provided to students who are significantly different from typical students have been inadequate (Ysseldyke & Algozzine, 1982). The ultimate tragedy of implementing REI would be if special education students were completely absorbed into the mainstream without adequate support. In such a situation they would primarily be taught to maintain behavioral control and would leave school with few functional skills, entering a community that has little use for them. It is imperative that funds and other resources for special services be protected to ensure that students with special needs are provided the additional assistance they require in the least restrictive environment. It is equally clear, and legally mandated, that funds for special services should be used to support students with disabilities in regular classes whenever possible to help improve the quality of education for these students.

In addition to ensuring adequate support for students with disabilities, both regular and special personnel must be trained to understand and accept individual differences. Regular staff should respect all children and seek appropriate help through special services when needed to serve them. Special services staff can be trained to provide support to students and also to regular educators as colleagues and not as "expert" consultants. They should learn to understand and work within the regular system. To achieve this goal requires that a core of common skills and knowledge be provided during preservice training to *all* educators.

Special and regular educators can learn to appreciate the basic concepts of each discipline and to share a common language. Educators from each area would then be more likely to respect the skills and knowledge unique to the other. For example, all teachers should be able to modify curricular content or instructional strategies in order to adapt to individual learners. However, special educators must have expertise in employing these strategies and be willing to assist regular teachers to teach all students more effectively. On the other hand, regular teachers have academic content areas of expertise that most special educators lack. They can share this knowledge with special educators so that learners with disabilities can be better served. It would be detrimental to support the complete merger of special and regular school systems if the merger erases the hard-won protection of and benefits for students with disabilities. Persons who are disabled have specific, unique needs. The very nature of a disability dictates that individuals so affected will not achieve at the same rate or to the same extent that nondisabled people do without special intervention, and therefore, individualization is necessary.

Special education developed from the belief that individuals with disabilities could not respond adequately to typical educational or acculturation processes. These individuals were seen to "deviate physically, mentally, or emotionally from the normal to the extent that they require unique learning experiences, techniques, or materials" (Kelly & Vergason, 1985, p. 160). Pioneers in special education, such as Itard and Seguin, were curious about how well these individuals could learn and which instructional techniques were most effective. After the seminal work of these early "special educators," special education became even more "special." Services were provided in segregated facilities designed to meet the needs of each disability group. Unique methods were used to address the unusual characteristics of each specific disability. The emphasis was not necessarily to address the needs of the person, but to focus on correcting the perceived disability.

Many problems have been identified in the provision of special services. Most young children do not receive the early education that would help them overcome the problems they encounter as a result of their disability. School-age individuals with disabilities often do not receive an education that prepares them to succeed in school and in adult life (Edgar, 1987). Adults with disabilities are often unemployed or underemployed, and unhappy (Edgerton, 1984). Many of these problems may be alleviated by examining the individual and family to determine specific needs, exploring how the individual fits into the community, and determining methods to help the person become a participating member of society.

Special education developed as a result of "the requirement that all children attend school and the recognition that schools were not for everybody" (Ysseldyke & Algozzine, 1982, p. 39). That is, although students with disabilities were required to attend school, they were not successful in the regular classroom. Therefore, special classes, special schools, and even special residential facilities were created. This belief, that students with disabilities need special treatment, grew beyond a focus on the typical school years to encompass all individuals with disabilities no matter their age. Special education, along with other special services, developed unique clientele, terminology, and systems. In effect it became a separate system. However, as a separate system it has, in large part, failed in its purpose. By and large, people with disabilities still remain outside of the mainstream of the community and have not received the training required to become part of that community. Services must be provided and training must be conducted in integrated environments if people with disabilities are to become participating members of society.

Considerations for Lifelong Parent–Professional Partnerships

Susan Lehr made a number of salient points in the closing discussion of her chapter on parenting people with disabilities (chapter 12, this volume). Her first hope for the future is that professionals remember and exercise the Golden Rule when working with parents and their sons and daughters who are disabled—simply, we are people first, treat us as you wish to be treated.

Although both law and common practice require parents to participate in planning the education for their children and to agree to the program's goals, objectives, methods, and setting, many parents feel they are passive partners in the educational process. We hope that the future of special education for parents will consistently acknowledge that they wish to be active partners in the education of their offspring. In addition, parents possess a large amount of knowledge about their child, but they may need to be encouraged to share this information. Communicating to parents that their knowledge and contributions are of value is an excellent way to reinforce their sharing.

It is also apparent that parents can provide powerful support to one another. Parents of children with disabilities are the only true experts on how the presence of a disability affects family systems. Special educators of the future are advised to reinforce parent networks. Professionals work with large numbers of parents and can help parents contact one another to form relationships or support groups. The reassurance of another parent can be critical if a parent is hesitant to agree to a new, unknown program or placement. Research indicates that parents influence the degree of independence their children achieve. Parents may wish to protect their offspring from the perceived dangers of community based instruction or regular school campuses (Haring, K.A., Lovett, & Saren, 1991). Linking a hesitant parent with one who has experienced success with a program innovation is an excellent strategy. One of the main points that Lehr makes in chapter 12 of this volume is that parents are critical allies: Well-cemented parent-to-parent bonds are important foundations to family functioning, and the profession and those it serves are benefited greatly by committed parents. Lehr discusses several other truths that should influence how we involve and serve families in the future. First, the decisions parents make are principled and value driven; they may conflict with professional doctrine but they must be acknowledged, accepted, and used as the basis for working together to benefit the individual with disabilities. Second, professionals should not make assumptions about families or presume to speak for them. If the professional is willing to listen, the family will speak for themselves. Third, professionals should recognize and rejoice with families in their accomplishments, encourage their pride over the achievements or gains of the family member who is disabled, and share with them the enrichment of life experience in the presence of a disability. Finally, professionals should be honest with parents, who rely on professional knowledge. Perhaps the most obvious, but nevertheless the most important, message that should guide our future family services is that parents, above all, love their children.

Prospects for Achieving School Success

Wang's discussion of achieving school success for all students (chap. 5, this volume) provides a thought-provoking framework for exploring educational reform. Although we have made great progress in providing free public education for all children in this country, we have fallen short of the vision of school success for every child. Wang points out that an alarming number of students exit school without adequate literacy skills, unprepared to function in an increasingly complex society, and warns that with changing demographic patterns this trend will increase. The goal of the coming decade is to improve schools so that students with diverse learning characteristics, and related service and educational support needs, are successfully educated. By providing special programs for students who have difficulty learning without ensuring educational outcomes, we have perpetuated a subtle form of inequity. That is, we have compensated for learning differences by making school easier for less able students, thereby doing disservice to them.

Wang (chap. 5, this volume) believes that all students must complete a common curriculum or a basic education in order to be considered successful in school and offers suggestions for how schools can be restructured to achieve this goal. Clearly, some students will need more time and extraordinary instructional support to master the common curriculum, and school systems will need to be flexible. Wang's chapter provides a framework for building an information base that administrators, policymakers, and educators can use for making program improvement decisions. The challenge of the future is for school improvement efforts to provide all students with the best possible opportunities to succeed in learning through the systematic utilization of school resources while facilitating the development of students who have the most difficulty learning.

Supported Education of the Future

Supported education, the inclusion of people with disabilities in regular school and community settings with the support of special services to help them succeed in those environments, is the goal of special education in the future. The research reviewed in Breen's chapter (chap. 4, this volume) convincingly demonstrates the efficacy of behavior analysis and resulting direct intervention in supporting integrated school services. Progress toward the larger goal of supported education—the development of enduring relationships—is less amenable to behavior analytic measurement. Systematic behavior change programs can dramatically increase the rate of social initiation and duration of interaction between people with disabilities and their nondisabled peers. To what degree this translates into friendships and the quality or intensity of relationships is difficult to assess. As Breen pointed out, the assessment of friendship relationships must go beyond measuring single variables within sampled contexts. Chapter 3 of this volume, by T. G. Haring, Kennedy, and Breen, explores the broadening of measures to include multicomponent contextual variables in behavior analysis.

In light of this concern for the development of meaningful relationships, Nonoshita and N.G. Haring (chap. 2, this volume) stress the importance of developing systematic methods of teaching social competence. One of the main features of integration is meaningful interaction. Simply placing an individual in an environment does not ensure meaningful interaction with that environment or with the people in it. Further research must be conducted on (a) developing systematic instructional methodologies to build the social competence of people with disabilities, (b) identifying effective methods for increasing the awareness of people without disabilities about the abilities of people with disabilities, (c) and investigating efficient methods for improving the interaction skills of people with disabilities.

In reviewing the material presented by Wang (chap. 5), Breen (chap. 4), and Nonoshita and N.G. Haring (chap. 2), it is clear that research is needed to help us implement the concept of supported education. The goal of full inclusion is a lofty one and must include the determination of the following questions:

1. How do we ensure that students with disabilities meet the goals and objectives of their IEPs?
2. What type of training must be provided in preservice and in-service sessions to prepare teachers to serve all levels of children?
3. What are the critical variables in changing the attitudes and acceptance of people with disabilities by their nondisabled peers? (i.e., Does mainstreaming improve attitudes? What is the effect of pulling students with disabilities out of the mainstream to work on basic or critical skills, for example self-care, that can not be appropriately trained in the regular classroom? What are the most effective and unintrusive methods for supporting students with disabilities in regular classrooms? How must the structure of regular classrooms change for supported education to work? How appropriate is a highly academic regular secondary class for a student with severe disabilities? How many social interaction opportunities exist in such a setting?)
4. What administrative processes are useful in placing students, allocating staff and faculty, working with monies from different funding sources, negotiating with regular education faculty members, supervising special education staff, encouraging interdisciplinary teaming and collaboration, shifting a school district from a traditional to a full inclusion model, and evaluating outcomes?

T.G. Haring, Kennedy, and Breen (chap. 3, this volume) not only address methodological concerns but also put forth a philosophical basis for behavior analysis in the use of future support technologies. Although there are several ways to view the world, each of which is valuable, it is most compatible with the major tenets of behavior analysis to view events as part of the context in which they occur. Thus, the interrelationship between behavior and environment is of the utmost importance. "It is the dynamic interaction between behavior and environment, or more precisely, the functional relationships that are derived from the interaction, that constitute a behavioral analysis". Therefore, if a goal of special services is to integrate people with disabilities into the community, services and training should be provided in the community to analyze the interaction and to support the individual in that environment. Services and training provided apart from the natural environment diminish their contextual meaning.

For example, T.G. Haring, Kennedy, and Breen (chap. 3, this volume) see as a major future focus the building and maintenance of social relationships among people with and without disabilities. Development of such meaningful relationships is complex; they must be viewed in the context in which they occur and examined according to their specific meaning, which may be different for each social relationship. The authors see emerging research in the areas of task analysis, problem behaviors, and social relationships as highly contextualistic. The development of a contextual behavior analysis paradigm may be the most productive approach to address the emerging challenges facing special services.

Age-Specific Services

Bennett and Guralnick (chap. 7, this volume) describe the impact that advances in medical technology have had on the services provided to very young children. Improved medical technology has resulted in a dramatic reduction in neonatal mortality for very low birthweight and other at-risk infants. There is every reason to believe that such advances will continue at the same, or even faster, rapid pace. Current evidence indicates that these infants may be deprived of social stimulation while receiving intrusive medical care. How we meld new medical technology into a system that meets the needs and concerns of infants and toddlers and their families will be a major challenge in the future.

The authors of chapter 7 (this volume) stress the challenge to parents in their ability to care for a child at biological risk. This is especially evident during the transition from the hospital to home and the community. It is important that professionals interact with families in a positive manner to support them in providing a nurturing environment. Training that enhances the skills to provide this positive support should become an even greater part of the personnel preparation for early intervention professionals.

The services the infant and family receive come from a variety of professionals. To make these services effective and at the same time provide the support and security the child and family need in these difficult stages requires that service providers work together. This will necessitate that professionals collaborate to design and implement a plan that addresses the needs of the family. To accomplish this goal, special service providers must have an understanding of each professional's role and must develop positive working relationships.

Hanson and K.A. Haring (chap. 8, this volume) also stress the need for a transdisciplinary approach to service provision. As they emphasize, the services provided to young children are complex and involve a number of professionals and paraprofessionals representing a variety of disciplines. In the future it will become even more necessary for early childhood special service providers to share the responsibilities of evaluation and planning and to engage in role release. To achieve this transdisciplinary approach will require a change of focus in and improved personnel preparation at both the preservice and inservice levels.

Personnel must be trained to provide "best practice" early intervention that is individualized, conducted in a social context, focused on active learning, and functional. In order to achieve the goals of successful early intervention these services should be family focused, with appropriate goals provided in integrated settings through a collaborative effort by a variety of service providers. The provision of such appropriate services will be a major challenge in the future. This will become even more difficult as society becomes more culturally diverse, as more mothers work outside the home, and as more children are born and survive with significant biological risks.

Hanson and K.A. Haring (chap. 8, this volume) further delineate best practices in early intervention by describing the results of a survey designed to develop a national consensus on what these practices are. The experimental validation of the efficacy of the best practices identified will become a major research agenda of the future. In keeping with the main tenets of this volume, Hanson and K.A. Haring reinforce the importance of integrated normalized environments where young children with disabilities or at significant risk for developing disabilities have opportunities to improve their skills through meaningful interactions with peers who are normally developing.

Perhaps the most important point made in the curriculum chapter by Liberty (chap. 6, this volume) is that regardless of the model utilized, the content of a student's educational program should be based on individualized goals that are determined by the student's level of performance and needs. Keeping the concept of individualized programming at the forefront is helpful in solving the problems that are presented when trying to provide truly integrated educational, vocational, and residential options for people with disabilities.

Liberty's chapter (chap. 6, this volume) makes excellent additional contributions in describing extant curricula and their application to lifecycle services. It also discusses present applications of technology, specifically computers, to assist in the integration of people with disabilities. Currently, computer software provides excellent opportunities for self-paced drill and practice so that students with academic delays can be served in age appropriate regular classes that meet their remediation needs. Something as simple and widely applicable as word processing frees the student with disabilities from being entrapped by his or her inadequacies in mechanics of written expression. Computer technology can provide protheses for speech production and locomotion as well as the microtechnological core of other adaptations for physical and sensory disabilities. Presently, it is cost-prohibitive to provide individualized computer technologies that are adaptive and can be used with ease by all in need. Assuring that every person who is disabled and can benefit from adapted or computer technology is provided those opportunities is a challenge for future special services.

In concluding her chapter, Liberty (chap. 6, this volume) does an excellent job of projecting how curricula will improve in the future by addressing pragmatic integration, decision making, adult adjustment options, interactive curricula, friendship curricula, and holistic curricula.

Liberty concludes with the hope that in the future people with disabilities will collaborate with people without disabilities in developing public policy, as well as research and service delivery agendas.

The prevention of students from dropping out of school in adolescence, be they special education students or students at risk for failure, is a strong future agenda item addressed in the Richards, Lovett, and Gaylord-Ross chapter (chap. 9, this volume) on integrated services for adolescents with disabilities. The chapter suggests that better collaboration between regular and special education may improve meaningful school outcomes. The authors summarized eight considerations to improve educational practices for students with disabilities (Weisenstein & Elrod, 1987). The first consideration is that training should be geared toward a utility of skills that are generalizable to novel situations. Second, the educator should assure that nonnatural reinforcers are faded and replaced by reinforcers that are naturally occuring. The third consideration is that students need to develop critical thinking skills while in school to achieve later successful adult adjustment. Related to critical thinking is the fourth consideration, improving creative problem-solving skills and the ability to plan in secondary education. The fifth consideration is that students be taught prevocational skills such as promptness and accuracy of work within the academic and social learning school setting. The whole concept of internal control is key in each consideration and is summed up in the sixth and seventh considerations, which are related to the development of cognitive behavior modification. The sixth concern addresses the use of self-talk and self-monitoring to improve time on-task. The seventh consideration is metacognition, or teaching students to "learn how to learn"; this encompasses strategies such as planning, scheduling, monitoring, rehearsal, self-questioning, revising, reviewing, and evaluating one's performance. These cognitive considerations can increase self-knowledge and responsibility for one's learning, which enhance one's performance in every setting. The final consideration is training motivational skills. Recent research (Bryan, 1991) indicates that positive beliefs concerning self-efficacy and the individual's attribution (i.e., believing that one's actions contribute to one's success) are powerful mediating variables to facilitating successful learning.

Research has yet to support the effectiveness of these strategies for persons with severe disabilities. However, the Richards et al. chapter (chap. 9, this volume) outlines numerous considerations for the education of students with more intense special needs. The chapter also includes a lengthy discussion of the vocational needs of adolescents with disabilities and offers recommendations for ways in which secondary schools should address them. The chapter concludes with an excellent discussion of transitional services. Recent amendments to the EHA, now called the Individuals with Disabilities Education Act (IDEA), mandate that a transition plan be in place for every student with disabilities 16 years of age or older. It is clear that this mandate provides the impetus for improving the functionality and appropriateness of secondary special services in the future.

The chapter on adult services by Lovett, Richards, and Gaylord-Ross (chapter 10, this volume) elaborates on the concept of systems change that was briefly defined in chapter 1. The authors aptly refer to the long history of segregation and institutionalization under traditional systems and discuss how political and economic forces maintain outdated systems and obstruct conversion to consumer-oriented integrated systems. The underlying theme of this volume is that systems change is needed at every level to assure integrated lifecycle services for people with disabilities. In order for adults who are disabled to function as contributing members of society, a number of systems must change, for example, the health departments, social services, public schools, adult services, Medicaid/ Social Security, vocational rehabilitation, and postsecondary/higher education. The adult chapter also summarizes six recommendations made by Whitehead (1989) that will assist us in providing integrated community-based services in the future. They are as follows:

1. Policies and procedures should be established to ensure that funds are available for community services.
2. Advocates for integrated services should participate in developing proposals for change and then monitor changes in state and federal regulations.
3. Procedures should be established to ensure that all qualified/eligible persons are enrolled and receive full benefits from national assistance programs.
4. Disincentives to employment should be eliminated.
5. Procedures should be established to ensure that agencies coordinate financial support efforts.
6. Formal cooperative agreements between agencies should be established to ensure the continuity of services when responsibility for an individual shifts from one agency to another.

In addition, chapter 10 (this volume) discusses the potential for self-advocacy to be a major force in adult services. In the future, self-advocacy will have profound impact on service providers, bureaucrats, and the families of people with disabilities (Taylor & Knoll, 1989). Chapter 10 concludes with a strong statement:

> A move toward integrated adult services requires the elimination of social, economic, and administrative barriers to community integration. It requires the design of services and supports to encourage rather than discourage involvement in community life and to cultivate rather than impede relationships between people with and without disabilities. There is no doubt that the concept and implementation of integrated services pose a challenge to those who work in the

field of special services, a challenge to the families of persons with disabilities, and most of all, a challenge to individuals with disabilities themselves. We must be prepared to meet these challenges and make the most of this opportunity to ensure that adults with disabilities have the opportunities they deserve and the choices that are their right.

The chapter by Pierce (chap. 11, this volume) on integrated services for elders with disabilities brought up several troubling issues concerning the quality of generic geriatric services. This is an issue at every age and level of service delivery, as pertinent in infant/toddler, preschool, school, and adult services as it is for those provided to elders. Pierce questions whether or not we want elders with disabilities to participate in low-quality "typical" senior citizen centers. Clearly, we do not; and in the same vein, placing young children who are disabled or at risk in low-quality "typical" day-care centers is not appropriate simply because they are integrated.

Pierce's chapter (chap. 11, this volume) echoes the theme identified throughout this volume: How do we ensure collaboration between special and generic services? Research and model development, again, are critical considerations for the future. Pierce identified a number of specific research agendas to be addressed in the future:

1. Exploration of what is true choice making: Is doing nothing an allowable retirement choice?
2. How integrated are generic services for elders?
3. What constitutes a healthy retirement?
4. What are appropriate leisure activities for elders?
5. How can a general geriatric agenda, such as Elderhostel, be merged with one for elders with disabilities?

Clearly, the larger issues of integrated services for elders with disabilities are relatively unresearched and present numerous challenges for the future.

Conclusion

In conclusion, the future is bright for realization of the goals discussed in this volume. We anticipate that society in general will change greatly as the attitudes of nondisabled community members change to ones of acceptance and understanding. These attitude shifts will foster better cooperation between professions so that special services become truly transdisciplinary in nature. With these modifications in perceptions, the overall accessibility of our society will improve for persons with disabilities.

Advances in medical technology will continue to prevent and ameliorate disabling conditions. These include the following:

1. The isolation of genotypes for prevention of multiple dystrophy, muscular sclerosis, cystic fibrosis, Huntington's chorea, and other syndromes.
2. Provision of adequate prenatal care, early prenatal testing (such as CVS), and genetic counseling.
3. Improvements in neonatology to prevent further damage from occurring in the NICUs.
4. Refinement in medication for central nervous system related disorders and the development of substances to prevent neuronal damage and enhance regeneration of cells.
5. Improved relations between the medical profession and members of other disciplines as well as families.
6. Improved training of medical doctors concerning the obsolescene of the medical model for developmentally disabled persons.
7. Medical acceptance of the value of behavioral data in medication decisions particularly for seizure and behavior disorders.
8. The development of some type of national health insurance to assure that all citizens have equal access to medical technology.

Advances in technology in general will also enhance the future for persons with disabilities. It is anticipated that at minimum the following will take place: (a) technology will be available to all who could benefit, regardless of its cost or the degree of individualization needed; (b) there will be dramatic improvements in the compatibility of computer systems; (c) the speed, weight, and responsiveness of protheses designed to ameliorate sensory and physical disabilities will be improved; (d) adaptations for all forms of transportation will improve wheelchairs, sensors, and mobility aids; and (e) sophistication in robotics and refinements in synthesized voices will enhance the independence of people with disabilities. These improvements in medical and technological areas will coincide with the advances in instructional methods described throughout this book. Professionals must be prepared and service systems must be altered to ensure the accessibility of medical, technological, and instructional innovations for people with disabilities.

In the future we hope to see a service system that supports all people regardless of background or ability. A system designed by people with disabilities and their families as well as by professionals from generic and special services. A system that meets the needs of individuals to enhance their involvement in communities. Such a system is a very worthwhile goal. Let us dedicate ourselves to continue to work systematically toward that lofty goal.

References

Bryan, T. (1991, April). Social Skills in Students With Learning Disabilities: Why? When? and How? Paper presented at the International Conference of the Council for Exceptional Children, Atlanta, GA.

Edgar, E. (1987). Secondary programs in special education: Are many of them justifiable? *Exceptional Children*, *53*, 555–561.

Edgerton, R.B. (1984). *Lives in process: Mentally retarded adults in a large city*. Washington, DC: American Association on Mental Deficiency.

Haring, K.A., & Lovett, D.L. (1990). The adult adjustment of special education graduates: A follow-up study. *Journal of Special Education*, *23*, 463–477.

Haring, K.A., Lovett, D.L., & Saren. D. (1991) Parent perspectives of their adult offspring with disabilities. *Teaching Exceptional Children*, *24*(2), 6–10.

Haring, N.G., & McCormick, L. (1990). *Exceptional children and youth* (5th ed.). Columbus, OH: Charles E. Merrill.

Kelly, L.J., & Vergason, G.A. (1985). *Dictionary of special education and rehabilitation* (2nd ed.). Denver, CO: Love.

Lipsky, D.K., & Gartner, A. (1989). *Beyond separate education: Quality education for all*. Baltimore: Paul H. Brookes.

Reynolds, M.C., Wang, M.C., & Walberg, H.G. (1987). The necessary restructuring of special and regular education. *Exceptional Children*, *53*, 391–398.

Stainback, W., & Stainback, S. (1989). A rationale for the merger of special and regular education. *Exceptional Children*, *51*(2), 102–111.

Taylor, S.J., & Knoll, J.A. (1989). Community living and the education of students with severe disabilities. In R.Gaylord-Ross (Ed.), *Integration strategies for students with handicaps* (pp. 321–327). Baltimore: Paul H. Brookes.

Weisenstein, G.R., & Elrod, G.F. (1987). Transition services for adolescent age individuals with mild mental retardation. In R.N. Ianacone & R.H. Stodden (Eds.), *Transition issues and directions* (pp. 38–48). Reston, VA: Council for Exceptional Children.

Whitehead, C. (1989). Influencing employment through federal and state policy. In W.E. Kiernan & R.L. Schalock (Eds.), *Economics, industry, and disability* (pp. 270–360). Baltimore: Paul H. Brookes.

Ysseldyke, J.E., & Algozzine, B. (1982). *Critical issues in special and remedial education*. Boston: Houghton Mifflin.

Index

MIX
Papier aus verantwortungsvollen Quellen
Paper from responsible sources
FSC® C105338

If you have any concerns about our products,
you can contact us on
ProductSafety@springernature.com

In case Publisher is established outside the EU,
the EU authorized representative is:
Springer Nature Customer Service Center GmbH
Europaplatz 3, 69115 Heidelberg, Germany

Printed by Libri Plureos GmbH
in Hamburg, Germany